STUDY GUIDE AND SELF-ASSESSMENT

FOR

THE AMERICAN PSYCHIATRIC PRESS

TEXTBOOK OF

PSYCHIATRY

STUDY GUIDE AND SELF-ASSESSMENT

FOR

THE AMERICAN PSYCHIATRIC PRESS

TEXTBOOK OF

PSYCHIATRY

Mark R. Lovell, Ph.D.
Michael D. Franzen, Ph.D.

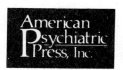

1400 K STREET, N.W.   WASHINGTON, DC 20005

Contents

Section IV: Psychiatric Treatments

Section V: Special Topics

Preface

This book has been written to accompany *The American Psychiatric Press Textbook of Psychiatry*, edited by John A. Talbott, M.D., Robert E. Hales, M.D., and Stuart C. Yudofsky, M.D. The *Study Guide* has been constructed to maximize the benefit from reading the *Textbook*. It is our goal that this book will be useful to medical students, residents, and clinicians seeking to acquire, update, or assess the base of knowledge necessary to treat patients with neuropsychiatric conditions.

This book consists of between 15 and 20 multiple-choice questions per chapter. Each question is accompanied by a brief answer taken from the *Textbook*. These answers represent condensed versions of the discussions found in the *Textbook* and are designed to highlight important features of each chapter. To promote optimal utilization of the *Study Guide*, the following recommendations are made. First, each chapter contained in the *Textbook* should be read carefully before attempting to answer questions from the corresponding chapter in the *Study Guide*. This should promote a more thorough understanding of the material than could be gained by selected reading of the *Textbook* or from reading the *Study Guide* alone. Next, it is suggested that readers attempt to answer all of the chapter questions before checking the accuracy of their answers. Finally, we recommend that the answers be verified by referring to the corresponding answers accompanying each chapter. This provides readers with direct feedback as to their specific choices and allows for correction of mistaken assumptions. Readers are then encouraged to refer to the *Textbook* for a more complete discussion of the particular subject area under review. We are hopeful that the *Study Guide* will contribute to your understanding and appreciation of the extensive and intriguing data base required to evaluate and treat patients with psychiatric disorders.

Mark R. Lovell, Ph.D.
Michael D. Franzen, Ph.D.

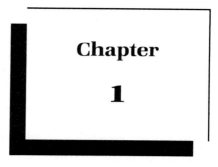

Chapter 1

Neuroscience and Psychiatry

DIRECTIONS: Each of the statements or questions is followed by five suggested responses or completions. Select the one that is the best choice or most complete answer in each case.

1.1 Which of the following statements regarding the neuron is true?

    A. The neuron relies on extracortical cells for the manufacture of neurotransmitter substances.

    B. The structure and physiology of all neurons are similar.

    C. Neurons do not normally undergo mitosis.

    D. Damaged neurons are replaced via cellular genesis.

    E. The synthesis of protein structures takes place in the dendrites.

1.2 Which of the following is a proper definition of the dendrites?

    A. The dendrites are small tubular protuberances at the front of the cell body that act as receptors for neurotransmitters.

    B. Dendrites store neurotransmitters until such time as the cell is excited and the neurotransmitters are released.

    C. Dendrites are the simple proteins that serve as precursors to the more complex neurotransmitters.

    D. Dendrites are mechanical transfer apparati for returning the discharged neuron to its resting potential.

    E. Dendrites are enzymes released into the synaptic cleft to decompose used neurotransmitters.

1.3   Catecholamine neurotransmitters include:

    A.   protein peptides
    B.   elemental ionic cations
    C.   elemental ionic anions
    D.   dopamine and beta-endorphins
    E.   dopamine, norepinephrine, and epinephrine

1.4   Which of the following regarding co-localization is true?

    A.   Co-localization generally involves a classical neurotransmitter and a neuropeptide.
    B.   Co-localization involves the linkage of two neurons in a single task.
    C.   Co-localization never involves two classical neurotransmitters.
    D.   The two substances involved in co-localization have an antagonistic relation.
    E.   When one neuron is injured, its co-localized neuron takes over its function.

1.5   Intracellular second messengers:

    A.   are chemical messengers that repeat and reinforce the information contained in the chain of cellular depolarization
    B.   activate enzymes that then affect the metabolism or function of the neuron
    C.   are transmitted through the cell membrane via ion channels
    D.   are released into the synaptic cleft following release of the main neurotransmitters
    E.   can be visualized with staining techniques

1.6   Reticular core neurons:

    A.   are implicated in the highly specific tasks of visual recognition memory
    B.   when damaged, show focal neurological signs
    C.   are essential to the executive and planning operations of cognitive functions
    D.   are geographically clustered in the brain stem
    E.   modulate neuronal function in vast areas of the nervous system

1.7 The effects of norepinephrine are:

    A. generally excitatory
    B. mediated in the brain by two types of receptors
    C. nonspecific for central nervous system receptors, but specific for peripheral receptors
    D. nonspecific for peripheral central nervous system receptors, but specific for central receptors
    E. generally inhibitory

DIRECTIONS: For each of the statements or questions below, one or more of the alternative answers is correct. Choose answer:

    A if only 1, 2, and 3 are correct
    B if only 1 and 3 are correct
    C if only 2 and 4 are correct
    D if only 4 is correct
    E if all are correct

1.8 The neuron is composed of the following parts:

    1. cell body or soma
    2. dendrites
    3. axon
    4. synapses

1.9 Which of the following regarding the axon is true?

    1. It is a tubular extension along which electrical impulses flow to the nerve terminal.
    2. A single neuron has only one axon.
    3. The length of an axon may vary from less than one millimeter to more than a meter.
    4. The axon makes a direct physical contact with the postsynaptic neuron.

1.10 Which of the following regarding the innervation of the axon is true?

    1. The innervation of the axon is idiosyncratically and perhaps randomly organized.
    2. Excitatory inputs are generally located at the distal end of dendrites.
    3. The axon is innervated by chemical contacts with surrounding neuronal cells.
    4. Inhibitory inputs are generally located at the proximal end of the dendrites and around the soma.

1.11   What describes the regulation of catecholamine synthesis?

1. Catecholamine synthesis is regulated by genetic feedback.
2. Catecholamine synthesis is unregulated—the level of catecholamines is regulated by enzymatic decomposition of endproducts.
3. Catecholamine synthesis is regulated by glandular secretions.
4. Catecholamine synthesis is regulated by the dampening effect of excess catecholamine on the activity of catecholamine precursors.

1.12   What describes the role of nerve terminal vesicles?

1. They protect catecholamines from enzymatic degradation.
2. They help synthesize protein peptides.
3. They allow discrete quantities of transmitters to be released when needed.
4. They help regulate the ionic disequilibrium of the action potential.

1.13   Which of the following regarding neuropeptides is true?

1. Neuropeptides are involved in the enzymatic degradation of catecholamines.
2. Neuropeptides help maintain the resting potential of a neuron.
3. Neuropeptides are synthesized in various extracellular sites.
4. Neuropeptides are generally synthesized in the neuronal cell body.

1.14   The activity of second messenger systems:

1. occurs over much longer time frames than that of ion channel openings
2. is associated with transient alterations in the metabolic state of the neuron
3. modifies ion channels via phosphorylation
4. is usually modulatory

1.15   Serotonin-releasing neurons are:

1. widely involved in central nervous system innervation
2. localized in the raphe nuclei
3. associated with the regulation of rapid eye movement sleep
4. associated with the modulation of pain sensitivity

1.16   GABAergic neurons:

1. mediate the effect of many sedatives, anxiolytics, and anticonvulsants
2. are implicated in the dyskinetic symptoms of Huntington's disease
3. may be involved in the appearance of the symptoms of tardive dyskinesia
4. are found in the peripheral but not the central nervous system

DIRECTIONS: Each of the following questions consists of lettered headings followed by a list of numbered alternatives. Select the single lettered heading that is most closely associated with the appropriate numbered alternative. Each lettered heading may be chosen only once.

Psychoactive drug

A.   Haloperidol
B.   Benzodiazepines
C.   Tricyclic antidepressants

Description of effect

1.17   effect a time-dependent desensitization of beta-receptors
1.18   exert their effect via potentiation of GABAergic effects
1.19   produce a marked increase in the turnover of dopamine

ANSWERS

1.1   The answer is **C**.

The neuron is a relatively self-sufficient structure that is able to synthesize the cellular components necessary for independent life. The basic function of neurons is to play some role in the processing of information. In general the synthesis of neurotransmitter substances takes place in the body of the cell. Neurons can differ widely in both structure and function. However, accompanying this wide range of specialization is an inability to undergo mitosis. Therefore, the supply of neurons in a mature brain is finite. Injury resulting in destruction of cells cannot be ameliorated by the production of replacement cells, as is possible in other organs.

1.2   The answer is A.

At the anterior end of each neuron soma is a set of cylindrical growths that act as the primary receptors for chemical information released by a presynaptic neuron. The number of dendrites is related to the function of the neuron. Neurons that relay information with few processing duties tend to have a small number of dendrites. Neurons that serve an integrative function have numerous dendrites synapsing on multiple neurons.

In the presynaptic neuron, boutons, which are terminal pouchlike containers for neurotransmitters, release the transmitters when their neurons are sufficiently depolarized. These transmitters cross the synapse and attach themselves to receptor sites on the dendrites. If a sufficient number of transmitter molecules attach to the dendrites, the receptor neuron reaches action potential and transient depolarization occurs in that cell as well.

1.3   The answer is E.

The catecholaminergic system is perhaps the most studied and best understood of the neurotransmitter systems. Dopamine, norepinephrine, and epinephrine are all catecholamines. In fact, dopamine, norepinephrine, and epinephrine are all steps in a single synthetic path. The first step is production of dopamine. In cells that contain dopamine-beta-hydroxylase, norepinephrine is produced. Cells that also contain phenylethanolamine N-methyl transferase will produce epinephrine. Despite this similarity of synthetic operations, these three catecholamines can have very different effects on the nervous system.

1.4   The answer is A.

Recent information has challenged the assumption that each neuron had only one transmitter associated with its activity. There are several instances in which a classical neurotransmitter has been found to coexist with a neuropeptide in the same neuron. There are even instances that involve two classical neurotransmitters in the same cell. These co-localized transmitters probably play complementary roles in the function of the neuron. It may be that the classical transmitter is released in response to normal impulse flow, while the neuropeptide is released during periods of increased cell activity. Co-localization may play a role in the specialization of functions served by a single neurotransmitters.

1.5 The answer is B.

Receptor transduction events may be initiated by ion channel activity or by the transmembrane activation of enzymes generating intracellular second messengers. The effect of these second messengers is to momentarily change the metabolic, functional condition of the neuron. They perform this function by activating enzymes to catalyze the intraconversion of other enzymes or ion channels. The time frame of the effects of second messengers is much longer than that of ion channel's effects on receptor responses. Examples of second messengers are cyclic adenosine monophosphate and cyclic quanylic acid.

1.6 The answer is E.

The components of the reticular core have direct relevance for psychiatry, especially the pathways of the noradrenergic, serotonergic, dopaminergic, and catecholaminergic systems. Most of the neurons in the reticular core probably do not involve specific informational processes, but instead act in a modulatory fashion on other neuronal activity. Their effect is most important in the cortical and limbic regions. Because they are not involved in processing specific information, disruption in these systems does not result in focal or hard neurological signs. Instead disruptions in the reticular core neurons are more likely to result in abnormalities of drive, affect, arousal, or cognitive functions.

1.7 The answer is B.

The neurons in the reticular core that use norepinephrine as the primary transmitter are known as the noradrenergic system. The principal noradrenergic nucleus is the locus ceruleus at the base of the fourth ventricle. The release of norepinephrine can result in either excitation or inhibition, depending on the type of receptor to which the norepinephrine binds itself. For example, stimulation of alpha-1 receptors results in neuronal excitation, while stimulation of alpha-2 receptors results in neuronal inhibition.

1.8 The answer is E.

The neuron has four component parts: the soma, dendrites, axon, and synapse. The soma or cell body contains the nucleus of the neuron. Here the neurotransmitters and necessary proteins are manufactured.

The dendrites are tubular extensions of the soma that act as the receptor sites for neurotransmitters. The axon is a long extension from the soma to the terminal end. Electrochemical inpulses travel the length of the axon following depolarization of the cell membrane secondary to reception of a sufficient quantity of neurotransmitter. When the impulse reaches the terminal end, the boutons release more neurotransmitter, which then repeats the process with the new postsynaptic neuron. The synapse is actually a functional part of the neuron, and not an actual morphological component. The synapse is the gap between the terminal end of the presynaptic neuron and the dendrites of the postsynaptic neuron. Neurotransmitters pass through here on their way to the postsynaptic dendrites. Excess neurotransmitter is degraded here by the action of enzymes.

1.9   The answer is **A**.

Although each neuron has only one axon, some axons such as those for nigrostriatal dopaminergic neurons, may have numerous branches in order to innervate multiple neurons at the postsynaptic site. Electrochemical impulses flow down from the soma to the terminal. The length of an axon can vary from less than a millimeter to more than a meter. The axon does not make actual physical contact with the postsynaptic dendrites, but instead relies on extracellular fluid to carry the transmitter to the receptor sites.

1.10   The answer is **C**.

The innervation of the axon is highly organized and logically represented. The distal end of the dendrites usually contains excitatory inputs. Inhibitory inputs are usually located in the proximal end of the dendrites and around the soma. Therefore, inhibitory inputs play a major role in the ability of a neuron to generate an action potential in a given instance. When the inhibitory inputs are activated, the difference between the voltage of the interior of the cell and that of the extracellular environment becomes larger, thus requiring depolarization to produce the action potential. This requires more excitatory neurotransmitters to bind to receptor sites before the cell "fires."

1.11   The answer is **D**.

The regulation of catecholamine production is necessary in order to avoid wasteful and inefficient overproduction of catecholamines and the subsequent degradation of the excess quantity. The produced catecholamines are stored in the nerve terminal vesicles. The excess that exists in solution in the terminal itself inhibits the activity of tyrosine hydroxylase, the rate-limiting step in the synthetic pathway that produces catecholamines. Therefore, fewer catecholamines are produced. When the nerve "fires" and the vesicles release their catecholamines into the synapse, the excess catecholamines enter the now depleted vesicles, removing their inhibition of tyrosine hydroxylase and resulting in a temporary increase in catecholamine production.

1.12   The answer is B.

Vesicles are small membraneous sacs located in the nerve terminal. An energy-dependent process stores catecholamines in the vesicles. The vesicles play two major roles in the function of catecholamines. First, by storing the catecholamines until needed, the vesicles protect them from degradation by monoamine oxidase. Reserpine interferes with this process, resulting in catecholamines remaining in the terminal where they are degraded. This depletes the supply of catecholamines. The second role of the vesicles is that by storing a discrete quantity of catecholamine until release following attainment of the action potential, a regular, reliable quantity of catecholamine is released each time, helping to regulate some aspects of neurotransmission.

1.13   The answer is D.

Neuropeptides are not involved in the degradation of transmitters, nor are they involved in maintaining the resting potential of the cell. The classical transmitters are synthesized in the nerve terminals, but the neuropeptides are synthesized in the neuronal cell body. This is because the peptides are small proteins that are synthesized under the direction of messenger ribonucleic acid. The neuropeptides are then stored in a vesicle that migrates down the axon to the nerve terminal.

1.14   The answer is E.

The effects of second messenger systems occur over a period of several hundred milliseconds as opposed to the receptor-mediated ion channel openings that occur as extremely brief and discrete activities. The responses to second messenger systems can cause either temporary changes in the metabolic condition of the neuron or modification of the ion channels. Therefore the second messenger systems are usually thought of as having a modulatory effect.

1.15   The answer is E.

Neurons that release serotonin are localized in a nucleus in the raphe nuclei. The raphe nuclei are located around an aqueduct in the midbrain. From there, the serotonin-releasing neurons innervate almost all areas of the central nervous system. Depending on characteristics of the receptors, serotonin may have differential effects. One type of these receptors is implicated in the effect of the anxiolytic buspirone. Other effects of serotonin include regulation of rapid eye movement sleep, regulation of aggression in the limbic system, and modulation of pain sensitivity.

1.16   The answer is A.

GABAergic neurons have many implications for clinical psychiatry. Many sedatives, antianxiety drugs, and anticonvulsants activate the GABA receptors in the course of causing their clinical effects. GABAergic neurons may be short axoned, as in the case of the cortex, hippocampus, and limbic structures, or may be long-track projecting neurons such as those that project from the caudate-putamen to the globus pallidus and the substantia nigra. Disruption of GABAergic neurons is involved in the development of the dyskinetic symptoms of Huntington's disease. Loss of GABAergic output from the striatum occurs in tardive dyskinesia.

1.17   The answer is C.
1.18   The answer is B.
1.19   The answer is A.

The immediate effects of antidepressants include potentiation of noradrenergic and serotonergic neurotransmission by blocking reuptake. However, the clinical effects of antidepressants may not occur for a period of two to three weeks following initiation of the drug regimen. Recent research indicates that the long-term effects of tricyclic antidepressants include a time-dependent desensitization of cortical–limbic beta-receptors and enhanced noradrenergic transmission.

Benzodiazepines have a favorable ratio of anxiolytic effects to sedation effects. They also are less likely to cause respiratory depression, making them safer than barbituates for some of the same problems. Withdrawal effects are also less than for barbituates. The pharmacological effect of benzodiazepines appears to be in the potentiation of GABAergic neurons without actually increasing the number of GABA receptive sites.

Neuroleptics such as haloperidol seem to have their pharmacological effect by producing an increase in dopamine turnover. Haloperidol may block brain receptors for dopamine. In laboratory animals, the effects of drugs that enhance dopaminergic transmission (such as stereotyped behaviors and emesis) can be blocked by administering neuroleptics.

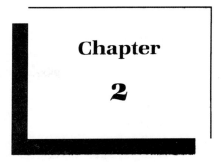

Chapter 2

Genetics

DIRECTIONS: Each of the statements or questions is followed by five suggested responses or completions. Select the one that is the best choice or most complete answer in each case.

2.1 Genetic investigation in psychiatry has several goals. Which of the following is not among these goals?

    A. to validate the criteria for and boundaries of diagnostic entities
    B. to identify the forms of mating that will produce a disorder
    C. to develop methods of preventing psychiatric disorders
    D. to establish the nongenetic component of psychiatric syndromes
    E. to establish the genetic component of psychiatric syndromes

2.2 The lifetime morbid risk statistic is meant to obviate which problem with investigations of the degree to which a syndrome is familial?

    A. Family risk studies usually ignore environmental etiological factors.
    B. Family risk studies do not take into account the degree of occurrence in normal controls.
    C. Blind diagnosis is usually not possible in family risk studies.
    D. Family risk studies generally use nonrepresentative hospitalized cases.
    E. Some family members may not have exhibited the syndrome at the time of the investigation.

2.3 An important problem in evaluating family risk studies is that the rates of inherited psychiatric syndromes may be influenced by:

    A. intrauterine environmental variables

    B. learned or "copy-cat" behavior in relatives of affected individuals

    C. assortative mating

    D. the extent to which the affected individual has responsibility for the upbringing of the offspring

    E. the socioeconomic status of the family

2.4 Adoptive studies have four general forms. All of the following are examples of adoption studies except:

    A. the study of adopted-away children of a disordered parent

    B. the study of children of nondisordered parents adopted into a family with a disordered parent

    C. the study of the adoptive and biological relatives of disordered adoptees

    D. the study of dizygotic twins reared apart

    E. the study of monozygotic twins reared apart

2.5 High-risk studies do not investigate:

    A. differences between afflicted adults and low-risk, nonafflicted adults

    B. presymptomatic differences between high-risk and low-risk individuals

    C. early manifestations of psychopathology in subjects who later develop the disorder

    D. childhood psychopathological syndromes as related to the psychiatric abnormalities of the parents

    E. environmental variables associated with development of the disorder

2.6 Major problems in the execution and interpretation of high-risk studies do not include:

    A. the effect of assortative mating

    B. the large sample required for statistical significance

    C. the difficulty of identifying nonspecific pathological environmental stressors

    D. difficulty in determining the degree of penetrance of a gene

    E. the difficulty of elucidating the influence of environmental variables when the genetically predisposed individuals cannot be specified

2.7 Which of the following statements regarding the results of genetic studies of schizophrenia is not true?

   A. There are elevated risks in first-degree relatives.
   B. Schizophrenia is more common in biological relatives of schizophrenic adoptees than in biological relatives of controls.
   C. All four types of adoption studies have resulted in similar results.
   D. Premorbid predictors of schizophrenia have been identified.
   E. Although the adoption study method provides evidence for a genetic contribution to schizophrenia, the cross-fostering method generally supports the environmental hypothesis.

DIRECTIONS: For each of the statements or questions below, one or more of the alternative answers is correct. Choose answer:
   A   if only 1, 2, and 3 are correct
   B   if only 1 and 3 are correct
   C   if only 2 and 4 are correct
   D   if only 4 is correct
   E   if all are correct

2.8 High-risk studies examining the characteristics of children of schizophrenic mothers have shown that:

   1. high-risk infants show more anxious attachment behavior by age one year
   2. high-risk children are less attentive and more passive in play at age two years
   3. high-risk infants show more sensorimotor deficits by age one year
   4. high-risk children are more likely to exhibit idiosyncratic thought patterns by age three years

2.9 In a twin study, evidence for the existence of pathogenic genes is found if:

   1. the concordance rate of the disorder is equal for monozygotic twins and siblings
   2. the concordance rate of the disorder is higher for monozygotic twins than for dizygotic twins
   3. the concordance rate of the disorder is lower for monozygotic twins than it is for dizygotic twins
   4. the concordance rate for dizygotic twins is equal to that for siblings

2.10 Monogenic and polygenic disorders may be distinguished:

1. by the fact that monogenic disorders usually produce discontinuously different symptom patterns
2. by the percent of offspring affected by the disorder
3. by the fact that polygenic disorders usually produce continuous distributions of the degree of symptomatology
4. exclusively by the degree of penetrance

2.11 Which of the following regarding the investigations of genetic components of affective disorders is true?

1. There is an approximately 65 percent concordance for monozygotic twins.
2. The concordance for monozygotic and dizygotic twins is approximately equal.
3. Adoption studies of major mood disorders have inconsistent results.
4. The monozygotic twin concordance rate for major depression is higher than for bipolar affective disorder.

2.12 The study of twins in anxiety disorders indicates:

1. a higher concordance for monozygotic twins with panic disorder and/or agoraphobia than for dizygotic twins
2. no significant differences for generalized anxiety disorder for monozygotic versus dizygotic twins
3. a higher concordance for monozygotic twins with obsessive–compulsive disorder than for dizygotic twins
4. approximately a 31 percent concordance for panic disorder and/or agoraphobia among monozygotic twins

2.13 General approaches to uncovering the genetic basis of disease include:

1. identifying an abnormal gene product
2. identifying an etiologically specific treatment
3. identifying the location of an abnormal gene
4. identifying a specific genotype-phenotype relation

2.14 Family studies of anorexia nervosa have shown:

1. an increased rate of familial anorexia
2. an increased rate of familial bulimia
3. an increased rate of familial subclinical anorexia nervosa
4. an increased risk for affective disorders among first-degree relatives

2.15 Adoption studies in alcohol indicate that:

1. alcoholism in biological parents predicts alcoholism only in adopted-away male offspring
2. alcoholism in biological parents predicts alcoholism in adopted-away children regardless of sex of the child
3. alcoholism in the environment does not increase the rate of alcoholism in adoptees
4. the presence of alcoholism in an adopted parent predicts alcoholism in the adoptee

2.16 Components of genetic counseling include:

1. diagnosis
2. estimating risk of recurrence
3. evaluating the aims, intelligence, and emotions of the counselee
4. helping the counselee understand the risk of occurrence in the context of the burden of the disorder

DIRECTIONS: Each of the following questions consists of lettered headings followed by a list of numbered alternatives. Select the single lettered heading that is most closely associated with the appropriate numbered alternative. Each lettered heading may be chosen only once.

Type of adoption study

A. Adoptee study method
B. Cross-fostering
C. Adoptee's family method
D. Monozygotic twins reared apart

Description

2.17 is the study of children born of nondisordered parents adopted into a disordered family
2.18 is the study of children adopted away from a disordered parent
2.19 is the study of adoptive and biological relatives of a disordered individual
2.20 requires calculation of concordance for disorder in twins

ANSWERS

2.1 The answer is **B**.

Genetic investigations in psychiatry attempt to describe the genetic contributions to psychopathology. There are many strategies to assist in this attempt. The strategies are related to the different goals of genetic investigations. One goal is to specify the genetic component of the etiology of psychiatric disorders by determining whether the disorder is genetically caused or by determining the genetic contribution (the type of genetic representation, dominant or recessive, and the location and product of the genes involved). Another goal is to specify the nongenetic component of the disorder and thereby establish whether any subtypes of the disorder are nongenetically caused and the form of interaction between genetic and environmental variables in the production of the disorder.

Another goal is to validate the criteria for the diagnosis, including for the subtypes of the disorder. Meeting this goal will help determine the level of severity of the disorder which is most hereditary and whether different clinical entities are related by virtue of being different manifestations of the same genotype. Related goals are to establish genetic variations in psychological symptoms and variations in nonpathological personality traits. Finally, the ultimate goal of genetic investigations is to develop methods of preventing or treating disorders based on a knowledge of the factors responsible for the emergence of the disorder. Identifying the forms of mating that will produce the disorder is not a goal of genetic investigations

2.2 The answer is **E**.

The lifetime morbid risk is an estimate of the eventual rate of illness present among relatives of an individual with the same illness. Family risk studies involve interviews with family members or reviews of medical records in order to determine how many of them carry the same diagnosis as the identified patient. Because some disorders will not be present in family members who are at risk to develop the disorder, this set of procedures may underestimate the actual rate of the disorder. The methods used for calculating this statistic require some knowledge of the cumulative incidence for a given disorder.

2.3 The answer is **C**.

As with any form of empirical investigation, there are some limitations to the methods used to evaluate family risk for a given disorder. One of the most important problems is related to the concept of assortative mating. Individuals with a certain disorder may choose to marry partners with similar characteristics including symptoms of the disorder. This tendency may inflate estimates of the extent to which the disorder in the identified subject is responsible for the appearance of the disorder in the offspring because both parents may be contributing to the appearance. Another problem is related to the environment shared by the family members. This shared environment may be partly responsible for the appearance of the disorder in the offspring.

2.4 The answer is D.

Adoption studies can be quite useful in any attempt to estimate the relative contributions of heredity and environment to the incidence of a disorder. When children remain in the biological family of origin, one cannot be sure whether concordance of the disorder among siblings is due to the genetic material inherited from the parent or to the influence of the shared environment. When children are adopted away, concordance is more readily interpreted.

There are four general types of adoption studies: 1) the study of adopted away children of a parent with the disorder, 2) the study of children born of nondisordered parents raised by disordered adoptive parents, 3) the study of the adoptive and biological relatives of a disordered adoptee, and 4) the study of monozygotic twins raised apart. The study of dizygotic twins raised apart does not contribute much knowledge because of the confound between different genetic material and different environments.

2.5 The answer is A.

High-risk studies investigate the role of a risk factor such as genetics or exposure to teratogenic factors in producing a disorder in an individual. These studies do not investigate the differences between disordered adults and low-risk nondisordered adults. However, these studies do investigate the presymptomatic differences between the high-risk individuals and control individuals in order to see if these differences predict later development of the disorder. These studies also seek to uncover early manifestations of psychopathology in children who later develop the same disorders as their parents. Another avenue of investigation for these studies is to identify the childhood syndromes that are genetically related to the adult disorder and to identify the environmental variables associated with the development of the disorder in the genetically predisposed group.

2.6   The answer is **D**.

High-risk studies are empirical investigations of the characteristics of individuals who, because of genetic variables or environmental exposures or experiences, are likely to be afflicted with a certain disease or disorder. In this sort of study the effect of the environment is either controlled or studied in relation to the eventual occurrence of the disorder.

Researchers who wish to conduct high-risk studies face several major problems in the execution and interpretation of such studies. One problem is that there may be a systematic bias due to co-parent psychopathology resulting from assortative mating, the tendency for people with a certain disorder to marry other individuals who may also have some form of the disorder. Another problem is that in order to reach statistical significance in the study of low prevalence disorders, large sample sizes are required. A third problem is related to the difficulty of identifying nonspecific environmental stressors whose effect may be cumulative. Finally, a major problem occurs when the individuals who are genetically predisposed cannot be clearly identified, making it difficult to determine the influence of environmental variables on the occurrence and course of the disorder.

2.7   The answer is **E**.

It is more likely that schizophrenia is a syndrome rather than a single disease. This fact makes genetic studies difficult. However, because of the importance of understanding schizophrenia, there have been a number of investigations of the genetic contributions to schizophrenia. Studies examining the risk of schizophrenia in first-degree relatives of schizophrenic patients have found that the risk for first-degree relatives is higher than for individuals from the general population. Twin studies of schizophrenia have consistently shown that there is a greater concordance of schizophrenia in monozygotic twins than there is in dizygotic twins. Some important premorbid predictors of schizophrenia have been identified in the offspring of schizophrenic individuals.

All four types of adoption studies have been conducted in the area of schizophrenia, and all four types support the genetic hypothesis. For example, the adoptee study method has produced findings that indicate there is an increased incidence of schizophrenia in the adopted-away offspring of schizophrenic mothers compared with adopted-away offspring of control mothers. Use of the adoptee's family study method indicates that schizophrenia is more common in the biological relatives of schizophrenic adoptees than in the biological relatives of control adoptees.

2.8   The answer is **A**.

High-risk studies of schizophrenia have included investigations of the characteristics that differentiate the offspring of schizophrenic subjects from the offspring of control subjects and investigations of premorbid features that predict eventual occurrence of the disorder in the offspring of schizophrenic parents. Anxious attachment behavior patterns and sensorimotor deficits occur more frequently in high-risk infants by the age of one year. By the age of two years, high-risk children are more likely to exhibit passive behavior in play and are less likely to be attentive during play activities. Although these pieces of evidence have been interpreted in favor of an inherited neurointegrative defect in schizophrenia, they might also be due to developmental delays secondary to the greater occurrence of obstetrical complications in schizophrenic mothers. The results of investigations of premorbid predictors of schizophrenia have shown that among children of schizophrenic patients the factors of obstetrical complications and the presence of soft neurological signs such as impaired balance, left/right confusion, and motor overflow predict the occurrence of schizophrenia in later life.

2.9   The answer is **C**.

Many psychiatric disorders have both genetic and environmental etiological factors thought to be important to the occurrence of the disorder. Unraveling the interacting influences can be a difficult task. Twin studies allow a unique opportunity to investigate the relative amounts of influence from the two classes of variables. The usual method is to investigate the relative concordance of the disorder in monozygotic twins versus dizygotic twins. The logic is that while dizygotic twins share an environment and some genetic material, monozygotic twins share all of their genetic material as well as their environment. If the concordance rate for monozygotic twins is higher than it is for dizygotic twins, and if the concordance rate for dizygotic twins is approximately equal that for siblings, then the results are generally interpreted as being in favor of the genetic hypothesis.

Although at first blush the twin study seems to be an ideal method for investigating the relative roles of environment and heredity, there are some drawbacks. For example, the environments of monozygotic twins raised together may be more similar than the environments of dizygotic twins raised together. Monozygotic twins are more often dressed alike and treated similarly than are dizygotic twins. Emotionally and attitudinally based behavior from parents and family members are more similar for monozygotic twins than for dizygotic twins. One other complication is that monozygotic twins may share more temperamental variables than dizygotic twins, resulting in the elicitation of more similar behavior from parents and others in the environment.

2.10   The answer is **A**.

An important consideration in the genetic investigation of psychiatric disorders is that some disorders may be the result of monogenic representation (influenced by one abnormal gene) and some may be the result of polygenic representation (influenced by more than one abnormal gene). There are two general strategies for investigating whether monogenic or polygenic representation is involved. Monogenically caused disorders tend to have expression in a dichotomous fashion: Either the associated characteristic is present or it is absent. Polygenically represented disorders tend to have expression in a continuous distribution of degrees of the associated characteristic. Another method for determining whether the disorder is monogenic or polygenic is to examine the percentage of disordered family members of the identified subject. If a disorder is monogenically represented in a dominant gene, then 50 percent of the offspring are going to acquire the disorder. Monogenic representation of a recessive gene results in 25 percent of the offspring being affected by the disorder. Polygenic disorders have a much more variable rate of occurrence in offspring and other relatives.

2.11   The answer is **B**.

Investigations of the genetic contributions of affective disorders have shown some interesting results. There appears to be a differential influence of genetics for bipolar affective disorder and major depression. For example, first-degree relatives of individuals with bipolar affective disorder have an elevated risk for both bipolar affective disorder and for major depression. First-degree relatives of individuals with major depression have an elevated risk only for major depression.

Twin studies of the major affective disorders indicate that the concordance for monozygotic twins is approximately 65 percent, while the concordance for dizygotic twins is approximately 14 percent. One study of twins indicates that the concordance rates for monozygotic and for dizygotic twins are higher for bipolar affective disorder than the respective rates for major depression. There have been only a few adoptee studies of major depression, and these have had inconsistent results.

2.12   The answer is **E**.

Only one twin study of anxiety disorders has been conducted using *Diagnostic and Statistical Manual of Mental Disorders (Third Edition)* diagnostic criteria. This study found a higher concordance for panic disorder and/or agoraphobia in monozygotic twins than in dizygotic twins. There were no significant differences in the respective concordance rates for generalized anxiety disorder. One study investigating obsessive-compulsive disorder found a significantly greater concordance rate for monozygotic twins than for dizygotic twins, a result that was in agreement with the results of a Japanese study.

2.13   The answer is C.

There are two general approaches for uncovering the genetic basis of disease: identification of an abnormal gene product and identification of the gene location. The first approach has been the traditional method for investigating the genetic bases of many different diseases that are associated with an accumulation of metabolites in a well-established biochemical pathway. The abnormal gene product such as a defective enzyme is detected and then the genetic coding for that product can be specified. Unfortunately, most neuropsychiatric disorders do not have identifiable biochemical pathways. Therefore, the approach that seeks to first identify the location of the abnormal gene and then specify the abnormal gene product may be applicable in these cases.

The usual method used in the second approach is called genetic linkage analysis. This method relies on the fact that the probability of crossing over or recombination of genetic material is inversely related to the distance between gene loci. When gene loci are close enough, they do not cross over independently and are said to be linked. If a gene responsible for a disorder is found to be linked to a maker gene whose location is known, the location of the gene for the disorder can be estimated.

2.14   The answer is E.

Although genetic studies of anorexia nervosa have not received the same attention and energy as have other psychiatric disorders, there have been some interesting results of the studies conducted. There appear to be increased rates of anorexia nervosa, bulimia, and subclinical anorexia nervosa in first-degree female relatives of anorectic patients. A potentially important result is that first-degree relatives of anorectic patients appear to be at greater risk for affective disorders, even greater than the risk for anorexia nervosa in those relatives. In some studies, the risk for affective disorders in relatives of anorectic patients equals the risk for affective disorders in relatives of patients with major depression. The studies conducted in the area of bulimia have not used standard diagnostic criteria and have given inconsistent results.

2.15   The answer is B.

There is a very strong family association in the occurrence of alcoholism. Alcoholism in parents predicts alcoholism in male offspring even when these offspring are raised by adoptive parents. It is unclear whether the same relation holds for the female offspring of alcoholic parents, since those studies have had inconsistent results. It does not appear that alcoholism in the adoptive environment influences the occurrence of alcoholism. Although a Swedish study found support for both a genetic contribution to alcoholism and environmental influence from variables such as the socioeconomic status of the father, again, there did not appear to be an influence of alcoholism in the adopted environment on eventual rate of alcoholism among the adoptees.

2.16 The answer is **E**.

As our understanding of the genetic contributions to medical disorders has increased, there have been increases in requests for genetic counseling. Some reasons for requesting genetic counseling include wanting to know about personal risk or risk for potential offspring if marriage or pregnancy is being considered. Or relatives of an individual with a disorder may seek information in order to assuage their guilt. A physician who conducts genetic counseling or even refers patients for genetic counseling should first have an understanding of the motivations behind the request.

Components of genetic counseling include making an accurate diagnosis; obtaining a complete family history; estimating the risk of recurrence; evaluating the aims, intelligence, and emotions of the counselee; helping the counselee understand the risk of recurrence in the context of the specific demands and sequelae of the disorder; forming a plan of action; and providing follow-up to the counselee. When applied to genetic counseling for psychiatric disorders, some of the stages cannot at present be thoroughly completed. For example, estimating the risk of recurrence in psychiatric disorders is a speculative endeavor. However, the counselor should attempt to provide each component to every individual to the extent that accurate information is available and the counselee has the cognitive and emotional resources to deal with the information.

2.17 The answer is **B**.
2.18 The answer is **A**.
2.19 The answer is **C**.
2.20 The answer is **D**.

Adoption studies allow the research to separate the influence of two major parental variables on the eventual occurrence of a disorder in offspring. The two influences are genetic material and childrearing practices (environmental). In general, some drawbacks of these strategies provide moderation of the interpretations of these studies. The first consideration is that relatively few children are adopted away at birth, and there is usually some early environmental influence from the biological parents. Second, the environment includes the intrauterine environment, which may be a significant factor in the transmission of certain disorders. Also, adoption does not occur on a random basis and the factors that influence a parent to give up a child as well as those that influence a parent to adopt a child may have a systematic effect on the occurrence of the disorder. Given those drawbacks, adoption studies still can provide some very useful information.

The adoptee study method involves the evaluation of adopted-away children of a disordered parent. If the rate of occurrence of the disorder for adopted-away children is the same as for children who stay with the disordered parent and higher than for the children of nondisordered parents, then the data are evidence that genetic factors play a substantial role in the transmission and occurrence of the disorder.

The flip side of the above strategy is to study the children born of nondisordered parents who are adopted into a family with a disordered parent. This is known as the cross-fostering strategy. If the children have an occurrence rate for the disorder that is similar to that for children of nondisordered parents adopted into nondisordered families, this can be seen as evidence for the genetic hypothesis. If these children have an occurrence rate similar to that for offspring of disordered parents, this can be seen as evidence for the environmental hypothesis.

Comparing the biological and adoptive relatives of children of disordered biological parents is known as the adoptee's family method. Higher rates of occurrence in the biological relatives indicate the relative influence of heredity.

Finally, the study of monozygotic twins raised apart allows a unique opportunity to investigate the relative influence of genetic and environmental variables. In this type of study a concordance rate instead of a simple rate of occurrence is calculated. The idea is to determine whether the concordance rate varies when environments vary, given that genetic material is thought to be constant. Higher concordance rates for monozygotic twins raised apart than for dizygotic twins raised apart is evidence for the genetic hypothesis.

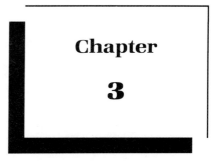

Chapter

3

Epidemiology of Mental Disorders

DIRECTIONS: Each of the statements or questions is followed by five suggested responses or completions. Select the one that is the best choice or most complete answer in each case.

3.1 The most widely used measure of agreement for reliability studies is:

    A. kappa
    B. percentage agreement
    C. consistency
    D. beta
    E. mu

3.2 Observer bias in epidemiological studies refers to:

    A. the same process as selection bias
    B. the process by which the examiner may probe more or less deeply to establish the presence of a risk factor helping to confirm the research hypothesis
    C. an unexamined characteristic being associated with both the suspected risk factor and the disorder
    D. the process by which the patient unknowingly provides the examiner with information that confirms the study's hypothesis
    E. none of the above

3.3   The central feature of the experimental method is:

    A.   random assignment of subjects
    B.   attention to interrater reliability
    C.   the use of statistical methods
    D.   total elimination of observer bias
    E.   the use of the observational method of study

3.4   In a classic study based on information from mental health treatment settings in New Haven in the 1950s, Hollingshead et al. found that:

    A.   the incidence rate for psychiatric illness was essentially the same for individuals of different social classes
    B.   the rate of psychiatric illness was highest in the more advantaged social classes than in the lower classes
    C.   patients in psychiatric treatment within a six-month period represented 10 percent of residents in the community
    D.   the rate of psychiatric illness was greater in lower social classes than in higher social classes
    E.   none of the above

3.5   Epidemiological studies of schizophrenia conducted in Europe have yielded prevalence rates ranging from:

    A.   2.5 to 5.3 per 1000
    B.   6.0 to 8.3 per 1000
    C.   10.0 to 12.6 per 1000
    D.   .05 to 1.1 per 1000
    E.   20.2 to 30.0 per 1000

3.6   Criterion validity refers to:

    A.   judgment by "experts" that the items that make up a test "make sense"
    B.   judgment that the items that make up a test cover the domain of knowledge relevant for the test's purposes
    C.   comparison of a test to another established test
    D.   the number of true cases who are detected by a test instrument
    E.   the ability of a test to predict who will develop the disorder at some point in time in the future

3.7 Which of the following epidemiological methods is primarily concerned with assessing the effect of preventive or therapeutic interventions designed to alter the development or outcome of illness?

    A. descriptive studies
    B. analytic studies
    C. historical studies
    D. experimental studies
    E. community diagnosis studies

DIRECTIONS: For each of the statements below, one or more of the alternative answers is correct. Choose answer:

    A if only 1, 2, and 3 are correct
    B if only 1 and 3 are correct
    C if only 2 and 4 are correct
    D if only 4 is correct
    E if all are correct

3.8 Which of the following are true regarding psychiatric epidemiology?

1. It is the quantitative study of the distribution of mental disorders in human populations.
2. It has been called the basic science of public health.
3. Population has been the traditional concern of epidemiologists.
4. Epidemiologists use quantitative methods to study populations.

3.9 The analytic level of epidemiological study focuses on which of the following areas?

1. assessing individual risks
2. identifying causes
3. historical study
4. population sampling

3.10 The use of prospective longitudinal studies involves:

1. the comparison of characteristics of individuals known to suffer from a psychiatric illness with those of individuals who do not suffer from psychiatric illness
2. the formation of a sample from the population who are younger than the typical onset for the disorder and assessment of risk factors
3. the use of experimental methods
4. reexamination after a reasonable length of time (usually one year) to determine who has developed the illness

3.11 Which of the following major sources of potential error can impede reliability in a diagnostic assessment?

1. information variance
2. observer variance
3. criterion variance
4. test–retest variance

3.12 International studies of affective disorders have found:

1. greater incidence of affective disorders in eastern block countries compared to the west
2. higher rates of affective disorders in Africa
3. a much higher prevalence of unipolar depression in adult males compared to females
4. generally consistent prevalence rates for studies of industrialized nations

DIRECTIONS: Each of the following questions consists of lettered headings followed by a list of numbered alternatives. Select the single lettered heading that is most closely associated with the appropriate numbered alternative. Each lettered heading may be chosen only once.

Level of epidemiological study

A. The experimental level
B. The analytic level
C. The descriptive level

Description

3.13 provides estimates of the rate of a disorder in the population
3.14 assesses the effect of preventive or therapeutic intervention
3.15 explores variations in rates among different groups in the population

ANSWERS

3.1   The answer is **A**.

The most widely used statistical measure of agreement for reliability studies is kappa. This measure corrects for the proportion of chance agreements to give an indication of agreement achieved beyond what would occur by chance alone. Calculation of the kappa statistic has been described for a variety of situations, including multiple examiners who produce multiple diagnoses for a given subject. Guidelines for interpreting kappa suggest that values above .75 are excellent, values between .40 and .75 are good, and values below .40 are poor.

3.2   The answer is **B**.

A researcher who is attempting to establish risk factors for a particular disorder by inquiring into the subject's past history may have clues that the subject is in the case or comparison group. As a result, the examiner may probe more or less deeply to establish the presence of a risk factor, thereby helping to confirm the study's hypothesis. This is referred to as observer bias and is especially problematic for studies in which retrospective assessments are used.

3.3   The answer is **A**.

The central feature of the experimental method is the random assignment of subjects to either the experimental intervention group or the control group, within the intervention. The process of randomly assigning subjects is expected to prevent selection bias and also to reduce possible confounding bias, because any unknown underlying causes would be equally distributed between the control and experimental groups, at least with large enough numbers. The practice of having examiners and subjects "blind" to their assignment in the groups is also expected to minimize observer bias.

3.4   The answer is **D**.

In a classic study based on information for mental health treatment settings in New Haven, Connecticut, in the 1950s, Hollingshead et al. found that the highest rate of psychiatric disorders occurred in the lowest social class, as compared with the higher social classes. More specifically, these researchers found a rate in the highest social class ranging from 5 to 7 per 1,000, compared with 17 per 1,000 in the lowest social class. This study had a major impact on public policymakers and was one of the pieces of information lending support for the Community Mental Health Act of 1963.

3.5 The answer is **A**.

Epidemiological studies of schizophrenia conducted in Europe have yielded prevalence rates from 2.5 to 5.3 per 1,000. These figures represent a definitive summary of literature in a variety of languages. The results of several studies outside of Europe are consistent with these findings.

3.6 The answer is **C**.

In the absence of a definitive standard for establishing accuracy in psychiatric diagnosis, current practice in psychiatry has been to use another, usually well-known test as a comparison instrument to establish criterion validity. In studies of criterion validity, several measures of interest have been developed: Sensitivity is a measure of the number of true cases who are detected by the instrument being validated; specificity is the number of true noncases who are accurately assessed by the new instrument. Another measure, positive predictive validity, estimates the number of positive subjects who are truly cases of the disorder.

3.7 The answer is **D**.

Experimental epidemiology, particularly preventive trials designed to modify presumed risk factors in high-risk subjects, is one way to establish that an association observed in nonexperimental studies between a risk factor and an illness have a cause-and-effect relationship. The question of whether or not an observed association between a possible risk factor and an illness is a cause-and-effect one plagues many epidemiological studies. Short of conducting experimental investigations designed to reduce the potential impact of a risk factor, other types of evidence (for example, observational) may be used to lend confidence that the association is meaningful.

3.8 The answer is **E**.

Psychiatric epidemiology is the quantitative study of the distribution of mental disorders in human populations. Population has been the traditional concern of the epidemiologist. Epidemiology is unusual among clinical disciplines in focusing on populations rather than on individuals, and this characteristic has led it to be called the basic science of public health. By providing quantitative methods to study populations, epidemiology provides an opportunity for precise estimation of the importance of risk factors, the performance of diagnostic tests, and the effectiveness of new treatments.

3.9   The answer is **B**.

The analytic level of study in epidemiology focuses on several types of information. First of all, epidemiologists are as interested in reducing the burden of illness in the population as clinicians are for the individual patient. Knowing the rates of illness for the population at large provides the epidemiologist with a powerful springboard to identification of groups in the population who have a high risk of developing the illness in the future. Once these high-risk populations are identified, it is possible to implement more focused studies to characterize the attributes that place members of the group at particular risk. In addition, statistical techniques developed by epidemiologist provide estimates of the magnitude of elevated risk. In the search for possible risk factors and efforts to establish their relative importance, epidemiologists have also been interested in historical trends. For example, there is suggestive evidence that depressive illness may be occurring more commonly in younger generations than previously.

3.10   The answer is **C**.

Prospective longitudinal studies provide several types of information with regard to the estimation of incidence rates. An excellent way to assess incidence rates in a population is to form a sample from the population who are younger than the typical age of onset for the disorder and to assess them for a variety of characteristics that may be potential risk factors to be considered in the study. After a reasonable amount of time has passed (typically one year) subjects can be reexamined to determine who has developed the illness. The incidence rate is then calculated with the number of new cases in the numerator and the total number of people at risk at the beginning of the time period in the denominator.

3.11   The answer is **A**.

Three major sources of potential error can make it difficult to achieve reliability in diagnostic assessments. Information variance refers to the fact that different examiners (or even the same examiner on different occasions) may solicit different information from the subject and therefore use a different data base for assessing potential disorders and classifying them. Observer variance suggests that different examiners may interpret the same information differently. Criterion variance refers to the problem that different examiners, even when using the same data base, may have different criteria for assigning a subject to a particular diagnostic group.

3.12 The answer is **C**.

Examining the world literature on prevalence of affective disorders, Boyd and Weissman (1981) found generally consistent prevalence rates for studies within industrialized nations. They reported the prevalence of unipolar depression as about 3 per 100 adult males and 4 to 9 per 100 females. However, in a study of two Ugandan villages using the Present State Exam, much higher rates were found: 14.3 per 100 for males and 22.6 per 100 for females. To date, these higher rates in Africa have yet to be satisfactorily explained.

3.13 The answer is **C**.
3.14 The answer is **A**.
3.15 The answer is **B**.

Descriptive studies provide estimates of the rate of disorder in a population. This level of study has focused on providing estimates of prevalence of a mental disorder in the community (community diagnosis), the identification of syndromes, and the study of individuals who have not yet entered psychiatric treatment.

The experimental level of study assesses the effect of preventive or therapeutic interventions designed to alter the development or outcome of the illness. Once possible risk factors have been identified, and a likely causal chain has been proposed, it is possible to design interventions and test the effectiveness of these treatments in reducing the clinical problem of interest.

The analytic level of study explores variations in rates among different groups to identify risk factors. This involves assessing individual risks of development of a disorder as well as searching for possible risks through the study of historical trends.

Chapter 4

Normal Growth and Development

DIRECTIONS: Each of the statements or questions is followed by five suggested responses or completions. Select the one that is the best choice or most complete answer in each case.

4.1 Which of the following statements is true?

    A. Growth refers to an organism's potential for change over time in response to environmental events.

    B. Growth refers to the movement of an organism toward its genetically determined abilities.

    C. Growth refers to the simple increase in tissue, size, or number of cells.

    D. Growth refers to the movement of an organism toward its genetically determined physical structures and concomitant functions.

    E. Growth refers to the changing structure of thought and behavior over time.

4.2 Which of the following is not true regarding the concept of epigenesis?

    A. Epigenesis posits a relation among stages of development.

    B. Under epigenesis, the child is "born" or becomes a new person at each stage.

    C. Under epigenesis, development is linear.

    D. Serial stages influence subsequent stages.

    E. Each stage is dependent on resolution of the experience of the previous stage.

4.3 Freud's psychoanalytic developmental theory encompasses which one of the following points?

    A. Childhood is a period of absent sexuality.

    B. The anxiety aroused by the birth experience underlies all symptom formation.

    C. Rationalization is a major defense mechanism of childhood.

    D. The watershed of childhood experiences is when a child first spends a significant portion of the day at school away from home.

    E. Psychopathology is the result of either a fixation or a regression, but both refer to earlier stages of development.

4.4 Which of the following groups is a correct list of Rene Spitz's organizers?

    A. smiling, fear of strangers, and signaling no

    B. smiling, verbalizing, and gesturing

    C. verbalizing, gesturing, and watching

    D. watching, listening, and smelling

    E. verbalizing, listening, and gesturing

4.5 Sleep electroencephalogram patterns follow which form?

    A. Infant sleep is characterized by a large proportion of Stages 3 and 4 sleep.

    B. The adult pattern of sleep is not formed until puberty.

    C. Sleep spindles are frequent at first, but taper off by the third or fourth month.

    D. When infants fall asleep, they pass rapidly from Stage 1 through Stage 4.

    E. Infants continue their pattern of three- to four-hour cycles of sleep and wakefulness until about one year of age.

4.6   Which of the following is not true regarding Piaget's sensory–motor stage of development?

A.   The sensory–motor stage occurs only after resolution of the concrete operations stage.

B.   Here, an object out of sight is considered by the child to be no longer existent.

C.   Sensory impressions are closely linked to motor activity. .

D.   There are six substages of development in the sensory–motor stage during which the infant learns to perceive the environment in a manner similar to others in the same culture.

E.   During this stage the infant learns to extend movements already started.

4.7   Neurodevelopmental, cognitive, and social data all suggest that:

A.   by age 7, all of the adult skills are present; all that is needed is practice in application

B.   between the ages of 6 and 9, there is a smooth upward curve of change

C.   there is a discontinuity at age 7

D.   the brain doesn't reach its adult form until age 14

E.   the period between ages 6 and 8 represents a quiet period of consolidation

4.8   Which of the following is not a part of Bowlby's theories?

A.   Attachment originates in inborn response systems.

B.   The visual characteristics and behavior of the infant keep the adult caretaker in interaction with the infant.

C.   The babylike characteristics are fairly consistent across species.

D.   The behavior and characteristics of babies have an evolutionary advantage.

E.   Attachment is stronger for blood relations than for social relations.

DIRECTIONS: For each of the statements or questions below, one or more of the alternative answers is correct. Choose answer:

    A if only 1, 2, and 3 are correct
    B if only 1 and 3 are correct
    C if only 2 and 4 are correct
    D if only 4 is correct
    E if all are correct

4.9 Which of the following is true regarding stranger anxiety?

1. Its development depends on an ability to engage in social discrimination.
2. It first appears between about four and six months of age.
3. Stranger anxiety is less likely to occur if a parent is present or if a toy is presented.
4. Its occurrence is a sign of maladjustment.

4.10 Stern's theory of development states that between seven and nine months the sense of self undergoes further organization to include:

1. a concept of a purposeful self
2. a concept of guilt
3. a concept of good versus bad
4. a capacity to share subjective experience

4.11 Which of the following statements regarding the concept of a private self are true?

1. This concept is elaborated between the ages of 3 and 5 years.
2. This concept doesn't emerge until adolescence.
3. Emergence of this concept allows more complicated interpersonal relations.
4. This concept precludes the expression of jealousy.

4.12 Which of the following statements regarding attainment of formal operations are true?

1. Only 10 percent of 14-year-olds attain formal operations.
2. Thirty-five percent of 16- to 17-year-olds attain formal operations.
3. Between 25 and 33 percent of adults attain formal operations.
4. Attainment of formal operations usually occurs with achievement of abstract intelligence at age 14.

4.13 In their studies of adolescents, the Offers have specified developmental routes, including:

1. continuous growth
2. surgent growth
3. tumultuous growth
4. hierarchical growth

DIRECTIONS: Each of the following questions consists of lettered headings followed by a list of numbered alternatives. Select the single lettered heading that is most closely associated with the appropriate numbered alternative. Each lettered heading may be chosen only once.

A. differentiation
B. integration
C. hierarchical reorganization
D. critical period

4.14 considers development to be not only linear but also as having changing structures over time

4.15 proposes that psychological and social systems mature into entities

4.16 states that development includes a process of concatenating information between and among the senses

4.17 states that an environmental releaser can stimulate the emergence of an inborn capacity only within a certain time frame

ANSWERS

4.1 The answer is **C**.

Developmental theory has several terms whose meanings may or may not be consistent with the meanings found in common parlance. In this area, the term *growth* is used to refer to the single increase in tissue, size, or number of cells. An increase in weight is referred to as growth. The term maturation is used to describe a condition whereby an individual changes in accord with his or her abilities, function, and structures. The term *maturation* has a somewhat less determinate meaning than other terms in developmental theory. The term *development* itself refers to those changes seen as a result of "maturation" as well as those changes that occur as the result of social or environmental variables.

4.2   The answer is B.

Development is sometimes seen as a series of stages through which an individual passes on the way to adulthood. Under the concept of epigenesis, each subsequent step is influenced by the steps that preceded it. In fact, before an individual can move on to the next step, the issues of the previous step must be resolved. Therefore, it can be seen that the relation among steps of development is linear and follows the same trajectory for all individuals.

4.3   The answer is E.

Psychoanalytic theories of child development derive from both a genetic view where retrospective inferences are used to organize a personal history and a developmental view where psychoanalysts conduct prospective observations of developing children. Freud thought that children were polymorphously perverse and that experiences could cause certain body zones to retain their sexual nature into adulthood. Libido theory specified the path that children were supposed to take to sexual maturity.

Freud thought that repression was a major defense mechanism in childhood. When repression did not take place successfully, anxiety broke to the surface signaling that dangerous thoughts were close to entering consciousness. The oedipal conflict and its resolution constitute a watershed of childhood development. Here the child is faced with conflicting feelings regarding the parents. Psychopathology can result either from a fixation at an early stage of development due to a failure to resolve the conflicts at that stage or from a regression to an earlier stage when under stress.

4.4   The answer is A.

Rene Spitz conducted direct observations of infants, resulting in a genetic field theory. He proposed the existence of three organizers that influenced and were influenced by the environment of the child. The first organizer is the smiling response, which the infant gives in response to certain visual stimuli and which evokes certain responses from the environment. The second organizer is the stranger response, which occurs at about seven months of age. This organizer marks the attachment of the infant to a significant other and the anxiety that is felt when some other person is too close to the child. The third organizer is the signal for no. The acquisition of this signal marks the beginning of the child as an individuated human being who can exert his or her own will separate even from the mother.

4.5   The answer is D.

In the period immediately following birth, the infant has a rapidly repeating short cycle (3.5 to 4 hours) of sleep and wakefulness. These periods of sleep are dominated by Stages 1 and 2 sleep, which are a light sleep. The sleep spindles don't appear until about three to four months of age. At about this same age, the infantile electroencephalogram patterns of sleep where Stage 1 rapidly changes into Stage 4 move to a pattern where the changes from State 1 to Stage 4 more closely resemble the electroencephalogram patterns found in adult sleep.

4.6   The answer is A.

Piaget's sensory–motor stage of development precedes the concrete operations stage and is actually a series of six substages during which the infant begins to perceive the environment in a manner similar to that used by others in the same cultural environment. This first stage of development is called sensory–motor partly because all sensory operations are tied to motor behaviors. In the first and second substages, objects that are out of sensory experience cease to exist for the child. Events are not perceived as being linked to events that surround the original event in space or time. It is only in the third substage that the child learns to follow the extension of movements already started and to realize that those movements are connected to the same series of events. During the fourth substage, the child discovers reversible actions—that if an object is covered from sight, it can be uncovered and found to be still existing as the same object. During the fifth and sixth stages the child achieves some notion of the permanence of the object.

4.7   The answer is C.

All investigation, whether social or neurobiological, provides evidence that there is a discontinuous shift that occurs at about age 7. At this age the brain attains its adult format and weight. The density of neuronal dendrites is greatest at this age. At this age children begin to realize that their own feelings and thoughts are important to other people. They also begin to understand the motivation of other people and start to be able to place themselves in "someone else's shoes." However, children at this age also may become rule-bound and moralistic, because they are able to apply rules that they learn only in a rigid manner.

4.8   The answer is E.

Bowlby suggested that the behavior and physical, visual characteristics of the infant evoke caregiving behavior in adults, thereby increasing the chances of survival of the infant. Bowlby developed his theory partly from a review of ethological studies. Bowlby states that certain characteristics of "babyness" are universal across species, for example, infants' tiny size, relatively large head with a prominent forehead, small face, large eyes, and chubby cheeks. By engaging in characteristic babylike behavior, the infant helps ensure that an adult caregiver will remain close in the environment. The exhibition of behavior by the infant and the response of the adult are genetically determined and show an evolutionary advantage by increasing the chances of survival of an organism that cannot care for itself. By this logic, all adults will respond in the same way to the infant regardless of the relation to the infant.

4.9   The answer is A.

The development of stranger wariness at about seven months is a sign of normal development. This is a period when the infant begins to develop a sense of self and also begins to have some sense of social discrimination. Earlier, corresponding to a period between four and six months of age, the infant seems to enjoy being handled by multiple people in the environment. Then the infant begins to show signs of interest but wariness when in the presence of strangers. Facial expressions of fear in response to strangers occur before the actual behavioral signs of fear, which may not appear until the age of eight months to one year. The expressions of fear can be reduced if the parent is close to the infant or if a toy is given to the infant.

4.10   The answer is D.

Stern's theory of development suggests that between seven and nine months of age, the infant's sense of self undergoes a reorganization such that the infant begins to have a capacity to share certain subjective experiences. For example, nine-month-old infants can pay attention to objects that are watched by the mother. These infants will follow the pointed finger of the mother and then check the facial expression of the mother to see if they are attending to the correct object. Babies at this age also begin to realize that it is possible to share internal feelings by some form of expression.

4.11   The answer is **B**.

Somewhere between the ages of three and five years, the child begins to realize that there is a private self that cannot be observed by others. Concomitant with this realization is an increase in the complexity of relationships with others. The child begins to use the concept of secrets, singular to a certain relationship. At the same time, the child begins to develop rivalry, jealousy, and envy. Peer relationships begin to include cooperative play and shared fantasies. At this time the child also begins to use language to express emotions.

4.12   The answer is **A**.

Formerly, it was thought that abstract thought began at age 14. However, recent evidence suggests that as little as 10 percent of 14-year-olds have achieved abstract thought or formal operations. Only 35 percent of 16- to 17-year-olds have achieved formal operations. Even in the group of adolescents considered gifted, only 60 percent have achieved abstract thought. However, this figure compares favorably to the general adult populations where it is estimated that between 25 percent and 33 percent can be said to have achieved formal operations.

4.13   The answer is **A**.

The Offers have studied patterns of growth in adolescents. They have specified three general routes of growth for adolescents. The first category is called continuous growth and it refers to conditions whereby a minimum of major separations, deaths, or severe illnesses occur. Children who experience continuous growth have parents who encourage independence.

Children who experience surgent growth tend to be late bloomers. They are less action oriented than the children who experience continuous growth. They also are more likely to experience periods of depressed affect or anxiety. They tend to be less introspective.

Children who experience tumultuous growth come from backgrounds that are less stable than those of the other two groups. They tend to experience self-doubt and report more conflict with their families. Children from this group prefer art, humanities, and social sciences over professional and business careers.

4.14   The answer is **C**.
4.15   The answer is **A**.
4.16   The answer is **B**.
4.17   The answer is **D**.

Hierarchical reorganization is an idea that suggests that development is not necessarily just linear, but also can be conceived of as being composed of stages with changing structures over time. These changing structures allow changes in organization that are not totally dependent on prior stages for their existence. Therefore the functions and adaptations of each stage are not easily predicted from those of the earlier stage.

Differentiation is a central theme in development. The social and psychological systems of an organism differentiate into separate entities. In addition, the infant learns to differentiate sensory information.

On the other hand, integration, another broad theme of development, takes place between and among the senses. At first the child uses the hand to grasp an object only if both the object and the hand are in the same visual field. Later, the child learns to reach for an object that is seen, even if the hand is out of sight, but can be felt. Still later the child learns to link complex series of behavior into single chains without much conscious sensory evaluation of the motor behavior.

The concept of the critical period comes from ethological research. Under this idea, environmental releasors elicit the demonstration of developmental capacities that, although genetically inborn, are available only during a certain period of time. For example, there appears to be a critical period for the emergence of imprinting in birds. This concept appears to be more applicable to lower animals and less applicable to mammals.

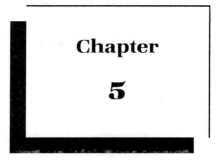

Theories of the Mind and Psychopathology

DIRECTIONS: Each of the statements or questions is followed by five suggested responses or completions. Select the one that is the best choice or most complete answer in each case.

5.1 Which of the following statements is correct concerning the topographical model?

    A. The mind is divided into conscious, preconscious, and unconscious.

    B. The bulk of psychic life can be described as being conscious.

    C. Primary process is governed by the reality principle and secondary process is governed by the pleasure principle.

    D. This model emphasizes the existence of the collective unconscious.

    E. None of the above.

5.2 Which of the following is not true regarding the psychoanalytic view of dreams?

> **A.** This viewpoint emphasizes the unconscious fulfillment of infantile wishes.
> **B.** This viewpoint emphasizes the use of displacement, condensation, and symbol formation.
> **C.** Dreams have a manifest and a latent component.
> **D.** Dreams always use standard symbols.
> **E.** None of the above.

5.3 Which of the following are true regarding the system preconscious?

> **A.** It is primarily motivated by the pleasure principle.
> **B.** The topographical model implies an anatomical correlation in the brain.
> **C.** It follows Aristotelian logic.
> **D.** The system preconscious and system conscious work by rules of primary process.
> **E.** None of the above.

5.4 Which contemporary of Freud is credited with legitimizing the study of hysteria?

> **A.** Charcot
> **B.** Adler
> **C.** Jung
> **D.** Jackson
> **E.** Rank

5.5 Pavlov's famous experiment with dogs illustrated the following process:

> **A.** operant conditioning
> **B.** classical conditioning
> **C.** instrumental conditioning
> **D.** negative reinforcement
> **E.** the use of "cognitive maps"

5.6 The explanation that learning theory might give to the psychoanalytic phenomenon of transference is:

> **A.** stimulus satiation
> **B.** stimulus discrimination
> **C.** extinction
> **D.** stimulus generalization
> **E.** shaping

DIRECTIONS: For each of the statements below, one or more of the alternative answers is correct. Choose answer:

    A if only 1, 2, and 3 are correct
    B if only 1 and 3 are correct
    C if only 2 and 4 are correct
    D if only 4 is correct
    E if all are correct

5.7 Which of the following are true of the structural model?

1. The mind consists of id, ego, and superego.
2. This model invalidates the topographical model.
3. In this model, the focus begins to shift away from drives and toward defenses.
4. This model emphasizes that the ego arises mainly from parental role models.

5.8 Which statements are true regarding defense mechanisms?

1. All defense mechanisms are basically variations of repression.
2. Defense mechanisms are mostly unconscious.
3. The presence of defenses is pathological.
4. Defense mechanisms are associated with fantasied actions.

5.9 Which of the following are correct?

1. Sullivan emphasized interpersonal factors in a complex theory of development.
2. Kohut emphasized deficiencies in development over internal drive conflicts in his theory of narcissism.
3. Successful efforts have been made to explain some of psychoanalytic theory in terms of learning theory.
4. Jung emphasized the balance of archetypal symbols in his theory of dream interpretation.

DIRECTIONS: Each of the following questions consists of lettered headings followed by a list of numbered alternatives. Select the single lettered heading that is most closely associated with the appropriate numbered alternative. Each lettered heading may be chosen only once.

Defense mechanism

- **A.** Introjection and identification
- **B.** Projection
- **C.** Reversal
- **D.** Denial
- **E.** Splitting
- **F.** Sublimation
- **G.** Repression

Description

5.10 is an invalidation of an unpleasant or unwanted piece of information, and living one's life as if it didn't exist

5.11 is said to be active when the ego functions to achieve maximum satisfaction of drives with minimum anxiety and minimum disruption of the environment

5.12 translates the aim of an instinct into its opposite

5.13 are normal mechanisms of growth as well as defenses—important objects are "taken in" to avoid the pain of their loss or separation

5.14 involves the fantasy of spitting, throwing, or in some other way hurling from ourselves some acceptable mental content

5.15 is the means by which we keep aspects of mental content separate

5.16 keeps unwanted affects, memories, or drives from consciousness

ANSWERS

5.1 The answer is **A**.

From his prepsychoanalytic era, Freud recognized that the bulk of psychic life lay outside of consciousness. It was his major contribution to psychiatric thinking that unconscious mental life was elaborated. In his conceptualization of the topographical model, Freud introduced the three "areas" of mind: conscious, preconscious, and unconscious. The enduring significance of the topographical model was to define unconscious processes as the field of psychiatric investigation and treatment.

5.2 The answer is **D**.

According to Freud, dreams were the outstanding example of unconscious mental activity. Dreamers reported what Freud called "the manifest dream." This was the conscious rendition of the dreamer's experience during the dream. In addition, Freud theorized that every dream contained several elements: day residue, which was the memories of the events of the preceding day that retain unconscious emotional charge; and nocturnal stimuli, which may be noises from the area where the dreamer is sleeping or an enteroceptive awareness of bodily processes. These relatively conscious processes are blended together with unconscious wishes and with their associated memories from childhood. Together, they constitute the "latent dream." In the process of sorting through the day residue and the nocturnal stimuli, the associated files to repressed unconscious childhood (or infantile) wishes were stimulated.

The process of turning the latent dream into the manifest dream is referred to as "dream work." To the initial actions of condensation, displacement, and symbol formation is added the transformation of the dream after the dreamer awakes.

5.3 The answer is **C**.

The system preconscious and the system conscious work by the rules of secondary process. Here the basic motivating force is the "reality principle," according to which gratification is delayed for other purposes. What has been called "Aristotelian logic" is followed, time moves in forward linear direction, contradictions may not exist simultaneously, and thinking is more concerned with the content and logic of ideas than with their emotional intensity. The topographical model does not imply a direct anatomical correlation in the brain between primary and secondary process with mental activity, although Freud always left the possibility open.

5.4 The answer is **A**.

Charcot legitimized for Freud the study of patients suffering from hysteria. Charcot rejected the notion that these patients were either malingering or that they had a "wandering uterus," and emphasized the link between their symptoms and traumatic events and the importance of symbolism in the disorder. Further, he demonstrated the role that hypnosis played in the treatment of hysteria.

5.5 The answer is **B**.

Pavlov's famous experiments with dogs illustrated how a stimulus not intrinsically or ordinarily associated with a response may be used to induce that response. He demonstrated that the organism "learns" to associate the once-neutral stimulus with a stimulus that always (or unconditionally) produces the response. For example, Pavlov showed that a dog will salivate when presented with food, because of an "unconditioned" physiological reflex response. If a bell is rung before the food is presented, the dog will "learn" to salivate when it hears the bell. This process has been called classical or respondent conditioning.

5.6 The answer is **D**.

Stimulus generalization may be seen as the explanation that learning theory gives to the phenomenon referred to in psychoanalytic circles as "transference." The process of stimulus generalization refers to the response of the organism, during conditioning, to other stimuli that resemble the original stimulus in some way. Transference would represent stimulus generalization gone amok, with an ordinarily innocuous stimulus from the analyst being erroneously generalized to a traumatic stimulus from the patient during childhood.

5.7 The answer is **B**.

In the structural model, Freud proposed the division of the mind into id, ego, and superego. The ego was a synonym for the mental self, the agency which exerted control over drives and defenses. The ego owes its origin to and starts out from its activity of perception. In the course of perceiving, the ego discerns differences between the internal and external, pleasurable and unpleasurable, and so forth. Thus the ego starts out as a function of the body that defines the mental image of the body. It is important to emphasize that the structural point of view and the topographical point of view are neither incompatible nor exactly complementary. Under the influence of structural theory, the attention of psychoanalysis moved away from instinctual drives to the workings of each individual ego as it dealt with drives and anxiety to achieve maximum adaptation.

5.8 The answer is **C**.

In order to function smoothly, the ego has to have a set of automatic operations with which to deal with the competing memories, perceptions, external realistic needs, drives, and anxieties that it faces. These automatic operations by which the ego balances its competing interests are known collectively as defense mechanisms. Defenses are unconscious ways of getting rid of unpleasant mental content, whether they are memories, wishes, drives, or affects. Defenses are carried out by the individual as internal, automatic workings of the ego that reveal the style with which the individual copes with unwelcome mental content. It is important to realize that defenses not only ward off unacceptable mental content, but are themselves mental content consisting of fantasies of their own.

5.9 The answer is **E**.

For Harry Stack Sullivan, personality was a hypothetical construct; what was real and actual was relationships. Everything therefore had to be interpreted through the lens of interpersonal relations.

Kohut emphasized deficiencies in development over internal drive conflicts in his theory of narcissism stressing that the development of a cohesive self is more important than the vicissitudes of instincts.

An example of attempts to explain aspects of psychoanalytic theory in terms of learning theory is the explanation of transference as stimulus generalization or the tendency for the organism to respond to other stimuli that resemble an original stimulus.

Jung emphasized the balance of archetypal symbols in his theory of dream interpretation. He conceptualized archetypes as innate ideas or preformating that readies us for real experiences. According to Jung, the dream reveals imbalances in the unity of the self and is understood by identifying the archetypal meaning of the symbols in question.

5.10 The answer is **D**.
5.11 The answer is **F**.
5.12 The answer is **C**.
5.13 The answer is **A**.
5.14 The answer is **B**.
5.15 The answer is **E**.
5.16 The answer is **G**.

Denial is the invalidation of an unpleasant or unwanted piece of information, and the living of one's life as though this piece of information did not exist. Denial is a more severe form of repression. It denies access to consciousness, but is more costly in terms of reality testing because a piece of reality is not only ignored (as in repression) but is actually invalidated. Thus reality testing is diminished. The persistent refusal to be swayed by the evidence of reality is an indicator that denial is at work.

Anna Freud added sublimation to the list of defense mechanisms as a normal ego function. Sublimation is said to be taking place when the ego functions to achieve maximum satisfaction of drives with minimum anxiety and minimum disruption of the environment.

Reversal is the process by which the aim of an instinct is translated into its opposite, as in activity changing into passivity or passivity changing into activity. Reversal has also been used as an explanation of how sadism and masochism can alternate with each other.

Introjection and identification are normal mechanisms of growth as well as defenses. Important objects are "taken into" the self to avoid the pain of their loss or separation. This is particularly intense in cases of ambivalently regarded objects. Identification is more or less healthy, more or less part of normal growth and development, and more or less pathological, depending on the type.

Projection is a complex defense mechanism that can operate at a more primitive or advanced level. Projection involves the fantasy of spitting, throwing, or in some other ways hurling from themselves some unacceptable mental content. The schematic prototype would be "I don't hate him, he hates me." In this example, the affect is disowned and is, through displacement, projected onto someone else. This defense mechanism is used to its extreme in paranoia.

Splitting is hypothesized to be the means by which we keep aspects of mental content separate. Initially, this consists of keeping pleasurable affects, memories, and the "good objects" separate from unpleasurable affects, memories, and the "bad objects."

Repression is the defense that keeps from consciousness unwanted affects, memories, or drives. Repression requires a permanent countercathexis established against the unwelcome mental content into awareness. The countercathexis takes place on an unconscious basis. When something is successfully repressed, it is barred from access to consciousness, but it is also no longer amenable to further modification by the ego and can take on a life of its own in the form of symptom complex or a portion of character structure.

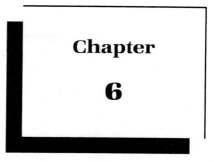

Chapter

6

Psychiatric Interview, Psychiatric History, and Mental Status Examination

DIRECTIONS: Each of the statements or questions is followed by five suggested responses or completions. Select the one that is the best choice or most complete answer in each case.

6.1 The single most important method of assessing and understanding a psychiatric disorder is:

    A. the mental status examination
    B. the psychiatric interview
    C. projective testing
    D. a complete battery of psychological testing
    E. self-report questionnaires

6.2 The basis for the therapeutic alliance is the:

    A. patient's motivations for working with a psychiatrist
    B. psychiatrist's friendly and concerned manner
    C. psychiatrist's dynamic understanding of the patient
    D. patient's infant relationship with his or her mother
    E. psychiatrist's mannerisms during the interview

6.3 The process by which the patient reflects an attitude or behaviors that run counter to the therapeutic objectives of the treatment is:

- **A.** resistance
- **B.** countertransference
- **C.** obstinate behavior
- **D.** ego differentiation
- **E.** free association

6.4 "I want" messages refer to:

- **A.** unconscious wishes of the therapist to change the patient
- **B.** the therapist's need to see the patient as healthier than he or she really is
- **C.** the psychiatrist's assertion to move on to other areas of inquiry when the patient is focused on a single theme
- **D.** a conscious attempt on the part of the patient to frustrate the therapist
- **E.** none of the above

DIRECTIONS: For each of the statements below, one or more of the alternative answers is correct. Choose answer:

- **A** if only 1, 2, and 3 are correct
- **B** if only 1 and 3 are correct
- **C** if only 2 and 4 are correct
- **D** if only 4 is correct
- **E** if all are correct

6.5 In setting up an initial diagnostic interview with the patient, the psychiatrist:

1. arranges an appointment at a time convenient to the patient
2. defers discussing his or her clinical impressions garnered in the phone conversation until he or she sees the patient
3. tells the patient how much time they will have for the interview
4. defers talking about the cost of the evaluation until he or she sees the patient

6.6   The psychiatrist should not reveal information the patient has shared in confidence without the patient's permission except when:

1. the psychiatrist feels that the spouse should know
2. the patient is a preschooler and the psychiatrist discusses the interview with the mother
3. the psychiatrist uncovers a delusion of jealousy
4. the psychiatrist determines that the patient is a danger to himself or others

6.7   During the initial interview, the psychiatrist:

1. assumes a primary posture for listening
2. remains silent for long periods of time if the patient becomes silent
3. encourages the expression of feelings
4. focuses the first 50 minutes on the history of the present illness

6.8   During the concluding part of the interview, the psychiatrist should:

1. inform the patient about the amount of time remaining
2. ask the patient if he or she has any questions
3. request permission to contact the patient's personal physician
4. use *Diagnostic and Statistical Manual of Mental Disorders (Third Edition, Revised)* terminology to share his or her clinical impressions

6.9   Transference reactions are:

1. unconsciously determined
2. inappropriate in the present
3. projections onto the psychiatrist
4. treated as real in therapy

6.10   Hypnopompic and hypnagogic hallucinations are associated with:

1. psychosis
2. normal sleep
3. night terrors
4. narcolepsy

6.11   Childhood symptoms reflecting emotional distress include:

1. night terrors
2. nail biting
3. enuresis
4. impotence

DIRECTIONS: Each of the following questions consists of lettered headings followed by a list of numbered alternatives. Select the single lettered heading that is most closely associated with the appropriate numbered alternative. Each lettered heading may be chosen only once.

Facilitative message

A. Self-disclosure
B. Positive reinforcement
C. Checklist questions
D. Open-ended questions

Description

6.12 reflects a topic that the psychiatrist is interested in exploring but leaves it to the patient to choose which areas he or she believes are relevant

6.13 involves the psychiatrist's signaling approval of the patient's discussion of a relevant topic

6.14 involves the psychiatrist's providing the patient with a potential list of responses on a given topic

6.15 refers to the psychiatrist's sharing of personal information during the course of the interview

ANSWERS

6.1 The answer is **B**.

The psychiatric interview is the central vehicle for assessment of the psychiatric patient. The patient presenting for psychiatric evaluation is seeking help, and the psychiatrist is the medical expert trained to diagnose and treat the patient. In the context of the psychiatric interview, the patient reveals what is troubling him or her. The psychiatrist listens and makes responses that are geared to obtaining as clear an understanding of the patient's problems as possible. The psychiatrist arrives at a diagnostic formulation of the patient's difficulties at the end of the interview. The more accurate the diagnostic assessment, the more appropriate the treatment plan is.

6.2   The answer is **D**.

The therapeutic alliance is the process by which the patient's mature, observing ego is used with the psychiatrist's analytic abilities to advance their understanding of the patient's difficulties. The basis for this alliance is the trusting relationship established in early life between the child and his or her mother, as well as other significant trusting relationships from the patient's past. The establishment of this trust is extremely important because without such an alliance, the patient cannot reveal his or her innermost thoughts and feelings.

6.3   The answer is **A**.

Resistance is a theoretical construct that reflects any attitude or behaviors that run counter to the therapeutic objectives of the treatment. Freud originally described several types of resistance, including conscious resistance, ego resistance, id resistance, and superego resistance.

Conscious resistance occurs for a variety of reasons such as a lack of trust of the psychiatrist, the patient's shame in relating certain events, or fear of rejection by the psychiatrist.

Ego resistance may take the form of repression whereby, for mostly unconscious reasons, the same psychodynamic forces that led to the patient's symptoms keep him or her from developing an awareness of the underlying conflict. Transference resistance is a second form of ego resistance, whereby the patient projects undesirable feelings onto the psychiatrist and attributes these feelings to the psychiatrist. A third type of ego resistance is secondary-gain resistance. This may occur when the patient's symptoms elicit nurturing responses from others, thereby meeting the patient's dependency needs.

Id resistance refers to the patient's repeatedly bringing up the same material in therapy in the face of repeated interpretations of the behavior by the psychiatrist.

Superego resistance occurs most often with obsessional, depressed patients who because of guilt feelings, exhibit a need for punishment. Hence, the patient continues to exhibit symptoms that serve to punish him or her.

6.4   The answer is **C**.

"I want" messages refer to the psychiatrist's assertion to move on to other areas of inquiry during the psychiatric interview when the interview has failed to progress because of the patient's need to focus on a single theme. By asserting the need to move on, the psychiatrist avoids building up his or her own resentment toward the patient and averts the acting out of these frustrations.

6.5   The answer is **A**.

The initial telephone contact sets the stage for subsequent psychiatric interviews. During this contact, the psychiatrist exhibits the capacity to be an expert listener who will work with the patient to understand the patient's difficulties. Rapport begins with this initial contact.

In addition to actively listening to the patient's problem, the psychiatrist advises the patient about what to expect during the initial interview. The patient is informed about the minimum amount of time that the interview will take, the hourly cost of the interview, the charge for missed appointments, and whether or not the psychiatrist will be available to treat the patient. The psychiatrist inquires about available times that will be best for the patient, and a time is set that is mutually agreeable.

6.6   The answer is **C**.

The psychiatrist is bound by medical and ethical principles to not divulge any information that is revealed by the patient without the patient's consent. If the patient refuses to give permission to divulge this information, whether it is to the referring physician or in filling out an insurance form, the psychiatrist must respect the patient's wishes. Only when patients are in danger of harming themselves or others by virtue of their psychiatric illness is the psychiatrist obliged to divulge information. In addition, information may be divulged to the parent in the event that the patient is a child.

6.7   The answer is **B**.

The most important element in the psychiatrist's initial interview of the patient is to allow the patient to tell his or her story in an uninterrupted fashion with the psychiatrist assuming an attentive listening posture. The psychiatrist often wants to draw the patient's attention to the affective concomitants of the patient's verbalizations. One way this is done is by rephrasing the patient's response in such a way that emphasizes the feelings that accompany a reported event.

6.8   The answer is **D**.

During the concluding portion of the interview, the psychiatrist indicates the time remaining. He or she also asks the patient if there are any remaining areas that the patient has not talked about, and whether or not the patient has any questions. If records and other information are available, the psychiatrist requests written permission to obtain this information.

6.9   The answer is **A**.

Transference is the process by which the patient unconsciously projects his or her emotions, thoughts, and wishes related to significant past figures onto people in present life and onto the psychiatrist. Whereas these reactions may have been appropriate in the context of the original relationship, they are inappropriate when applied to figures in the present, including the psychiatrist. It is important that the psychiatrist recognizes transference as distortions and does not respond to them in kind.

6.10   The answer is **C**.

Hypnagogic and hypnopompic hallucinations are perceptual experiences associated with normal sleep and with narcolepsy. Hypnagogic refers to the drowsy state that precedes sleep and hypnopompic refers to the semiconscious state preceding awakening.

6.11   The answer is **A**.

In addition to investigating the child's presenting psychiatric problem and past psychiatric history, the psychiatrist should explore a variety of areas when interviewing a young child, including social adaptation, intellectual and educational development, relationships with important figures and friends (past and present), and the child's involvement in recreational activities. The psychiatrist should also explore areas relating to discipline and types of punishment that have been used, as well as any significant personal losses that the child has suffered.

Symptoms reflecting emotional distress in young children include enuresis, nail biting, night terrors, and excessive masturbation.

6.12   The answer is **D**.
6.13   The answer is **B**.
6.14   The answer is **C**.
6.15   The answer is **A**.

An open-ended question reflects a topic that the psychiatrist is interested in exploring but leaves it up to the patient to choose the most relevant and important areas of this topic. Examples of this type of question are "Can you describe your crying spells?" and "These crying spells seem to have been troubling you for some time. Can you tell me more about them?"

The use of positive reinforcement by the psychiatrist involves the signaling of approval of the patient's discussion of a relevant topic. Through the use of this facilitative message, the psychiatrist encourages the patient to describe sensitive topics and feelings without demeaning the patient for his or her response. This type of encouragement will likely lead to the patient's verbalizing other emotional states when these areas are explored.

Checklist questions on the part of the psychiatrist spell out the list of potential responses for a patient when he or she is unable to describe or quantify a topic to the degree that the psychiatrist believes is necessary. Examples of this type of question include "When do you feel nervous?" and "How often do you wake throughout the night?"

Self-disclosure refers to the psychiatrist's sharing of personal information such as thoughts, feelings, or actions that he or she believes will be helpful to the patient, in the context of psychotherapy. Requests by the patient for the psychiatrist to reveal himself or herself are best treated in the context of understanding the individual patient. In some cases, self-disclosure may lead to the patient's increased trust in the psychiatrist. However, such requests may be a form of resistance in other patients.

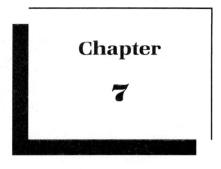

Chapter

7

Psychiatric Classification

DIRECTIONS: Each of the statements or questions is followed by five suggested responses or completions. Select the one that is the best choice or most complete answer in each case.

7.1 The concept of mental disorder as defined by the *Diagnostic and Statistical Manual of Mental Disorders (Third Edition-Revised) (DSM-III-R)* is best described as:

    A. a clinically significant behavioral or psychological syndrome that is associated with present distress or increased risk of suffering, death, pain, or loss of freedom

    B. a clinical condition that represents a highly distinct entity with distinct boundaries between it and other disorders and normality

    C. a clinical condition that can be described as being deviant in that the behavioral syndrome creates a conflict between the individual and society

    D. a clinical condition that often represents an expectable response to a particular event such as the death of a loved one

    E. none of the above

7.2 Which of the following statistical indices provides a measure of agreement between clinicians, correcting for chance variance?

    A. Spearman's r
    B. the kappa statistic
    C. Cohen's beta statistic
    D. the mu statistic
    E. the F statistic

7.3 Which of the following best describes face validity as it pertains to psychiatric classification?

    A. the extent to which a disorder seems reasonable as a descriptor of a particular entity and allows professionals to communicate about the disorder
    B. the extent to which the defining features of a diagnostic category are unique to that category
    C. the extent to which a diagnostic category is useful for predicting the treatment response of a particular disorder
    D. the extent to which a diagnostic category allows us to understand the etiologic process of the disorder
    E. none of the above

7.4 Which of the following is not an index of procedural validity?

    A. sensitivity
    B. predictive power
    C. generalizability
    D. specificity
    E. All of the above are indices of procedural validity.

7.5 Which of the following represents the first use of a standardized psychiatric assessment instrument in the United States?

    A. Wing's Present State Exam
    B. the Mental Status Schedule
    C. the Beck Depression Inventory
    D. the Schedule for Affective Disorders and Schizophrenia
    E. the Rorschach Inkblot Test

7.6 Which of the following is not one of the four controversial diagnostic categories proposed as "needing further study" in *DSM-III-R*?

    A. self-defeating personality disorder
    B. late luteal phase dysphoric disorder
    C. masochistic personality disorder
    D. paraphilic coercive disorder
    E. sadistic personality disorder

7.7 *DSM-IV* is expected to be published in:

    A. 1990
    B. the year 2000
    C. 1988
    D. 1993
    E. there are no plans for further revision of the *DSM*.

DIRECTIONS: For each of the statements below, one or more of the alternative answers is correct. Choose answer:

    A if only 1, 2, and 3 are correct
    B if only 1 and 3 are correct
    C if only 2 and 4 are correct
    D if only 4 is correct
    E if all are correct

7.8 Which of the following statements represent(s) the purposes of having a diagnostic system in the field of psychiatry?

    1. A diagnostic system provides a language with which mental health professionals can communicate.
    2. A diagnostic system helps in defining the characteristics of a particular disorder and how it differs from other conditions.
    3. A diagnostic system promotes an understanding of the causes of the disorder.
    4. A diagnostic system such as *DSM-III-R* provides a focus on specific etiologies of a disorder.

7.9 *DSM-III-R* was developed only three years after the publication of *DSM-III* because:

    1. New data had accumulated that suggested the need for changes in many *DSM-III* definitions.
    2. Some of the *DSM-III* criteria were found to be unclear.
    3. *DSM-III* criteria were found to be inconsistent across diagnostic categories.
    4. *DSM-III* criteria were found to be contradictory in some cases.

7.10 Which of the following statements is (are) true concerning diagnostic reliability?

1. The reliability obtained by test–retest methods is generally lower than reliability assessed by joint assessments.
2. The reliability of a diagnostic category puts an upper limit on its validity.
3. When reliability is assessed on the basis of unitary case material, it is generally lower than if assessed on the basis of live interviews.
4. The most powerful way to establish reliability is to ask clinicians to diagnose a series of cases independently.

7.11 Which of the following is (are) true regarding the United States–United Kingdom Diagnostic Project?

1. The study was designed to explore the reasons why affective disorders were much more commonly diagnosed in England than in the United States.
2. The study found that schizophrenia was more likely to be diagnosed in England than in the United States.
3. The study found that international diagnostic differences were mainly due to differing clinical concepts in the two countries rather than to differences in actual patients.
4. The data from this study are limited because of a failure of the study to use a structured diagnostic interview as a measure of psychopathology.

DIRECTIONS: Each of the following questions consists of lettered headings followed by a list of numbered alternatives. Select the single lettered heading that is most closely associated with the appropriate numbered alternative. Each lettered heading may be chosen only once.

Diagnostic classification system

A. *DSM-I*
B. *DSM-II*
C. *DSM-III*
D. *DSM-III-R*

Description

7.12 was published in 1965 to coincide with the World Health Organization's eighth revision of the *International Classification of Diseases*

7.13 was the first system to provide descriptions for the mental disorder categories it listed

7.14 was published to provide more consistent criteria across diagnostic categories

7.15 was the first system to use a multiaxial classification system

ANSWERS

7.1 The answer is **A**.

In *DSM-III-R* each of the mental disorders is conceptualized as a clinically significant behavioral or psychological syndrome or pattern that occurs in a person and that is associated with present distress (a painful symptom) or disability (impairment in one or more important areas of functioning); a significantly increased risk of suffering death, pain, or disability; or an important loss of freedom. In addition, this syndrome must not be merely an expectable response to a particular event, for example, the death of a loved one. Whatever its original cause, it must currently be considered a manifestation of a behavioral, psychological, or biological dysfunction in the person. Neither deviant behavior (for example, political, religious, or sexual) nor conflicts that are primarily between the individual and society are mental disorders unless the deviance or conflict is a symptom of a dysfunction in the person.

7.2 The answer is **B**.

In 1960, Cohen proposed the use of the kappa statistic for indexing agreement among clinicians, correcting for chance agreement. The values of kappa vary from -1.0 (total disagreement) to $+1.0$ (perfect agreement), with a kappa of 0 indicating no more than chance agreement. It is generally agreed that a kappa value of .70 and above is quite good, between .50 and .70 is fair, and below .50 is poor.

7.3 The answer is **A**.

Face validity is the extent to which, on the face of it, the definition of a disorder seems reasonable as a description of a particular clinical entity and allows professionals to communicate about the disorder. For example, the list of symptoms that define the *DSM-III-R* category of major depression has significant face validity since the clinicians generally agree that these are the signs and symptoms they see in their patients who are depressed.

7.4 The answer is **C**.

There are basically three important indices on which a new test or procedure can be evaluated, using some standard test or procedure as the criterion: sensitivity, specificity, and predictive power. The sensitivity of a diagnostic procedure is calculated as the percentage of "true" cases it correctly identifies as having the diagnosis (that is, its true positive rate). The specificity is the percentage of noncases that it correctly identifies as not having the diagnosis (its true-negative rate). Finally, the predictive power of a test is the percentage of total cases in which the test agrees with the standard, that is, the total number of cases that both tests agree have the diagnosis, plus the total number of cases that both tests agree do not have the diagnosis, all divided by the total number of cases.

7.5 The answer is **B**.

The use of standardized psychiatric assessment instruments began in this country in 1961 with Spitzer et al.'s Mental Status Schedule and in England a few years earlier with Wing's Present State Examination. Since that time, a large number of standardized interview schedules for psychiatric assessment have been developed.

7.6 The answer is **C**.

During the development of *DSM-III-R*, the proposed inclusion of four categories was particularly controversial. These categories are paraphilic coercive disorder, late luteal phase dysphoric disorder, self-defeating personality disorder, and sadistic personality disorder. Although the advisory committees that worked on the definitions of these disorders and the Work Group believed that sufficient research and clinical evidence existed regarding the validity of each of these categories to justify its inclusion in the revised manual, critics argued that evidence as to the validity of these disorders was lacking and that there was potential for misuse of the diagnostic categories.

Arguments against the proposed category of paraphilic coercive disorder included the possible misuse of this diagnosis in the legal arena to win lighter punishment for rapists, and this category was dropped from the manual on the grounds that not enough data had accumulated to warrant its inclusion. The other three categories were objected to mainly on the grounds that they would be misused in a way that would be harmful to women.

The controversies surrounding these four categories were resolved by including them in an appendix to *DSM-III-R* entitled "Proposed Diagnostic Categories Needing Further Study."

7.7   The answer is D.

DSM-III and *DSM-III-R* have had a major impact on psychiatry in this country and abroad. *DSM-IV* is expected to be published in 1993 to coincide with the publication of the 10th revision of the *International Classification of Diseases* by the World Health Organization.

7.8   The answer is A.

Having a diagnostic classification system serves three general purposes, as well as many specific clinical, administrative, legal, and research ones. First, such a system provides a language with which all mental health professionals can communicate. Generally agreed upon names for the various mental syndromes serve as a shorthand method of describing the entities that mental health professionals deal with, enabling efficient communication.

Second, in order to study the natural history of a particular disorder and develop an effective treatment, it is necessary to define the characteristics of a disorder and have an understanding of how it differs from other, similar disorders. To the extent that a relationship between diagnosis and treatment has been established for a particular category, the proper diagnosis of a person's condition can indicate the most effective treatment.

Finally, the ultimate purpose of classification is to develop an understanding of the causes of the various mental disorders. Knowing the cause of a disorder usually leads to the development of an effective treatment. The etiology or pathophysiologic process for most of the mental disorders in *DSM-III-R* is unknown, except for the organic mental disorders and those few nonorganic disorders (for example, post-traumatic stress disorder, conversion disorder, adjustment disorder) for which the etiology is included in the definition. Therefore, in *DSM-III* and *DSM-*

III-R, a descriptive approach to classification has been taken that includes definitions of the various disorders without reference to their etiology, except for those disorders mentioned above whose etiology or pathophysiologic process is unknown. This largely atheoretical approach has enabled clinicians of varying theoretical orientations to use this descriptive classification. In other words, clinicians can identify these conditions and still preserve their own approaches to understanding and treating them.

7.9   The answer is E.

Work on *DSM-III-R* was begun in 1983, just three short years after the publication of *DSM-III*. Although at the time some questioned the seeming haste in working on a revision, the scientific literature was already replete with articles reporting the results of studies using the *DSM-III* diagnostic criteria to select samples of patients, and articles reporting studies of the reliability and validity of the categories themselves. New data had accumulated that indicated the need for change in some of the *DSM-III* definitions, and experience with the criteria had revealed many instances in which they were not entirely clear, were inconsistent across diagnostic categories, or were even contradictory.

7.10   The answer is A.

The extent to which a diagnostic category has reliability is the extent to which it can be used consistently to classify individuals with a given psychiatric disorder. The reliability of a diagnostic category puts an upper limit on its usefulness (validity).

In the test–retest method, each clinician independently conducts his or her own interview, one after the other. This is the hardest test of diagnostic reliability, but the one that can be argued to most closely approximate real life, since it is applied to real patients. Reliability assessed by this method is generally lower than that obtained by joint assessments because of the increase in information variance (that is, variability in the information available to each interviewer).

The easiest but least powerful way to assess reliability is to ask two clinicians to diagnose independently a series of cases based on written case records or audiotapes or videotapes of diagnostic interviews. When reliability is assessed on the basis of written case material, it is generally lower than that assessed on the basis of "live" interviews. The reasons for this are not clear, since the complete standardization of materials guarantees the elimination of information variance.

7.11   The answer is **B**.

In the 1960s two major cross-national studies were conducted that bear on the validity of psychiatric diagnoses. The purpose of the first of these, the United States–United Kingdom Diagnostic Project (the "U.S.–U.K. study"), was to explore the reasons for the fact that affective disorders were much more commonly diagnosed in England than in the United States while the reverse was true for schizophrenia. The results of this study indicated that the international diagnostic differences were mainly due to differing clinical concepts in the two countries rather than to differences in the actual patients in the United States and England.

7.12   The answer is **B**.
7.13   The answer is **A**.
7.14   The answer is **D**.
7.15   The answer is **C**.

In 1965 the American Psychiatric Association decided that a new edition of the *DSM* should be published to coincide with the World Health Organization's eighth revision of the *International Classification of Diseases*.

The first version of the American Psychiatric Association's diagnostic manual was published in 1952 and was called the *Diagnostic and Statistical Manual, Mental Disorders*. Later it became clear that further revision of this manual was needed. The major significance of this book was that for the first time descriptions were provided for the mental categories it listed.

Work on *DSM-III-R* was begun in 1983, just three years after the publication of *DSM-III* . New data had accumulated in this time period to suggest the need for changes in some of the *DSM-III* definitions. Experience with the criteria had revealed many instances in which the criteria were not entirely clear, were inconsistent across diagnostic categories, or were even contradictory. *DSM-III-R* was developed to provide more consistent and less contradictory information across diagnostic criteria.

In addition to other differences between *DSM-III* and earlier diagnostic systems, *DSM-III* was the first diagnostic system to include a multiaxial system for evaluation.

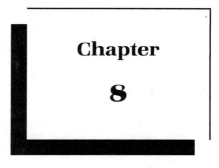

Chapter

8

Psychological Assessment: Tests and Rating Scales

DIRECTIONS: Each of the statements or questions is followed by five suggested responses or completions. Select the one that is the best choice or most complete answer in each case.

8.1 The type of test validity that refers to the test's relationship to independent ratings of an individual's performance in a particular area is:

    A. face validity
    B. criterion validity
    C. content validity
    D. construct validity
    E. congruent validity

8.2 The most widely used omnibus psychological test instrument developed for measurement of symptoms is:

    A. the Rorschach Inkblot Test
    B. the Thematic Apperception Test
    C. the Minnesota Multiphasic Personality Inventory
    D. the California Personality Inventory
    E. the Draw-a-Person Test

8.3 The diagnostic instrument most widely used to assess thought disorder is:

  A.   the Wechsler Adult Intelligence Scale–Revised
  B.   the Beck Depression Inventory
  C.   the Rorschach Inkblot Test
  D.   the Dysfunctional Attitude Scale
  E.   the Draw-a-Person Test

8.4 Which of the following is one primary advantage of tests representative of the interpersonal tradition of personality assessment?

  A.   This system may be able to predict not only the kind of interpersonal style that the patient expresses, but also the response that the patient's style is likely to elicit from others.
  B.   This system is not based on a theory of personality.
  C.   This system has not been based on the assessment of psychopathology and hence is more readily used with "normal" populations.
  D.   This system has lent itself more readily to the validation of personality constructs than have more traditional approaches.
  E.   None of the above are advantages of the interpersonal approach.

8.5 The primary role of neuropsychological assessment in clinical psychiatric settings is:

  A.   the identification of how psychodynamic issues affect cognitive processing
  B.   the identification of behavioral deficits most likely associated with established patterns of organic impairment
  C.   the identification of cognitive processing styles
  D.   an experimental approach that may have utility in guiding subsequent revisions of the *Diagnostic and Statistical Manual of Mental Disorders (Third Edition-Revised) (DSM-III-R)*
  E.   none of the above

8.6 What is the single most important rationale for the use of psychological tests that provide information on psychodynamic issues?

  A.   These instruments are highly structured and allow for the assessment of specific behavioral factors.
  B.   The data that these instruments provide are easily adapted to *DSM-III-R* criteria.

C. These instruments are easily administered and therefore are more useful in clinical psychiatric settings than are omnibus measures.

D. These instruments may provide information about personality dynamics and structure that are outside the conscious awareness of the examinee.

E. These instruments are easily administered and interpreted by nonprofessional staff.

8.7 The most widely used assessment procedure to evaluate patients for dynamic factors is:

A. the Draw-a-Person Test
B. the Bender Visual–Motor Gestalt Test
C. the Schedule for Affective Disorders and Schizophrenia
D. the Thematic Apperception Test
E. the Rorschach Inkblot Test

8.8 An assessment instrument that is recommended to assess coping style is:

A. the Luria–Nebraska Battery
B. the Wechsler Adult Intelligence Scale
C. the Minnesota Multiphasic Personality Inventory
D. the Hamilton Anxiety Rating Scale
E. the Bender Visual–Motor Gestalt Test

8.9 The test considered to be the prototype of psychological assessment instruments to measure stress and coping with stress is:

A. the Jenkins Activity Survey
B. the Beigel Manic State Rating Scale
C. the Thematic Apperception Test
D. the Minnesota Multiphasic Personality Inventory
E. the Schedule for Affective Disorders and Schizophrenia

DIRECTIONS: For each of the statements below, one or more of the alternative answers is correct. Choose answer:

A if only 1, 2, and 3 are correct
B if only 1 and 3 are correct
C if only 2 and 4 are correct
D if only 4 is correct
E if all are correct

8.10 Which of the following factors has (have) been particularly important in prompting changes in psychological assessment procedures for individuals suspected of having psychiatric difficulties?

1. the development of a behaviorally anchored diagnostic system
2. the application of single models of therapies developed for use with different patient populations
3. the proliferation of assessment geared to provide treatment information on specific patient groups
4. the proliferation of psychodynamically based therapies with the advent of *DSM-III*

8.11 Which of the following factors should be considered to be the "heart" of modern psychodiagnostic strategies?

1. a return to the idiographic approach to psychiatric research
2. a focus on differential therapeutics
3. a shift to more psychodynamic treatment approaches
4. a need to tailor psychological assessment to specific aspects of the referral question

8.12 The measurement of personality traits is important in developing a treatment plan because:

1. traits may exacerbate or be related to certain symptoms
2. traits may be the focus of intervention
3. traits may either help or hinder the development of a therapeutic relationship with the patient
4. the assessment of traits usually provides the impetus for the implementation of behavioral treatment strategies

8.13 Which of the following is (are) a potential difficulty with an approach to the assessment of personality disorders that is guided solely by *DSM-III* or *DSM-III-R* criteria?

1. *DSM-III* was a temporary document that was replaced soon after it was published.
2. These approaches do not allow for identification of specific symptoms.
3. Axis II criteria have not been theoretically or empirically derived.
4. *DSM-III-R* does not allow for the specification of variables such as severity of stressors or level of adaptive functioning that may be important in guiding diagnosis and treatment.

DIRECTIONS: Each of the following questions consists of lettered headings followed by a list of numbered alternatives. Select the single lettered heading that is most closely associated with the appropriate numbered alternative. Each lettered heading may be chosen only once.

Psychodiagnostic instrument

A. Minnesota Multiphasic Personality Inventory
B. Wechsler Adult Intelligence Scale–Revised
C. Luria–Nebraska Battery
D. Schedule for Affective Disorders and Schizophrenia
E. Beck Depression Inventory

Description

8.14 is a self-report measure based on a cognitive model of psychological adjustment/maladjustment
8.15 is an omnibus self-report measure administered in one to two hours and computer scored
8.16 is a frequently used neuropsychological test battery that provides information on 11 areas of cognitive functioning
8.17 is a frequently used test that yields 11 separate test scores and also provides summary measures of verbal and perceptual performance
8.18 is a semi-structured interview rating scale designed to provide sufficient information to classify patients into relatively homogeneous subgroups for the purpose of research

ANSWERS

8.1 The answer is **B**.

Validity is assessed in three ways: 1) content validity, 2) criterion-related validity, and 3) construct validity. Content validity is said to be present only if the content of the test can be said to adequately sample the area of interest. For example, an intelligence test must contain items that tap a number of different areas of intellectual functioning in order to meet acceptable standards for content validity.

Criterion-related validity refers to the test's relationship to independent criteria of an individual's ability in a particular area (concurrent validity) or to the ability of the test to make predictions about future behavior (predictive validity). For example, a test of the severity of depressive symptoms would achieve concurrent validity if performance on the test was found to relate closely to trained observers' ratings of depressive symptoms. Predictive validity would be demonstrated if scores on the measure were found to relate to the likelihood of response to treatment of the depressive symptoms.

Construct validity is achieved by demonstrating that the test measures a theoretical area of interest.

8.2   The answer is **C**.

The Minnesota Multiphasic Personality Inventory (MMPI) is probably the most widely used test instrument designed to sample from a broad area of psychiatric symptoms. Although labeled as a personality test, the MMPI was constructed to measure what are currently considered to be *DSM-III* Axis I conditions. This measure's popularity is related to its ease of administration and scoring, its extensive normative data base, and its inclusion of validity scales that provide information on the test-taking attitude of the patient.

8.3   The answer is **C**.

The presence or absence of delusional thinking, thought disorder, or hallucinations is assessed throughout the course of the psychiatric interview and mental status exam. However, often the patient may be unwilling to reveal frankly delusional thinking and more subtle forms of thought disorder may not be evident during the interview. The Rorschach Inkblot Test is often used to provide information on thought disorder. In this test, which consists of 10 relatively ambiguous stimuli cards, the patient is asked to state what the individual percepts look like. The patient's responses are then scored for location, form, movement, color, shading, and content. The resulting responses can then be interpreted via several existing scoring and interpretation systems.

8.4   The answer is **A**.

The interpersonal tradition dates back to Timothy Leary's circumplex model, in which the expression of all interpersonal styles is related to two major axes of power and affiliation. Theoretically, the system is able to predict not only the kind of interpersonal style that the patient exhibits but also the type of behavior that this style is likely to elicit from others. This approach to assessment differs from many other psychological tests in that it is theoretically guided and is based on a model of psychopathology rather than on the validation of personality constructs.

8.5   The answer is B.

The primary role of neuropsychological assessment in clinical psychiatric settings can best be described as the identification of behavioral deficits that are often associated with established patterns of organic impairment. More specifically, neuropsychological testing is often useful in providing information on dementia in the elderly, toxicity in substance abuse, and learning disabilities in children and adolescents. The assessment armamentarium of the clinical neuropsychologist is extensive, and a number of procedures are available for the evaluation of neuropsychological functioning. At the present time, efforts are being made to develop broadly based batteries of tests as well as more intensive procedures for the measurement of specific functions.

8.6   The answer is D.

The single most important rationale for the use of psychological tests that provide information on psychodynamic issues is that these instruments may provide clinical material that is outside of the conscious awareness of the individual. Since the stimuli that make up so-called projective tests such as the Rorschach Inkblot Test and the Thematic Apperception Test are ambiguous, the patient is less likely to respond in an attempt to provide the perceived "correct" response and therefore may provide information on unconscious determinants of behavior.

8.7   The answer is E.

The most widely used assessment instrument to assess ego functions and dynamic factors is the Rorschach Inkblot Test. Several scoring systems have been developed over the years. Most recently, Exner has developed a scoring system that attempts to integrate the best aspects of earlier systems. This system yields information on self-image, defensive structure, reality testing, affective control, impulsive acting out, and degree of thought organization.

8.8   The answer is C.

An assessment procedure that is recommended to measure coping style is the MMPI. Elevations on scales 3, 4, 6, and 9 indicate externalizing defensive style. Elevations on scales 1, 7, and 0 suggest an internalizing defensive style. The MMPI also allows for assessment of an individual's coping style through evaluation of the Validity Scales (scales L, F, and K). Elevations on the L and K scales relative to the F scale elevation suggest a defensive test-taking attitude.

8.9 The answer is **A**.

In measuring both stress and ability to cope with stress, one can assess the stimuli, the individual's response to the stimuli, or the interaction of the individual with the stressful stimuli. The prototype of psychological tests that measure stress and coping with stress is the Jenkins Activity Survey since it focuses on the cognitive and perceptual characteristics of the individual that mediate responses to stress. This instrument has been demonstrated to have predictive validity in studies of reaction to coronary heart disease.

8.10 The answer is **B**.

A number of converging factors have prompted a change in psychological assessment procedures over the last decade. First, in psychiatry extensive attention has been given to the development of a behaviorally anchored diagnostic system. This change has been prompted by the need for a explicit criterion-based diagnostic system for psychopharmacologic research. With the introduction of *DSM-III*, diagnosis has become more behaviorally explicit and reliable.

Second, with the proliferation of treatments, some of which are specific for specific conditions (that is, exposure in vivo for phobias and antipsychotics for thought disorder), careful diagnosis has become important for providing optimal treatment within the context of each individual's unique situation. Past psychiatric practice was characterized by the application of the same therapy to all patients rather than the matching of specific treatments for specific problems. This practice is now clearly wrong because it deprives the patient of the most effective treatment and wastes psychiatric resources.

8.11 The answer is **C**.

Differential therapeutics are at the heart of the assessment process and provide the rationale for the differential diagnosis. In the absence of treatment specificity, there is little justification for an extensive focus on diagnosis. The recent proliferation of psychological and clinical psychiatric treatment approaches has spawned a growing literature on the assessment of various characteristics that are thought to be important to the understanding and treatment of the specific psychiatric conditions. This emphasis means that assessment is more likely to need to be tailored to specific aspects of the referral to and the salient dimensions of information that constitutes the differential.

8.12   The answer is **A**.

In developing a treatment plan for the individual patient, the psychiatrist must assess personality traits for various reasons. First, personality traits may be the focus of intervention. Second, traits may exacerbate or be related to the incidence of certain symptoms (for example, depression). Third, traits may either help or hinder the development of a therapeutic relationship with the patient.

8.13   The answer is **B**.

There are several problems with the relatively new approach of assessing personality disorders solely by *DSM-III* and *DSM-III-R*. First, *DSM-III* was a temporary document, replaced by *DSM-III-R*, which necessitated changes in any instrument geared to *DSM-III*. Second, and more important, Axis II in both *DSM-III* and *DSM-III-R* is neither a theoretically or an empirically derived compilation of personality traits that lead to or constitute psychopathology. It is a somewhat arbitrary collection of traits thought to be important markers of psychopathology. Thus, any instrument guided solely by *DSM-III* or *DSM-III-R* will leave serious questions of internal consistency, content validity, and construct validity unanswered.

8.14   The answer is **E**.
8.15   The answer is **A**.
8.16   The answer is **C**.
8.17   The answer is **B**.
8.18   The answer is **D**.

Beck and his colleagues have argued for the acceptance of cognitions such as hopelessness, helplessness, and worthlessness as essential for understanding of depression. This cognitive theory has been sufficiently well elaborated to lead to the development of rating scales sensitive to these cognitions and to the design of a treatment approach to address them. The Beck Depression Inventory is probably the most widely used self-report inventory of depression. The 21 items of the inventory were selected to represent symptoms commonly associated with depression. The ratings of each item consist of a forced choice of one of four possible answers in order of symptom severity.

The MMPI is the most widely used omnibus self-report measure. This instrument, which is composed of 578 true–false questions, can be administered in one to two hours and can be scored and interpreted by computer.

A widely used battery of procedures has been developed from the work of Luria. In its present form, the Luria–Nebraska Battery covers 11 areas of motor function, rhythm (and pitch) skills, tactile and visual functions, receptive and expressive speech, writing, reading, arithmetic, and memory and intelligence. The complete exam consists of 269 items that yield raw scores in each of the 11 areas. Three additional scores for right and left hemisphere impairment and a pathognomonic score are also computed. These 14 raw scores are plotted as T scores for interpretation purposes.

Although a large number of tests have been developed to assess intelligence in adults, the most commonly used test has been the Wechsler Adult Intelligence Scale (WAIS) and the more recently developed Wechsler Adult Intelligence Scale–Revised (WAIS-R). The WAIS-R consists of 11 subtests, 6 of which tap verbal abilities and 5 of which tap performance (nonverbal) abilities. Scores on the individual subtests can be combined to yield Verbal, Performance, and Full Scale IQ scores.

The Schedule for Affective Disorders and Schizophrenia was developed in the 1970s as a semi-structured interview to gather information pertinent to the classification of psychiatric disorders. Its primary purpose was to provide sufficient information to classify patients into relatively homogeneous subgroups for the purposes of research.

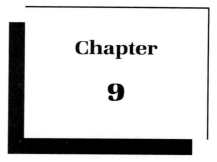

Chapter

9

Laboratory and Other Diagnostic Tests in Psychiatry

DIRECTIONS: Each of the statements or questions is followed by five suggested responses or completions. Select the one that is the best choice or most complete answer in each case.

9.1   Which of the following is not a clue suggestive of organic mental disorders?

    A.   history of drug or alcohol abuse
    B.   family history of inherited metabolic disease
    C.   fluctuating mental status
    D.   focal neurologic signs
    E.   psychiatric symptoms before the age of 30

9.2   The final criterion for choosing the type of laboratory and diagnostic testing is:

    A.   the results of the physical exam
    B.   clinical judgment
    C.   results of the neurologic mental status exam
    D.   the presence or absence of psychotic symptoms
    E.   lack of history of psychiatric illness

9.3   Possible contraindications to a lumbar puncture do not include:

    A.   raised intracranial pressure
    B.   presence of intracranial mass
    C.   current use of anticoagulants
    D.   negative results from blood work
    E.   skin infection around the lumbar puncture site

9.4   Appropriate laboratory tests for the presence of environmental toxins should be conducted:

    A.   when the probability of exposure is high
    B.   when anorexia and sleep disturbance are present
    C.   when behavioral abnormalities cannot be otherwise explained
    D.   as a routine matter
    E.   in the case of abrupt mental status changes

9.5   Common substances obtained to test for the presence of drugs do not include:

    A.   urine
    B.   blood
    C.   breath
    D.   cerebral spinal fluid
    E.   hair

9.6   The electroencephalogram is used primarily in the evaluation of:

    A.   epilepsy, other neurologic disorders
    B.   manic–depressive cycles
    C.   schizophrenia
    D.   dementia
    E.   response to neuroleptic medication

9.7   Evoked potential studies can be useful in:

    A.   diagnosing schizophrenia
    B.   the differential between some organic and functional complaints
    C.   evaluating the exaggerated startle response in post-traumatic stress disorder
    D.   evaluating complaints of impotence
    E.   the differential between histrionic and borderline personality disorders

9.8 In a young confused adult patient, the finding of diffuse delta waves in an awake electroencephalographic recording would be most consistent with:

    A. seizure disorder
    B. episodic explosive disorder
    C. chronic schizophrenia
    D. major depression with melancholia
    E. delirium

9.9 When using the monamine oxidase (MAO) inhibitor phenelzine in the treatment of depression, levels of platelet MAO inhibition that have been suggested to be most associated with a beneficial response to the phenelzine are:

    A. 30 to 40 percent MAO inhibition
    B. 40 to 50 percent MAO inhibition
    C. 50 to 60 percent MAO inhibition
    D. 70 to 80 percent MAO inhibition
    E. greater than 80 percent MAO inhibition

DIRECTIONS: For each of the statements or questions below, one or more of the alternative answers is correct. Choose answer:

    A if only 1, 2, and 3 are correct
    B if only 1 and 3 are correct
    C if only 2 and 4 are correct
    D if only 4 is correct
    E if all are correct

9.10 The field of laboratory testing in psychiatry will be determined by:

    1. quality assurance and liability issues
    2. research findings in clinical psychiatry
    3. research findings in the neurosciences
    4. economic realities

9.11 Which of the following statements regarding magnetic resonance imaging (MRI) are true?

1. MRI results indicate decreased blood flow to the frontal brain regions of schizophrenic patients.
2. MRI provides better definition of lesions in demyelinating disease than does computed tomography.
3. MRI provides better visualization of bone and small calcifications than does computed tomography.
4. Small frontal lobes have been reported using MRI in patients with schizophrenia compared with controls.

9.12 Pretreatment lithium evaluation commonly includes:

1. complete blood count
2. serum electrolytes
3. blood urea nitrogen
4. serum creatinine

9.13 Laboratory and diagnostic test(s) for pretreatment evaluation of electroconvulsive therapy that is (are) no longer commonly used include:

1. blood chemistries
2. urinalysis
3. electrocardiogram
4. spinal X rays

9.14 Various radioisotopes are presently used in which brain imaging procedure(s)?

1. single photon emission computed tomography
2. regional cerebral blood flow
3. positron emission tomography
4. magnetic resonance imaging

9.15 Which of the following statements regarding the dexamethasone suppression test (DST) are true?

1. The DST is better able to differentiate between depressed patients and controls than between depressed patients and patients with other psychiatric disorders.
2. Serum cortisol levels within 24 hours after oral dexamethasone administration of less than 5 µg/dl is considered abnormal.
3. Recent weight loss can result in false positive results.
4. A normal DST result allows a clinician to rule out a major affective disorder.

9.16 Possible indications for obtaining tricyclic antidepressant (TCA) blood levels do not include:

1. questionable patient compliance
2. poor response to traditional doses of a TCA
3. patients who experience side effects at very low doses
4. patients for whom a slow titration is required

9.17 Limitations to the use of the dexamethasone suppression test include:

1. a sensitivity in the range of only 45 percent
2. a specificity of 90 percent in normals but much lower in psychiatric patients
3. artifactual contamination from medical illnesses or weight loss
4. possibly lethal side effects

ANSWERS

9.1 The answer is **E**.

Although there is not total agreement as to the clinical presentations that are suggestive of organic disorders, there is some consensus as to a few signs that are usually associated with an organic condition. These signs should not be viewed as diagnostic but should instead alert the clinician to the possible presence of an organic condition that should then be investigated.

These signs include the emergence of psychiatric symptoms after the age of 40, during a major medical illness, or when taking drugs known to cause mental symptoms. Other signs include a history of alcohol or drug abuse or of taking multiple over-the-counter medications, physical illness that results in organ damage, and a family history of inheritable brain disease or metabolic disease. Mental signs that should alert the clinician to possible organic disease include altered state of consciousness, fluctuating mental status, cognitive impairment, and episodic or recurrent course, and the presence of visual, tactile, or olfactory hallucinations. Associated physical signs include signs of organ malfunction that affect the brain, focal neurologic signs, diffuse subcortical dysfunction, or signs of cortical dysfunction.

9.2   The answer is B.

There are several signs that when present may alert the clinician to the need for laboratory testing. However, because of the costs to the patient (in time and money) as well as the side effects and risks associated with certain laboratory tests, not all of these tests should be done with every patient. The clinical presentation of a patient will not provide an understanding of the etiology, but will instead usually provide a differential that must then be evaluated with the use of selected laboratory tests. There are many considerations in the choice of laboratory and diagnostic tests including legal and monetary concerns. However, the final consideration should be that of good clinical judgment.

9.3   The answer is D.

The lumbar puncture and examination of the cerebral spinal fluid can help provide information regarding the diagnosis of central nervous system syphilis, meningitis, encephalitis, or subarachnoid hemorrhage. The lumbar puncture can allow the clinician to obtain a white blood cell count; sugar, chloride, and protein determinations; and serological and bacteriological studies. However, the procedure is a painful one, and the decision to perform one should not be taken lightly. Common contraindications to the lumbar puncture include raised intracranial pressure, the presence of an intracranial mass such as brain tumor, abscess, subdural hematoma, or intracerebral hemorrhage, skin infection around the lumbar puncture site, or the use of anticoagulants in the patient. Negative results from blood work do not constitute a contraindication for performing a lumbar puncture.

9.4   The answer is A.

Behavioral abnormalities are associated with exposure to a large number of environmental toxins. Environmental toxins include the heavy metals, insecticides, pesticides, and solvents. It should be remembered that behavioral abnormalities are associated with other etiological events. For example, anorexia and sleep disturbance can be associated with exposure to environmental toxins, but these symptoms can also be associated with many other etiologies. Testing for exposure to environmental toxins should be conducted when there is a high probability of exposure to the toxins as determined by the history.

9.5   The answer is D.

Drug screening procedures are available for a wide range of illicit substances. These procedures can be conducted in the form of testing for the presence of numerous substances or in the form of a test for a single substance. Unfortunately, drug screening tests can have large numbers of false positives as the result of sensitivity to prescription drugs, operator error, equipment contamination, or sample mislabeling. Commonly used body specimens in testing for recent substance use include saliva, blood, urine, breath, or in some cases, a sample of hair. Cerebral spinal fluid is not commonly used to test for exposure to drugs.

9.6   The answer is A.

The electroencephalogram (EEG) is used primarily in the evaluation of epilepsy and other neurologic disorders such as neoplasm, trauma, stroke, or metabolic disease. Although research has reported abnormalities of the EEG in psychiatric disorders such as schizophrenia, these changes are nonspecific and are not contributory to diagnosis except to exclude neurologic disorders. The clinical use of the EEG involves visual inspection of the EEG tracings in order to uncover abnormalities such as dysrhythmias, asymmetries, suppressions of amplitude, or slowing of wave functions.

9.7   The answer is B.

In evoked potential (EP) testing a discrete sensory stimulation is presented to the patient and the electrical response of the brain is measured and recorded. The stimulation can be visual, as in a flashing light; auditory, as in the production of a noise; or somatosensory, as in application of stimulation to the body of the patient. In each case, the stimulation is repeated several times and the resulting brain responses are averaged into a characteristic wave form known as the EP. The EP is useful in diagnosing certain demyelinating diseases such as multiple sclerosis. It can also be useful in the differentiation of organic from functional complaints such as hysterical blindness. Other psychiatric illnesses have experimentally shown EP abnormalities. However, the specificity of these abnormalities is not sufficient to allow a recommendation that EPs be used in their diagnosis.

9.8   The answer is **E**.

The electroencephalogram (EEG) is a method of estimating brain process activity by recording the transient changes in surface electrical activity. Most EEG laboratories use the International 10–20 System of scalp electrode placement, although some labs may use some other standard system of electrode placement. The electrodes detect electrical activity that is presumed to originate mainly in the uppermost cortical cells. Although the EEG tracings by themselves may not provide information that is specific enough to allow diagnosis, when the tracings are combined with information from the clinical presentation and history, the EEG may help provide support for diagnostic hypotheses. For example, a finding of diffuse delta waves on an awake EEG recording would be most consistent with a diagnosis of delirium.

9.9   The answer is **E**.

Because the metabolism rate of different drugs may be differential for patients as a function of weight, age, and the presence of other drugs, effective dosage levels for these drugs will vary. Rather then relying solely on the ingestion dosage, it may be beneficial to measure the levels of the drugs in the blood of the patient. One instance where this is true is in adjusting the dosage level of the monoamine oxidase (MAO) inhibitor phenelzine. Laboratory techniques for measuring monoamine oxidase inhibition are still being developed. However, it appears that maximal therapeutic effects of phenelzine are achieved when blood platelet MAO inhibition is equal to or greater than 80 percent. It is unclear whether this test would be useful for other MAO inhibitors.

9.10   The answer is **E**.

The use of laboratory testing in clinical psychiatry is in a stage of development and change. Several factors are likely to affect application of laboratory testing methods in the clinical practice of psychiatry. These factors include research findings in clinical psychiatry, research findings in the basic neurosciences, changing economic realities, and issues involved with quality assurance and liability.

9.11   The answer is **C**.

Magnetic resonance imaging (MRI) is a noninvasive technique that allows visualization of interior body structures. At present, MRI is a time-consuming procedure that requires the patient to remain still during the entire period of the imaging. In time, the MRI may come to complement or even replace the computed tomographic (CT) scan. MRI does not provide better visualization of bone and calcification than does the CT scan. Nor does it allow for the visualization of decreased blood flow to the frontal lobes of schizophrenic patients. It is a measure of structure and not of brain processes. However, the MRI does provide better visualization of the lesions in demyelinating disease than does the CT scan. MRI has also indicated that the frontal lobes may be smaller in schizophrenic individuals than in normals.

However, the MRI cannot be viewed as a panacea for visualization of brain structures in all patients. Because of the high level of cooperation required of patients over an extended period of time, the MRI may not be useful in the evaluation of anxious or agitated patients. Because the MRI effects changes in the magnetic field surrounding a patient, it is contraindicated in patients with metal surgical clips, metal skull plates, or cardiac pacemakers. The MRI does not use ionizing radiation and may therefore be preferred to the CT or X ray when repeated scans are necessary.

9.12   The answer is **E.**

Although lithium is extremely useful in the treatment of several disorders, most notably in the treatment of bipolar affective disorder (manic), it can have multiple untoward effects. These adverse side effects include deleterious effects on the thyroid gland, kidneys, heart, and developing fetus. In addition, lithium may cause a benign elevation of the white blood cell count. Therefore pretreatment diagnostic workups prior to use of lithium include a complete blood count, serum electrolytes, blood urea nitrogen, serum creatinine, thyroid function tests, urinalysis, an electrocardiogram, and possibly a 24-hour urine test for creatinine clearance. Common thyroid function tests include a thyroid-stimulating hormone, T_3 resin uptake, and T_4. Some authors have suggested a fasting blood sugar, urine for glucose and ketones, a 24-hour urine volume test, and a 12-hour dehydration test for urine osmolality. If the patient is a sexually active female of childbearing years, a pregnancy test may be in order. The selection of any of these tests depends on the clinical judgment of the treating physician.

9.13   The answer is **D.**

As with any pretreatment evaluations, the pretreatment evaluation for electroconvulsive therapy (ECT) is determined by the probability of certain side effects. The commonly completed laboratory and diagnostic tests include a complete blood count, blood chemistries, urinalysis, spinal X rays, and an electrocardiogram. Depending on the medical history, medical and neurological exam, or mental status exam, a computed tomographic scan and electroencephalogram might also be ordered. Spinal X rays used to be commonly ordered in the pretreatment evaluation for ECT. However, the use of succinylcholine in ECT procedures has lowered the risk of orthopedic complications, and spinal X rays are not currently part of the routine pretreatment evaluation.

9.14   The answer is **A**.

Radioisotopes of one type or another are presently used in the brain imaging techniques of single photon emission computed tomography (SPECT), regional cerebral blood flow (rCBF), and positron emission tomography (PET). SPECT can visualize the entire brain, including both the cortical and the subcortical regions. In SPECT, a radiopharmaceutical agent is introduced into the brain via incorporation in compounds such as isopropyl-amphetamine. The gamma radiation of the single-photon-emitting agent is then detected by rotating gamma-cameras around the head. In this way brain function can be studied. Different aspects of brain function that can be visualized using SPECT include brain blood flow and specific central nervous system receptor functions.

In PET scans, a positron-emitting agent such as fluorine-18 or carbon-14 is incorporated in a biologically significant substance such as glucose and thus is introduced into the brain. The distribution of the isotopes, and thus of the biologically significant substances, is then measured by a series of radioactivity-sensitive detectors that are arranged about the head. Depending on the biologically significant substance used, the PET scan can be used to evaluate brain blood flow, brain oxygen utilization, or other aspects of brain glucose utilization.

The rCBF measures blood flow to various parts of the brain by introducing a biologically inert substance such as radioactive xenon-133 into the body through inhalation or some other means. Blood then carries the radioactive substance to various parts of the brain. The amount of radioactive substance in various areas of the brain corresponds to the amount of blood flow to that part of the brain. Multiple detectors on the head of the patient pick up the differential amounts of radioactivity, providing the estimate of relative blood flow. The rCBF cannot provide estimates of subcortical blood flow.

In contrast to the SPECT, PET, and rCBF, magnetic resonance imaging does not use radioactive isotopes. Instead, a magnetic field is applied to the brain and the nuclei of hydrogen atoms become aligned with this field. The hydrogen atoms are then exposed to brief pulses of electromagnetic energy. At the termination of these pulses, they return to their previous alignment and emit characteristic quanta of energy. The energy is picked by sensors and is analyzed by a computer that then provides an image of brain structures. The resulting resolution has extreme clarity.

9.15 The answer is **B**.

The dexamethasone suppression test (DST) previously enjoyed more widespread use than it currently does. Its previous popularity was due to the excitement generated by early reports that it was sensitive to subtle changes in the function of the hypothalamic–pituitary–adrenal axis, a system that was implicated in depression. It was thought that the DST could serve as a useful marker for endogenous depression. The DST has been the focus of much of the biological psychiatric research conducted in the past few years. More recent research reports indicate that although the DST is sensitive to some of the changes accompanying psychiatric illness, the DST is better able to differentiate between depressed patients and healthy controls than between depressed patients and patients with other psychiatric illnesses. Another drawback is that recent weight loss can result in a false positive result.

9.16 The answer is **D**.

There is not complete agreement regarding the applicability of measuring plasma tricyclic antidepressant levels. However, the American Psychiatric Association Task Force on the Use of Laboratory Tests in Psychiatry has recommended the use of measuring plasma levels of tricyclic antidepressants in patients who have questionable compliance, have a poor response to normal dosage levels of drugs, experience side effects at very low levels, are at high risk for side effects (such as older patients or medically ill patients), or are extremely ill and need to obtain therapeutic blood levels in a relatively short period of time.

9.17 The answer is **A**.

The dexamethasone suppression test (DST) has an uncertain utility in the practice of clinical psychiatry. Generally the DST consists of a procedure whereby the patient receives an oral dose of dexamethasone at 11:00 P.M. Blood is then drawn at 8:00 A.M., 4:00 P.M., and 11:00 P.M. the next day. Usually the test results are considered to be abnormal when the postdexamethasone serum cortisol level equals or exceeds about 5 μg/dl. There are limitations to the DST. For example the sensitivity of the DST may be in the range of 45 percent. Although the specificity of the DST may be around 90 percent in healthy controls, it is much lower in individuals with other psychiatric illnesses. Also there is the possibility of contamination of the results from recent weight loss, medical illness, acute psychiatric hospitalization, certain medications, and individual differences in the metabolism of dexamethasone.

Chapter 10

Organic Mental Disorders

DIRECTIONS: Each of the statements or questions is followed by five suggested responses or completions. Select the one that is the best choice or most complete answer in each case.

10.1 Which of the following regarding the organic mental syndrome is not true?

    A. Its essential feature is a psychological or behavioral abnormality associated with brain dysfunction.
    B. Its specific etiology must be known.
    C. It can be due to a permanent brain dysfunction.
    D. It can be due to a temporary brain dysfunction.
    E. It can have a wide variety of clinical manifestations.

10.2 Which of the following statements regarding the prevalence or incidence of organic mental syndromes is true?

    A. As many as 5 percent of individuals over age 65 may have a severe dementia.
    B. At least 40 percent of those individuals over 80 years old may have a severe dementia.
    C. Among psychiatric disorders, the organic mental syndrome is relatively uncommon.
    D. The incidence of organic mental syndromes is well documented.
    E. The incidence of organic mental syndromes is likely to decrease in the future.

10.3 The clinical course of delirium includes:

  A. a slowly declining level of functioning
  B. cognitive impairment in the presence of an intact sensorium
  C. an irreversible decline in functioning
  D. relatively little behavioral abnormality
  E. frequent fluctuations in brain dysfunction

10.4 Which of the following statements regarding delirium is true?

  A. Environmental sensory deprivation may induce delirium.
  B. The verbalizations of a delirious patient should not be taken seriously.
  C. Delirium may be subacute and mild.
  D. About one-fourth of inpatients with delirium will die within three to four months.
  E. Delirium is often the result of psychosocial factors.

10.5 Which of the following statements regarding dementia is true?

  A. Dementia is an unavoidable consequence of aging.
  B. A cardinal feature of dementia is complaint of spatial–perceptual impairment.
  C. Aphasic symptoms are rare in dementia.
  D. Dementia has a wide variety of clinical manifestations.
  E. The demented patient rarely shows impaired judgment.

10.6 Which of the following statements regarding the relation of delusions to dementia is true?

  A. Although paranoid delusions are rare, delusions of grandiosity are common in dementia.
  B. Paranoid delusions may serve to account for unexplained events that are actually secondary to lapses of memory.
  C. In general, delusions are rare in dementia.
  D. Delusions in dementia appear to be secondary to metabolic dysfunction.
  E. Delusions in dementia rarely have a meaningful content.

10.7   Which of the following statements is not true regarding the characteristics of multi-infarct dementia (MID)?

    A.   MID is the most common form of dementia.
    B.   Patients with MID are more likely to be male and younger than patients with Alzheimer's disease.
    C.   Patients with MID are more likely to have focal neurological signs than are patients with Alzheimer's disease.
    D.   MID patients are more likely to be aware of their deficits than patients with Alzheimer's disease.
    E.   The clinical course of MID involves a stepwise progression of symptoms.

10.8   Which of the following statements regarding the organic mood syndrome is not true?

    A.   Fluctuating levels of arousal are not found in this disorder.
    B.   Widespread cognitive decline does not occur in this disorder.
    C.   The affective disturbance must be accompanied by at least two neurovegetative symptoms.
    D.   The mood disturbance in organic mood syndrome is relatively sustained.
    E.   The clinical presentation of an organic mood disturbance can easily be differentiated from that of affective disorders.

DIRECTIONS: For each of the statements or questions below, one or more of the alternative answers is correct. Choose answer:
    A   if only 1, 2, and 3 are correct
    B   if only 1 and 3 are correct
    C   if only 2 and 4 are correct
    D   if only 4 is correct
    E   if all are correct

10.9   Which of the following are typical features of the organic mood syndrome?

    1. insidious onset
    2. prior history of depression
    3. exacerbation by psychosocial features
    4. absence of cognitive impairment

10.10 Which of the following are causes of the organic amnestic syndrome?

1. trauma
2. psychosocial stress
3. infection
4. a history favoring development of learned helplessness

10.11 Which of the following are features of organic hallucinosis?

1. memory impairment
2. deficient abstract reasoning skills
3. marked affective dysfunction
4. a relatively clear sensorium

10.12 Which of the following statements regarding the organic personality syndrome is true?

1. The symptoms occur abruptly.
2. The symptoms may reflect an exaggeration of previous personality style.
3. The symptoms involve diametrical changes in personality.
4. The symptoms may occur slowly and subtly.

10.13 Which of the following statements regarding the differential between dementia and pseudodementia is true?

1. Pseudodemented patients are more likely to call attention to and be distressed by their symptoms.
2. The demented patient gives close but incorrect answers; the pseudodemented patient states, "I don't know."
3. The cognitive deficits in dementia are more likely to be pervasive and enduring.
4. Pseudodemented patients show the sundowning phenomenon.

10.14 Treatment of acute agitated delirium involves:

1. titrating external stimuli
2. identifying and removing the etiological agent
3. smaller doses of neuroleptics than those used for psychotic disorder
4. simple directive verbal interactions

10.15 The treatment of severe chronic dementia involves:

1. simplifying the amount of information presented to the patient
2. rapid titration of high-potency neuroleptics
3. minimal use of hypnotics and sedatives
4. daytime naps on an as-needed basis

DIRECTIONS: Each of the following questions consists of lettered headings followed by a list of numbered alternatives. Select the single lettered heading that is most closely associated with the appropriate numbered alternative. Each lettered heading may be chosen only once.

Organic mental disorder

A Pick's disease
B Creutzfeldt-Jakob disease
C Huntington's disease
D Wilson's disease
E Organic amnestic syndrome

Description

10.16 is characterized by choreiform movements and a progressive dementia
10.17 is caused by a slow virus, generally fatal
10.18 reveals at autopsy prominent gliosis, with massive atrophy in frontal and temporal regions
10.19 is an inherited disorder of copper metabolism that affects the liver and the putamen of the lenticular nucleus
10.20 can be secondary to alcohol-induced Korsakoff's syndrome

ANSWERS

10.1 The answer is **B**.

Organic mental syndromes are characterized by an abnormality of behavior or other psychological functioning associated with temporary or permanent brain dysfunction. The syndrome is called an organic mental *disorder* only when the organic etiology of the disorder can be shown or presumed. Brain dysfunction can be responsible for a wide variety of clinical manifestations across different people and in the same individual. Therefore, exact diagnosis of the organic mental syndrome can be a difficult task. The clinician must be familiar with the range of both organic and functional disorders and must conduct a careful evaluation in order to arrive at the correct diagnosis.

10.2 The answer is **A**.

In general, the incidence and prevalence of organic mental disorders are not precisely known. Most of the epidemiological investigations of these disorders have involved specific populations such as nursing home residents or medical inpatients. A recent survey of the general population revealed a prevalence of 1.0 to 1.3 percent; however, the instrument used to detect the disorders was not sensitive to a wide range of deficits and therefore the results may have seriously underestimated the true prevalence.

However, certain general statements can be made. It appears that the life-long incidence of organic mental disorders may be the highest of all of the psychiatric disorders. It is estimated that 5 percent of the general population over the age of 65 and 20 percent of those older than 80 years suffer from a severe dementia. An additional 10 percent of the general population over the age of 65 years may suffer from a moderate dementia.

10.3 The answer is **E**.

Delirium is characterized by frequent fluctuations in brain dysfunction. These fluctuations may occur from day to day or from minute to minute. The fluctuations in arousal, orientation, perception, and cognition reflect changes in the underlying etiologic agent. The fluctuations may also reflect changes in the patient's environment, such as when an increase in sensory stimulation results in a decline in functioning. The sensorium is generally disturbed, unlike in the case of dementia.

Behavioral abnormalities may be widespread. If left untreated, these symptoms may worsen, clear, or remain stable. However, because delirium usually reflects a serious underlying metabolic condition, treatment may be successful in removing the symptoms, or at least in avoiding mortality.

10.4   The answer is D.

While it is true that psychosocial or environmental events may exacerbate a delirious condition, the cause of a delirium is always organic. There is a high mortality rate associated with delirium. Approximately one-fourth of inpatients with delirium will die within three to four months. The mortality rate is due to both the etiology of the underlying disorder and the greater potential for status epilepticus and severe autonomic arousal.

Although the content of delirious verbalizations may not seem to make much sense, these verbalizations may contain useful information regarding the patient's beliefs and attitudes regarding his or her illness. Delirium is usually thought of as being acute and severe, but it can occur in a subacute and mild form, especially if caused by infection or as the result of medication reactions.

10.5   The answer is D.

Dementia has many different causes and many different manifestations. Signs of dementia may include impaired judgment, abstraction skills, attention, concentration, memory, and other cognitive functions. The late stages of dementia may show pathological suck, grasp, snout, and palmomental reflexes. Also in the late stages, different dementias tend to resemble each other as the type and severity of deficits increases. Word-finding difficulties and paraphasias may also occur. Dementia is the result of a neuropathological process and should not be considered a part of normal aging.

10.6   The answer is B.

In the early stages of dementia, the patient may refuse an evaluation because of a fear that his or her deficits will be exposed. These patients tend to deny that they have any problems. When things do go wrong, such as losing articles or disagreements with family members over past conversation or events, the patient may develop a delusional system to explain the situation. These delusions are paranoid in flavor. The patient may suspect family members of conspiring to steal his or her money. Or the patient may suspect that someone is breaking into the house and stealing the articles that have been misplaced.

10.7   The answer is **A.**

Multi-infarct dementia (MID) is the second most common form of dementia after Alzheimer's disease. Approximately 10 percent of dementia cases are diagnosed as MID at autopsy. The clinical presentation differs somewhat from Alzheimer's disease. The clinical course of MID tends to show stepwise deterioration of cognitive functions with focal neurological signs. The abrupt onset of cognitive deficits is followed by a gradual incomplete recovery. However, as these events (either embolic or thrombotic infarcts) continue, the cognitive deficits accrue to a manifestation of relatively widespread and lasting dementia. The patient with MID is usually younger than the patient with Alzheimer's. The MID patient is also more likely to have a history of hypertension and is more likely to be aware of his or her cognitive deficits. If the ischemic events affect the basal ganglia and periventricular white matter, the patient may show pseudobulbar signs of affective lability.

10.8   The answer is **E.**

The organic mood syndrome is not characterized by fluctuating levels of arousal or by cognitive decline. The impairment found in the organic mood syndrome is usually more circumscribed than that found in dementia and delirium. Despite the fact that the organic mood syndrome has an organic etiology, it can resemble a functional affective disorder in its clinical presentation. Therefore the history is required to determine the presence of an organic etiology. The impairment in organic mood syndrome is an organically induced mood disturbance that can be depression, mania, or a mixture of the two. It is a relatively sustained disturbance and must be accompanied by at least two neurovegetative signs, such as weight loss, psychomotor retardation or agitation, or sleep disturbance.

10.9   The answer is **E.**

The features of organic mood syndrome include insidious onset, prior history of depression, exacerbation of symptoms by psychosocial stressors, and absence of cognitive impairment. Therefore it may resemble a functional mood disturbance. The diagnosis of organic mood syndrome is more easily made when the onset is sudden and can be related to an identifiable organic event such as a cerebrovascular accident. Chronic cases of organic mood syndrome may be due to endocrinopathies, systemic diseases, or neurological diseases.

10.10   The answer is **B**.

The organic amnestic syndrome is characterized by an impairment in recent memory. Generally, there is no impairment in orientation, level of arousal, or immediate memory. Causes of this syndrome include trauma, infection, infarction, seizures, alcohol abuse, and drugs. The most common etiology of the organic amnestic syndrome is alcohol abuse resulting in Korsakoff's syndrome. Unfortunately, when the organic amnestic syndrome is due to Korsakoff's syndrome, treatment may not result in improvement of symptoms.

10.11   The answer is **D**.

In organic hallucinosis, the patient is relatively free of cognitive impairment. The cardinal feature is organically induced hallucinations. The etiologies of organic hallucinosis include tumors, trauma, encephalomeningitis, and temporal lobe epilepsy. Hallucinations may be visual, auditory, gustatory, olfactory, or tactile. Tactile hallucinations are more common in alcoholic hallucinosis than in other etiologies.

10.12   The answer is **C**.

When changes in behavioral style or attitudes can be ascribed to an organic etiology, then a diagnosis of organic personality syndrome can be considered. These changes may be an exaggeration of previous behavioral patterns such as in the case of the suspicious individual who becomes frankly paranoid. The changes may occur slowly or abruptly. Injuries of the superior convexities of the frontal lobes may result in a picture of amotivation. Temporal lobe epilepsy is another disorder that has recognizable personality concomitants. These behavioral manifestations may include hypergraphia, hyperreligiosity, and either hypo- or hypersexuality. Individuals with temporal lobe epilepsy may also exhibit an overconcern with philosophical matters.

10.13   The answer is **A**.

Pseudodementia is a condition in which depressed patients show some of the same signs of cognitive dysfunction we usually associate with dementia. However, a careful history and evaluation will point out differences that can be used to perform the differential diagnosis. Pseudodementia is more likely to occur in individuals who have a prior history of depression. The symptoms of pseudodementia are more likely to arise over a period of weeks or months, in contrast to Alzheimer's dementia, in which the symptoms develop slowly. Alzheimer's patients usually maintain occupational and social functioning until later in the course of the disorder. Pseudodemented patients withdraw from activity early in the course of the disorder. Alzheimer's patients may show the sundowning effect of doing worse in the evening, whereas pseudodemented patients may actually improve at night.

Pseudodemented patients show concern over their deficits and point them out to others. Alzheimer's patients try to cover and deny their impairments. Patients with Alzheimer's disease are also more likely to produce close but incorrect answers during an examination; pseudodemented patients will simply answer "I don't know" to questions in a mental status exam. The deficits in Alzheimer's disease are more likely to be global, whereas the deficits in pseudodementia are somewhat more circumscribed.

10.14 The answer is **E**.

Delirium usually represents an underlying system-wide disorder which needs to be treated quickly. While the etiology is being identified and treated, the amount of environmental stimulation presented to the patient should be titrated to a level that can be handled. For example, the visiting hours can be extended or decreased as necessary, and the amount of light and ambient noise can also be adjusted to promote optimal functioning. Interactions with the patient should be reassuring, simple, and directive.

10.15 The answer is **B**.

Some of the aspects of the treatment for dementia are similar to those for delirium. For example, people in the patient's environment should help provide orientation for the patient. Simple declarative speech should be the mode of verbal interaction with the patient. Only necessary information should be presented to the patient. The patient may express an increased need for daytime naps, but these should be kept to a minimum in order to promote maximum functioning. Hypnotics can confuse demented patients, and their use should be kept to a minimum. Anxiolytics can produce paradoxical agitation and should also be avoided. High-potency neuroleptics may produce extrapyramidal side effects even at low doses, and their use should be carefully monitored.

10.16   The answer is **C**.
10.17   The answer is **E**.
10.18   The answer is **A**.
10.19   The answer is **D**.
10.20   The answer is **B**.

Patients with Huntington's disease exhibit choreiform movements and a progressive dementia, usually starting at the end of the patient's fourth decade of life. Early symptoms may look like schizophrenia or an affective disorder, but the genetic component of this disorder makes diagnosis relatively certain. Perhaps because many patients with Huntington's disease have witnessed the course of the illness in older relatives with the disorder, suicide is common. Autopsy and computed tomographic results show generalized atrophy concentrated in the frontal lobes, caudate nucleus, and putamen. There are also deficiencies of gamma-aminobutyric acid associated with this disorder.

Creutzfeldt-Jakob disease is extremely rare. Only one case per one million is diagnosed each year. It appears to be the result of a slow virus that first shows its symptoms many years after inoculation. The symptoms, including mild dementia, myoclonic jerks, fasciculations, and emotional changes, usually appear between the ages of 40 and 60 years. However, once the diagnosis is made, there is a rapid decline, resulting in severe dementia and death within a year.

It is often difficult to perform the differential between Pick's and Alzheimer's diseases. Pick's disease is only one-fiftieth as common as Alzheimer's. At autopsy, Pick's shows a characteristic pattern of prominent gliosis, severe atrophy of the frontal and temporal lobes, and neurons swollen by Pick's bodies.

Wilson's disease involves an inherited defect in copper metabolism. The most severe effects of this metabolic deficiency are in the liver and in the putamen of the lenticular nucleus. Symptoms of disturbed behavior such as would accompany neurosis or psychosis usually occur before the cognitive symptoms. By the second decade of life, rigidity and tremor appear as well as cirrhosis of the liver and the pathognomonic sign of Kayser-Fleischer rings (golden-brown pigmentation) on the cornea.

The organic amnestic syndrome is an impairment in recent, but not immediate or remote, memory that can be traced to an organic etiology. Etiologies include trauma, seizure, tumor, infection, infarction, or drugs, but the most common etiology is that of Korsakoff's syndrome secondary to chronic alcohol abuse.

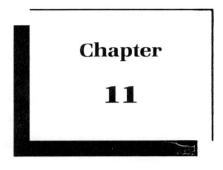

Chapter

11

Alcohol and Other Psychoactive Substance Use Disorders

DIRECTIONS: Each of the statements or questions is followed by five suggested responses or completions. Select the one that is the best choice or most complete answer in each case.

11.1 Which of the following findings is most often associated with phencyclidine intoxication?

    A. dilated pupils
    B. vertical nystagmus
    C. meiosis
    D. ophthalmoplegia
    E. all of the above

11.2 The highest risk factor for developing alcoholism is:

    A. being raised in a family with alcoholism
    B. being male and having a biologic parent with alcoholism
    C. having a mood disorder
    D. alienation from society
    E. low socioeconomic status

11.3 In the *Diagnostic and Statistical Manual of Mental Disorders (Third Edition-Revised)* all of the following are correct except:

    A. substance dependence has been broadened as a category
    B. tolerance and withdrawal are no longer sole criteria for dependence
    C. cocaine dependence has been added as a category
    D. fewer patients will be labeled as being dependent on a substance
    E. the term *psychoactive* has been added

11.4 Recent Epidemiologic Catchment Area studies have found:

    A. lifetime prevalence of substance use disorders of approximately 18 percent
    B. higher cocaine abuse than alcohol abuse
    C. increased prevalence in geriatric patients
    D. equal prevalence of alcoholism in men and women
    E. a major decline in alcoholism

DIRECTIONS: For each of the statements below, one or more of the alternative answers is correct. Choose answer:

    A if only 1, 2, and 3 are correct
    B if only 1 and 3 are correct
    C if only 2 and 4 are correct
    D if only 4 is correct
    E if all are correct

11.5 The advantages of methadone maintenance include which of the following?

    1. less need for clinic contact
    2. easy detoxification
    3. cessation of other substance abuse
    4. less criminal activity and unemployment

11.6 Marijuana has been associated with which of the following?

    1. delirium
    2. motor vehicle accidents
    3. delusional disorders
    4. amotivational syndrome

11.7 Which of the following withdrawal syndromes are most often associated with mortality?

1. alcohol
2. opiates
3. benzodiazepines
4. cocaine

11.8 Positive treatment outcome for alcoholism has been associated with the following factors:

1. low psychopathology
2. low antisocial problems
3. high socioeconomic stability
4. high family stability

11.9 Which of the following *Diagnostic and Statistical Manual of Mental Disorders (Third Edition-Revised)* diagnoses have been most often associated with cocaine abuse?

1. schizophrenia
2. affective disorders
3. panic attacks
4. attention deficit disorder

11.10 Indications for inpatient alcohol treatment include:

1. high motivation for treatment
2. major medical or psychiatric problems
3. ability to afford treatment
4. previous failed outpatient treatment

DIRECTIONS: Each of the following questions consists of lettered headings followed by a list of numbered alternatives. Select the single lettered heading that is most closely associated with the appropriate numbered alternative. Each lettered heading may be chosen only once.

Substance use disorder

A. alcohol
B. cocaine
C. sedative, hypnotic, or anxiolytic
D. amphetamines
E. phencyclidine
F. heroin

Description of symptoms of abuse

11.11   may start in conjunction with weight-loss treatment, energy enhancement, or serious intravenous drug use. Signs of abuse include tachycardia, pupillary dilation, loquacity, elation, and hypervigilance.

11.12   may be associated with the Wernicke-Korsakoff syndrome (truncal ataxia, ophthalmoplegia, and mental confusion) secondary to thiamine deficiency.

11.13   may lead to affective presentations ranging from intense euphoria to anxiety, stereotyped repetitive behavior, and bizarre aggressive behavior. Distorted perceptions, numbness, and confusion are also common.

11.14   produces a subjective "rush" when used intravenously that can be highly reinforcing. Physical signs of intoxication include pupillary constriction, decreased gastrointestinal motility, marked sedation, slurred speech, and impairment in attentional processes and memory.

11.15   can have tolerance developed in two to three weeks. Intoxication, withdrawal, withdrawal delirium, and amnestic disorders are similar to those of alcohol. Withdrawal may not be evident until 7 to 10 days after cessation of use.

11.16   can cause hyperalertness, euphoria, perceptual changes, disinhibition, enhanced sense of mastery, sexual arousal, and inflated self-esteem. The "rush" experience may be greatly intensified with intravenous or free-base use.

ANSWERS

11.1   The answer is **B**.

The psychoactive effects of phencyclidine (PCP, angel dust) usually begin within 5 minutes and plateau at approximately 30 minutes. Volatile emotional reactions are the predominant behavioral presentation. Physical signs of phencyclidine abuse include high blood pressure, ataxia, muscular rigidity, and at higher dosages, hyperthermia, involuntary movements, and coma. Dilated pupils and nystagmus, particularly vertical nystagmus, should heighten suspicion of abuse.

11.2 The answer is B.

Alcoholism is the result of a combination of an interaction between biological vulnerability and environmental factors such as childhood experiences, parental attitudes, and social and cultural factors. Twin and adoption studies have found that genetic factors significantly influence causation, but the mechanism of genetic transmission is as yet unknown. Monozygotic twins have approximately two times the rate for the concordance of alcoholism than do dizygotic twins, and the incidence is four times higher among male biological offspring of alcoholic fathers regardless of whether the child is raised by foster parents or by the biological father.

11.3 The answer is D.

Preliminary field tests have demonstrated that most of what would have been diagnosed as substance abuse by the *Diagnostic and Statistical Manual of Mental Disorders (Third Edition) (DSM-III)* would be diagnosed as psychoactive substance dependency by *DSM-III-Revised*. In *DSM-III-R*, the term *psychoactive* was added to substance abuse and dependency categories to differentiate psychoactive substance abuse from nutritional and other adverse drug reaction categories. In addition, it was proposed that psychoactive substance dependence be broadened to include at least three significant behaviors out of a nine-item list that includes psychosocial problems and a serious involvement with a psychoactive substance. The patterns of tolerance and withdrawal are no longer sole criteria for dependence in *DSM-III-R*. Several new categories have also been added to cover dependence on cocaine, phencyclidine, hallucinogens, and inhalants.

11.4 The answer is A.

The Epidemiologic Catchment Area Study, using standardized interviews in three U.S. studies, found that psychoactive substance abuse disorders ranked first among 15 *Diagnostic and Statistical Manual of Mental Disorders (Third Edition)* diagnoses, with an average of 13.6 percent of the general population sampled having a lifetime prevalence of alcohol abuse or dependence. In most cultures, men are overrepresented among problem drinkers, and in the United States this ratio is approximately

4 to 1. Most alcohol-related problems begin between the ages of 16 and 30, with the lowest percentage of problems beginning over the age of 50.

11.5   The answer is D.

Advocates of long-term methadone maintenance cite the benefits of decreases in opioid abuse, less criminal behavior, and less unemployment as advantages of this treatment strategy.

11.6   The answer is E.

Marijuana abuse has been associated with a number of adverse clinical features, including paranoias, depression, and motivational problems. In schools, jobs, or other situations in which mental clarity is required, marijuana may have detrimental effects. Numerous studies have outlined neuropsychological changes and deficits with marijuana use, though the effects can be highly variable. There is evidence that the ability to speak coherently, to form concepts, concentrate, and transfer information from immediate to long-term memory storage may be impaired by marijuana abuse.

11.7   The answer is B.

Alcohol morbidity and a disproportionate number of inpatient hospital days are associated with the effects of intoxication, withdrawal, or overdose. Withdrawal syndromes can be life threatening and are most dangerous when accompanied by medical problems such as pneumonia, liver failure, and subdural hematomas.

Seizures may be the first heralding sign of high-dose benzodiazepine withdrawal. Severe withdrawal may produce anxiety, psychosis, and possibly death from cardiovascular collapse.

11.8   The answer is E.

Treatment outcome studies of alcoholism indicate that a variety of treatments yield benefit and may be cost effective; however, few studies exist that differentiate which treatments are best for which kinds of patients. Thus far, outcome studies have found that patient factors such as family and job stability, less psychopathology, and a negative family history of alcoholism are more powerful predictors of positive prognosis than is type of treatment.

11.9   The answer is C.

Because of the lack of prospective studies in the area, it is very difficult to differentiate cocaine-induced psychiatric disorders from interactions with preexisting disorders. There may be a significant subset of patients who suffer from underlying affective disorders (cyclothymic or dysthymic). Other Axis I disorders may include substance abuse or attention deficit disorder.

11.10 The answer is C.

The choice of inpatient versus outpatient treatment for alcohol withdrawal depends on severity of symptoms, stage of withdrawal, medical and psychiatric complications, polydrug abuse, patient cooperation, ability to follow instructions, social support systems, and past history. For example, patients with organic brain syndrome, low intelligence, Wernicke's encephalopathy, dehydration, history of head trauma, neurological symptoms, medical complications, delirium tremens, seizures, alcoholic hallucinosis, or psychopathology that may require psychotropic medication are best treated in inpatient settings.

11.11 The answer is D.
11.12 The answer is A.
11.13 The answer is E.
11.14 The answer is F.
11.15 The answer is C.
11.16 The answer is B.

Amphetamine abuse may start in conjunction with weight-loss programs, energy enhancement, or more serious intravenous drug use. The symptoms of amphetamine use include tachycardia, elevated blood pressure, pupillary dilation, agitation, elation, loquacity, and hypervigilance. Adverse side effects include insomnia, irritability, confusion, and hostility.

Chronic alcohol abuse may be associated with the Wernicke-Korsakoff syndrome. This syndrome classically begins with abrupt-onset encephalopathy, with truncal ataxia, ophthalmoplegia, and mental confusion. The etiology of this syndrome involves thiamine deficiency secondary to dietary, genetic, or medical factors. Wernicke's encephalopathy may result in death or, more commonly, in Korsakoff's psychosis, a chronic amnestic disorder that classically presents with severe anterograde amnesia.

Volatile emotional affects are the predominant behavioral presentation with phencyclidine abuse. Affects range from intense euphoria to anxiety, stereotyped repetitive behavior, and bizarre aggressive behavior. Violent murders have been attributed to complications of phencyclidine abuse. Distorted perceptions, numbness, and confusion are also common.

Intravenous heroin intoxication produces a subjective euphoric "rush" that can be highly reinforcing. Tolerance to this high develops with repeated use. Physical signs of intoxication include pupillary constriction, decreased gastrointestinal motility, marked sedation, slurred speech, and impairment in attention or memory.

Tolerance to sedative hypnotic effects can develop in two to three weeks; however, anxiety effects may persist.

Intoxication, withdrawal, withdrawal delirium, and amnestic disorder symptoms are similar to those found with alcohol. Benzodiazepines have a much longer half-life than alcohol and may not be evident until 7 to 10 days following cessation of use.

The effects of cocaine intoxication range through euphoria, hyperalertness, perceptual changes, disinhibition, enhanced sense of mastery, sexual arousal, and improved self-esteem. These effects appear to depend on the dose and administration of the drug. The "rush" experience may be greatly intensified with intravenous or free-base use. Maladaptive behavioral changes include fighting, grandiosity, hypervigilance, psychomotor agitation, impaired judgment, and impaired occupational and social functioning.

Chapter 12

Schizophrenia, Schizophreniform Disorder, and Delusional (Paranoid) Disorders

DIRECTIONS: Each of the statements or questions is followed by five suggested responses or completions. Select the one that is the best choice or most complete answer in each case.

12.1   What is the estimated prevalence of schizophrenia in this country?

- **A.**   As many as .02 percent of the population of the United States suffers from schizophrenia.
- **B.**   Between 3 and 5 percent of the population of the United States suffers from schizophrenia.
- **C.**   The prevalence of schizophrenia is 2 percent in this country.
- **D.**   Between .5 and 1 percent of the population of the United States suffers from schizophrenia.
- **E.**   Between 8 and 10 percent of the population of the United States suffers from schizophrenia.

12.2 Clinicians are in general agreement that the best treatment approaches for schizophrenia involve:

    A. only medication and other somatic forms of treatment
    B. a combination of both medication and psychosocial care
    C. only medication; other forms of somatic treatment have not been found to be useful
    D. a psychoanalytic approach
    E. an operant behavioral approach

12.3 The major differential diagnosis in psychiatric settings involves separating schizophrenia from:

    A. schizophreniform disorder
    B. affective disorder, delusional disorder, or personality disorder
    C. schizophreniform disorder or delusional disorder
    D. personality disorder or organic mental disorder
    E. delusional disorder, organic mental disorder, or personality disorder

12.4 What is the most common form(s) of hallucinations in schizophrenia?

    A. visual
    B. tactile
    C. tactile and visual
    D. gustatory and olfactory
    E. auditory

12.5 Schizophrenic individuals seem to be protected from:

    A. cancer
    B. myasthenia gravis
    C. rheumatoid arthritis
    D. epilepsy
    E. diabetes mellitus

12.6 Identified risk factors for suicide in schizophrenic individuals include all of the following except:

    A. youth
    B. female sex
    C. unemployed status
    D. chronic relapsing course
    E. prior or current depression

12.7 Research studies indicate that the best form of treatment for delusional disorders includes:

    A. rapid titration of neuroleptic medication
    B. tact and clinical skill needed to convince the patient to enter therapy
    C. intensive psychoanalytically oriented therapy
    D. rigorous refutation of the delusional system
    E. there have been no studies conducted

12.8 Which of the following is not necessary for the diagnosis of delusional disorder in the *Diagnostic and Statistical Manual of Mental Disorders (Third Edition-Revised) (DSM-III-R)*?

    A. at least one month's duration of symptoms
    B. the presence of nonbizarre delusions
    C. history of poor premorbid social adjustment
    D. a fixed false belief in the presence of otherwise clear sensorium
    E. absence of hallucinations

12.9 The diagnosis of schizophreniform disorder requires which of the following?

    A. presence of symptoms for at least nine months
    B. presence of symptoms for at least six months
    C. active psychotic features
    D. absence of hallucinations
    E. none of the above

DIRECTIONS: For each of the statements or questions below, one or more of the alternative answers is correct. Choose answer:

    A if only 1, 2, and 3 are correct
    B if only 1 and 3 are correct
    C if only 2 and 4 are correct
    D if only 4 is correct
    E if all are correct

12.10 The character of symptoms in the delusional (paranoid) disorders includes:

    1. the presence of a dominant, well-systematized, encapsulated nonbizarre delusion
    2. accompanying affect that is appropriate to the delusion
    3. personality deterioration that is minimal
    4. only persecutory or grandiose delusions

12.11 A recent review of outcome in schizophrenia indicates which major point(s)?

1. a generally poor outcome in most cases
2. a large difference in outcome for first hospitalizations versus second hospitalizations
3. good outcome in 57 percent of the cases treated with antipsychotics
4. a slight improvement in outcome over the last century

12.12 Electroconvulsive therapy may be a useful treatment in schizophrenia if:

1. catatonia is present
2. a superimposed depression is present
3. onset is relatively acute (less than 18 months) with a lack of response to drugs
4. the patient has a chronic relapsing course

12.13 Kendler has shown that delusional disorder:

1. is more common in socially disadvantaged subjects
2. manifests itself in mid to late adult life
3. is more common in females than males
4. has a percentage of 60–75 percent patients who are married

12.14 According to *DSM-III-R*, a diagnosis of schizophrenia requires:

1. the ruling out of an organic mental disorder
2. continuous signs of the disturbance for at least nine months
3. the presence of characteristic psychotic symptoms for at least one week's duration
4. a substantial affective component to the symptoms

12.15 The United States–Great Britain Diagnostic Project demonstrated that:

1. schizophrenia is a culture-free diagnosis
2. schizophrenia was more commonly diagnosed in New York than in London
3. affective disorder was less commonly diagnosed in London than in New York
4. affective disorder was more commonly diagnosed in London than in New York

12.16   Age of onset in schizophrenia is earlier in:

1. men
2. women
3. disorganized subtype
4. paranoid subtype

12.17   According to Andreasen and Olsen, positive schizophrenia is characterized by which of the following?

1. bizarre behavior
2. prominent delusions
3. marked incoherence
4. attentional impairment

DIRECTIONS: Each of the following questions consists of lettered headings followed by a list of numbered alternatives. Select the single lettered heading that is most closely associated with the appropriate numbered alternative. Each lettered heading may be chosen only once.

A.   Paranoid schizophrenia
B.   Disorganized schizophrenia
C.   Catatonic schizophrenia
D.   Residual schizophrenia

12.18   refers to patients who once met the criteria for schizophrenia and now have continuing evidence of symptoms

12.19   has dominant symptoms of negativism, purposeless excitement, stupor, or mutism, among other symptoms

12.20   refers to patients who demonstrate incoherence, marked loosening of associations, or flat or grossly inappropriate affect

12.21   refers to patients who have a preoccupation with one or more systematized abnormal belief systems or frequent auditory hallucinations related to a single theme in the absence of a florid thought disorder

ANSWERS

12.1 The answer is **D**.

Estimates of the prevalence of schizophrenia indicate that between .5 and 1 percent of the population of the United States suffers from schizophrenia. The symptoms of schizophrenia first occur in young adulthood so individuals with this diagnosis generally have a lifetime of impairment. This fact has an extremely large effect on the individuals with schizophrenia as well as on their relatives.

Estimates from the early 1970s indicate that two percent of the U. S. gross national product is spent on the direct and indirect costs of this disorder. If the percentage figure applies to the economy of 1984, the total expenditure would amount to $73.2 billion dollars. Clearly, schizophrenia has a costly effect on the economy of this nation. The cost in human terms is no less expensive.

12.2 The answer is **B**.

The past few years have witnessed several reassessments regarding our views of schizophrenia, including that regarding which treatment is the best. Following the introduction of antipsychotic medication, there was a period of optimism that has subsequently dissipated. One of the initial effects of the use of antipsychotics was that many hospitals were able to discharge large numbers of schizophrenic patients. It soon became clear that although free of overtly psychotic symptoms, many of these patients were unable to function independently. In addition, many patients could only be discharged for short periods of time, resulting in a revolving-door phenomenon. More recent attempts to treat schizophrenia recognize that a multidimensional effort combining both medication and psychosocial approaches appears to be the most effective. Treatment approaches that use only one approach, whether it be medication or a strictly operant behavioral approach, are probably insufficient.

12.3 The answer is **B**.

In a psychiatric setting, the main differential diagnosis involves separating schizophrenia from affective disorder, delusional disorder, or personality disorder. Although schizophrenic patients may show affective symptoms, they do not meet the criteria for a full depressive or manic syndrome. Also, the affective features tend to develop after the appearance of the psychotic symptoms. Patients with schizophrenia have bizarre delusions in contrast to those patients with delusional disorder who have more realistic delusional systems and who do not have hallucinations. Patients with personality disorders have some of the poor social relations, odd speech, and bizarre ideation, but they do not have delusions, hallucinations, or grossly disturbed behavior. The diagnosis of schizophreniform disorder is given when the patient shows the symptoms associated with schizophrenia, but the duration is less than six months. The diagnosis is changed to schizophrenia when the symptoms persist for more than six months.

12.4   The answer is E.

The most common form of hallucination in schizophrenia is auditory, although visual hallucinations are possible, as are gustatory and olfactory, although the latter are usually seen in combination. The type and frequency of hallucinations may vary as a function of culture. Hallucinations are generally experienced as originating in the environment rather than in the mind. Tactile hallucinations may be experienced in the body as feelings of internal organs being pulled apart. The hallucinations may be simple, for example a flash of light or undifferentiated noise, or they may be complex, as in voices that speak whole sentences.

12.5   The answer is C.

Schizophrenic individuals have generally shown increased mortality when compared to the general population. In early studies, this was probably due to poor nutrition or prolonged institutionalization. Now the greater mortality is probably due to suicide and accidents. Early studies seemed to indicate that schizophrenic individuals were relatively protected from cancer, epilepsy, diabetes, allergies, and myasthenia gravis, but these findings have been explained as methodological errors. There is evidence that schizophrenic patients are relatively protected from rheumatoid arthritis.

12.6   The answer is B.

As many as 10 percent of schizophrenic individuals commit suicide. However, schizophrenic patients acccount for only two to three percent of all suicides. The danger is that, unlike other suicide patients, schizophrenic patients do not communicate their intentions and usually choose a highly lethal method. The risk factors for suicide in schizophrenia include male sex, age less than 30 years, unemployment status, a chronic relapsing course of illness, higher levels of education, prior depression, current depression, and recent discharge from an inpatient setting.

12.7 The answer is **E**.

There have been no systematic studies conducted to investigate the efficacy of various treatments for delusional disorder. However, clinical experience indicates that certain approaches may be useful. A combination of psychosocial and physical measures may be the best approach. The greatest problem in treating patients with delusional disorder is that they are suspicious and tend to be difficult to bring in to a psychiatrist. Tact and clinical skill are necessary to induce a patient with delusional disorder to initiate treatment.

Hospitalization may be necessary when the risk of physical danger is present. In some cases, involuntary hospitalization may be needed to prevent harm to the patient or others. However, this course of action may fuel the persecutory delusions. A useful approach may be to convince the patient that the depressive symptoms or anxiety is in need of treatment. The psychiatrist should refrain from either agreeing with or disagreeing with the delusions. The patient should be assured of confidentiality. Insight-oriented therapy is not recommended, nor is group therapy.

12.8 The answer is **C**.

The diagnosis of delusional disorder requires that the patient exhibit nonbizarre delusions lasting at least one month and involving situations that occur in real life. In addition, behavior is not odd or bizarre aside from the behavior related to the delusional system. There should also be an absence of schizophrenic symptoms such as hallucinations or disorganized behavior and speech. The central feature is a well-systematized nonbizarre delusion, that is, a fixed false belief, in the presence of an otherwise clear sensorium. Level of premorbid functioning may be variable.

12.9 The answer is **C**.

Diagnosis of a schizophreniform disorder requires the presence of active psychotic symptoms not due to an organic mental disorder and the ruling out of a brief reactive psychosis. The symptoms cannot last longer than six months. If the symptoms persist past six months, even if only in a residual form, the diagnosis is changed to schizophrenia.

Unfortunately, there is not much empirical support for this diagnosis as a separate entity, although these patients may have some brain computed tomographic abnormalities similar to those found in schizophrenic patients. However, it appears that the schizophreniform disorder falls between affective and schizophrenic disorders.

12.10   The answer is **A**.

The delusional disorders may be only a small group of disorders, but they are an important group. There are various types of delusional subtypes, but they all share three features: the presence of a dominant, well-systematized, and encapsulated nonbizarre delusion; exhibition of affect appropriate to the delusion; and minimal personality distortion.

12.11   The answer is **C**.

There are two major findings in a recent review of outcome in schizophrenia. The first is the large difference between outcome following first admissions and subsequent admissions. The second is a general, slight improvement in outcome over the course of a century. A rough grouping of outcomes results in estimates of 83 percent poor outcome in the 1900s, 60 percent poor outcome in the 1930s, 43 percent poor outcome in the 1950s, and 26 percent poor outcome in the 1970s.

12.12   The answer is **A**.

Convulsive therapy was originally used in the treatment of schizophrenia because of a mistaken idea that epilepsy and schizophrenia were incompatible. Originally, convulsions were induced using metrazol or camphor. Later, electrically induced convulsions (ECT) were used. Still later, it was discovered that ECT was more effective in the treatment of affective disorders than for schizophrenia. The use of ECT was found to be more effective in treating chronic institutionalized schizophrenic patients than was either psychoanalytically oriented therapy or milieu therapy, but it was less effective than the use of antipsychotics. Currently, ECT is thought to be useful in treating schizophrenia when catatonia is present or when a depressive disorder is superimposed.

12.13   The answer is **E**.

The incidence and prevalence of delusional disorder have not been well studied. Kendler reviewed the available reports and provided some generalizations. The results indicate that the delusional disorder accounts for between one and four percent of psychiatric admissions. Delusional disorder manifests itself in mid to late adult life and is more common among females than among males. It is also more common in socially disadvantaged patients in economic and education terms. This disorder appears to be more common in immigrants. Between 60 and 70 percent of these patients are married, but as many as one-third of them may be widowed.

12.14   The answer is **B**.

The diagnosis of schizophrenia has undergone several transmutations. The *DSM-III* and *DSM-III-R* both concentrate on aspects of history and behavioral presentation in making this diagnosis. According to the *DSM-III-R*, the diagnosis of schizophrenia requires:

1. The presence of characteristic psychotic symptoms for a period of at least one week's duration
2. Deterioration in social and occupational functioning and self-care
3. Ruling out a major mood syndrome, or only a brief mood syndrome in comparison to the schizophrenic symptoms
4. Continuous signs of the disorder for at least six months
5. With a history of autistic disorder, there must currently be prominent hallucinations and delusions
6. Ruling out an organic mental disorder

12.15   The answer is **C**.

The United States–Great Britain Diagnostic Project attempted to investigate cross-cultural patterns in the diagnosis of schizophrenia and affective disorder. Schizophrenia is a more common diagnosis in New York than in London, and manic–depressive disorder is a more common diagnosis in London than in New York. This difference in diagnostic rates appeared to be related to differences in conceptual and theoretical systems rather than to differences in actual prevalence. Therefore, schizophrenia appeared to be a culture-bound diagnosis. The results of this study helped provide the impetus for developing a reliable diagnostic method and led to the application of structured interview techniques in diagnosing schizophrenia.

12.16   The answer is **B**.

In general, schizophrenia tends to manifest itself in young adulthood. However, there appear to be some different patterns in the age of onset. For example, the age of onset tends to be younger in men than in women. The age of onset in disorganized schizophrenia—that subtype of schizophrenia with marked incoherence and gross behavioral abnormalities—tends to be younger than in other subtypes.

12.17   The answer is **A**.

Andreasen and Olsen have divided the common schizophrenic symptoms into categories of positive and negative symptoms. Positive symptoms include hallucinations, delusions, formal thought disorder (marked incoherence, derailment, tangentiality, or illogicality), and bizarre or disorganized behavior. Negative symptoms include marked poverty of speech or poverty of content of speech, affective flattening, anhedonia, asociality, avolition–apathy, and attentional impairment.

12.18   The answer is **D.**
12.19   The answer is **C.**
12.20   The answer is **B.**
12.21   The answer is **A.**

There are various subtypes of schizophrenic disorders. Paranoid schizophrenia is characterized by preoccupation with one or more systematized delusions or frequent auditory hallucinations with a single theme in the absence of a florid thought disorder, flat or inappropriate affect, or bizarre behavior.

Disorganized schizophrenia refers to patients who exhibit incoherence, marked loosening of associations, grossly disorganized behavior, or grossly inappropriate affect. In addition, these patients do not meet the criteria for paranoid or catatonic schizophrenia. This subtype tends to appear at an earlier age than the other subtypes.

The motor symptoms of rigidity or bizarre posturing in catatonic schizophrenia can also appear in other disorders, including affective and organic mental disorders. Therefore, the differential diagnosis needs to be carefully conducted. Other symptoms of catatonic schizophrenia include purposeless excitement, negativism, and stupor or mutism.

Undifferentiated schizophrenia is the diagnosis given to schizophrenic patients who do not meet the criteria for the paranoid, catatonic, or disorganized subtypes. Residual schizophrenia refers to schizophrenic patients who no longer have prominent psychotic symptoms, but who still show signs of blunted affect, social withdrawal, loose associations, eccentric behavior, or other evidence of lingering illness.

Chapter 13

Mood Disorders

DIRECTIONS: Each of the statements or questions is followed by five suggested responses or completions. Select the one that is the best choice or most complete answer in each case.

13.1 Modern approaches to the diagnosis of depression began with:

- **A.** Freud
- **B.** Kraepelin
- **C.** Adler
- **D.** Jung
- **E.** Sullivan

13.2 The major risk factor for bipolar disorder is:

- **A.** a family history of the disorder
- **B.** a premorbidly high level of neuroticism
- **C.** stressful life events throughout the course of the illness
- **D.** low socioeconomic status
- **E.** none of the above

13.3 Which of the following is not true regarding the catecholamine hypothesis of depression?

A. Depression and mania are believed to be linked to deficits or excesses of norepinephrine, respectively.
B. Overall, the evidence suggests that 3-methoxy-4-hydroxyphenylglycol (MHPG) levels are lower in depressed patients compared with normals.
C. Major differences exist between cerebrospinal fluid (CSF) metabolites of dopamine in depressed and normal individuals.
D. Animal studies have demonstrated important feedback regulatory interactions between peripheral sympathetic and central aminergic systems.
E. There is evidence that low CSF gamma-aminobutyric acid (GABA) levels may be related to the depressed state.

13.4 Research on neurotransmitter and drug receptors in the brain have found that:

A. antidepressants decrease the number of postsynaptic beta-adrenergic receptors while enhancing the serotonergic and alpha-adrenergic stimulation
B. chronic lithium use increases beta-receptor density while down-regulating serotonin receptors
C. there is emerging evidence that platelet alpha-2 adrenoceptors may be sensitized in some depressed patients
D. this line of research has not been found to be useful
E. none of the above

13.5 Anatomical studies of major depression and mania have found:

A. a tendency for left-sided brain lesions to be associated with mania
B. no differences in the incidence of mania and depression in patients with different brain lesions
C. a tendency for posterior lesions to be strongly correlated with major depression
D. a positive correlation between the degree of depression in stroke patients and proximity of the lesion to the left frontal pole
E. none of the above

13.6   According to Beck's cognitive theory, depression results from:

- **A.**   a lack of social skills
- **B.**   early maternal deprivation
- **C.**   a lack of social supports
- **D.**   the activation of depressogenic schemata
- **E.**   learned helplessness

DIRECTIONS: For each of the statements below, one or more of the alternative answers is correct. Choose answer:

- A   if only 1, 2, and 3 are correct
- B   if only 1 and 3 are correct
- C   if only 2 and 4 are correct
- D   if only 4 is correct
- E   if all are correct

13.7   The distinction between unipolar and bipolar affective illness has been supported by:

1. the efficacy of lithium therapy in bipolar illness
2. the finding that unipolar illness is almost never found in bipolar patients
3. evidence from genetic and family studies
4. the finding that cyclic forms of unipolar illness typically have a later age of onset than bipolar illness

13.8   Which of the following are true regarding the concept of endogeneity?

1. The concept was originally formulated by Kraepelin.
2. The concept was developed to define affective disorders that arose from internal causes.
3. The concept was developed to describe symptoms that are very responsive to environmental stimuli.
4. The concept has been used to describe the emergence of depressive symptoms in individuals without neurotic premorbid personalities.

13.9   Major risk factors for suicide among depressed patients include:

1. a diagnosis of chronic depression or a depression severe enough to require hospitalization
2. a history of previous suicide attempts
3. a family history of suicide
4. a change in status from inpatient to outpatient

13.10 Which of the following are true regarding seasonal affective disorder?

    1. Epidemiological evidence suggests that attacks of mania are more frequent in summer than at other times of the year.
    2. Patients with this disorder are predominantly women with bipolar II illness.
    3. The incidence of depression is relatively more common in the late spring.
    4. Onset of the disorder is most common beyond the fourth decade of life.

13.11 Which of the following are sleep abnormalities that have been found to be prevalent in major depression?

    1. short latency in time from sleep onset to the onset of rapid eye movement (REM)
    2. more REM sleep during the later part of the night
    3. an overall reduction in sleep
    4. decreased REM density

13.12 According to Abraham's psychoanalytic theory of depression, depression results from:

    1. the early withdrawal of maternal support
    2. dependence on others to provide gratification
    3. emotional difficulties at the oral phase of psychosexual development
    4. fixation at the anal stage of psychosexual development

DIRECTIONS: Each of the following questions consists of lettered headings followed by a list of numbered alternatives. Select the single lettered heading that is most closely associated with the appropriate numbered alternative. Each lettered heading may be chosen only once.

Mood disorder

    A. Cyclothymia
    B. Mood-congruent psychotic depression
    C. Dysthymia
    D. Mood-incongruent psychotic depression

Description

13.13 is characterized by depressive stupor or delusions and/or hallucinations with themes of personal inadequacy, guilt, punishment, or nihilism

13.14 is characterized by at least a two-year history of continual or numerous periods of depressive symptoms characteristic of major depression that do not meet the criteria for major depression

13.15 is characterized by at least a two-year history of numerous periods of depression and hypomania that do not meet the criteria for major affective disorder

13.16 is characterized by evidence of delusions or hallucinations that are not consistent with depressed mood

ANSWERS

13.1 The answer is **B**.

Modern approaches to the diagnosis of depression began with Emil Kraepelin, the German psychiatrist who pioneered classification of the psychiatric disorders. Following a medical model, Kraepelin focused on both longitudinal history and the pattern of current symptoms. Kraepelin proposed that manic–depressive illness constituted a genetic spectrum of disorders, including what are now called bipolar disorder, recurrent major depression, cyclothymia, and dysthymia. Kraepelin further differentiated manic–depressive illness from dementia praecox because the group he called manic depressive shared episodic course, a relatively benign prognosis, and a family history of the disorder. Schizophrenia was characterized by a chronic, deteriorating course.

13.2 The answer is **B**.

The major risk factor for bipolar disorder is a family history of the disorder, with 60 to 65 percent of afflicted patients having a positive family history of either unipolar or bipolar disorder. Although few studies have investigated the role of psychological factors in this illness, evidence suggests that stressful life events are more frequent prior to the first or second episode, but not later episodes. Bipolar patients generally do not demonstrate personality deviations and are essentially normal in their degree of neuroticism and introversion.

13.3   The answer is **C**.

The most cohesive of the early amine hypotheses of depression has been the catecholamine hypothesis. This hypothesis was built on the premise that depression and mania were biochemically opposite states. Depression was viewed as being associated with a functional deficit of catecholamines, principally norepinephrine, at critical synapses in the central nervous system. Mania was associated with a functional excess of these amines. Evidence is emerging that low CSF GABA levels may be related to the depressed state within given individuals, but this indicator is not specific for depression because low levels of GABA have also been found in certain schizophrenic subgroups.

Clinical symptoms suggest involvement of the peripheral autonomic nervous system, and data from animal studies demonstrate feedback regulatory interactions between the peripheral sympathetic and the central aminergic system. Overall, the evidence suggests that MHPG levels are lower in depressed patients than in controls.

13.4   The answer is **A**.

Neurobiological research suggests that the chronic use of a wide variety of antidepressant medications including classical tricyclics, atypical antidepressants, monoamine oxidase inhibitors, and electroconvulsive therapy tend to down-regulate postsynaptic beta-adrenergic receptors while enhancing the response to serotonergic and alpha-adrenergic stimulation. Chronic lithium also decreases beta-receptor density while down-regulating serotonin receptors in some regions of the brain.

13.5   The answer is **D**.

Anatomical studies of major depression and mania have found that lesions located in the frontal or temporal lobes are most frequently associated with mania or depression. Although current data are sparse, there is a tendency for left-sided lesions to be associated with depressions and right-sided lesions to be associated with manias. In their study of stroke patients, Robinson and his co-workers have found a positive correlation between the degree of depression and the proximity of the lesion to the left frontal pole.

13.6 The answer is **D**.

According to Beck, depression results from the activation of specific cognitive distortions, which have been found to be present in depressed individuals. Beck called these distortions "depressogenic schemata"— the template for screening, coding, assimilating, and responding to internal and external stimuli that are derived from early experiences. In Beck's formulation of depression, schemata relate to experiences concerning self-evaluation and interpersonal relationships. Once they have been activated by some stressor, they lead to an unrealistically negative view of themselves, the world, and the future. Beck called the negative view of these three aspects of experience the "cognitive triad."

13.7 The answer is **B**.

The unipolar–bipolar distinction has been supported by evidence from both clinical trials (primarily the efficacy of lithium in treating bipolar disorder) and genetic and family studies. Bipolar disorder is much more prevalent in the relatives of bipolar patients than in the relatives of patients with other disorders. Therefore, this distinction serves as the basis for the classification of the affective disorders in the *Diagnostic and Statistical Manual of Mental Disorders (Third Edition-Revised) (DSM-III-R)*.

13.8 The answer is **C**.

The endogenous–reactive dichotomy is particularly important because of its etiologic and treatment implications. The concept of endogeneity was first used in 1929 by the English psychiatrist Robert D. Gillespie, who originally applied the term to disorders that arose from internal causes and were unresponsive to environmental stimuli. As its usage evolved, the endogenous concept took on further implications, including depressions occurring in the absence of precipitating stress; depressions occurring in older people with stable, nonneurotic premorbid personalities; depressions that are very severe; depressions with psychotic symptomatology; and depressions characterized by a particular symptom complex.

13.9 The answer is **E**.

Major risk factors for suicide among depressed patients include a) a diagnosis of chronic depression or a depression severe enough to have required hospitalization, b) a history of previous suicide attempts, c) a family history of suicide, and d) a change in status from inpatient to outpatient. In addition, as is the case in the general population, depressed individuals at highest risk for suicide are unemployed males who are unmarried or live alone.

13.10 The answer is **A**.

With regard to seasonal affective disorder, modern-day epidemiological evidence shows that attacks of mania are more frequent in summer than at other times of the year. The incidence of depression is relatively more common in the late spring. Patients are predominantly women with bipolar II illness. As with other forms of affective illness, onset most often occurs in the second or third decade of life, although a number of cases have also been reported in children.

13.11 The answer is **B**.

Several abnormalities of polygraphically monitored sleep have been reported in major depression. For instance, short-latency in time from sleep onset to onset of REM sleep, reduced slow-wave sleep, and increased frequency of rapid eye movements during sleep (increased REM density) have been found. In addition, a shift in the temporal distribution of REM sleep so that more occurs in the early part of the night (shorter REM latency and longer first REM periods), and reduction of sleep with longer latency sleep onset, have been found.

13.12 The answer is **A**.

According to Abraham's psychoanalytic theory of depression, vulnerability to depression arose from emotional difficulties during the oral phase of psychosexual development. These difficulties generally took the form of withdrawal of early maternal support and love, resulting in a fixation of emotional development at the oral stage. As a consequence, a dependency on sources of oral gratification and on others to supply emotional gratification characterize the depression-prone individual. Abraham further proposed that depression in adulthood ensues when the vulnerable individual is faced with actual, perceived, or threatened loss.

13.13 The answer is **B**.
13.14 The answer is **C**.
13.15 The answer is **A**.
13.16 The answer is **D**.

In mood-congruent psychotic depression, the patient displays depressive stupor or delusions and/or hallucinations with mood-congruent content (that is, themes of personal inadequacy, guilt, punishment, and nihilism).

To obtain a *DSM-III-R* diagnosis of dysthymia, the patient must have at least a two-year history of continual or numerous periods of depressive symptoms characteristic of major depression that do not meet full severity and/or duration criteria for the syndrome.

By definition, dysthymia is a chronic condition. The typical age of onset varies from early teen years to late life. Dysthymic patients are at high risk of developing major depressive episodes as well as other psychiatric disorders.

To meet *DSM-III-R* criteria for cyclothymia, the patient must have at least a two-year history of episodes of hypomania and depression that do not meet criteria of major affective disorders. Depressed periods are typically characterized by depressed mood and by loss of interest, whereas hypomanic periods are characterized by periods of elevated, expansive, or irritable mood. Cyclothymia is typically characterized by brief (two to six days), alternating periods of elation and depression.

To receive a diagnosis of psychotic depression with mood-incongruent features, a patient must manifest delusions and/or hallucinations that are not consistent with depressed mood. For example, this may include delusions of persecution or control, thought broadcasting, or thought insertion.

Chapter 14

Anxiety Disorders

DIRECTIONS: Each of the statements or questions is followed by five suggested responses or completions. Select the one that is the best choice or most complete answer in each case.

14.1 Anxiety is a symptom common to several psychiatric disorders. Patients with panic attacks have characteristics that separate them from the anxiety disorders. These characteristics do not include:

    A. chronic feelings of uneasiness
    B. response to sodium lactate infusion
    C. familial aggregation
    D. development of agoraphobia
    E. response to antidepressants

14.2 Which of the following is not a condition under which a first panic attack is likely to occur?

    A. the context of a life-threatening situation
    B. the loss of a close interpersonal relationship
    C. separation from family
    D. during a period of relaxation following strenuous exercise
    E. while under the influence of mind-altering drugs

14.3 Panic attacks usually last:

    A. Less than 30 seconds
    B. Between one and three minutes
    C. Between 5 and 20 minutes
    D. Between 10 and 15 minutes
    E. Between 20 and 30 minutes

14.4 Which of the following is not a symptom category of generalized anxiety disorder?

    A. motor tension
    B. brief periods of shortness of breath
    C. autonomic hyperactivity
    D. apprehensive expectation
    E. vigilance and scanning

14.5 Which of the following has not been proposed as a biological theory of panic disorder?

    A. increased catecholamine levels
    B. overactivity of the locus coeruleus
    C. carbon dioxide hypersensitivity
    D. lactate panicogenic metabolism
    E. decreased dopamine levels

14.6 Which of the following statements regarding the psychoanalytic theories of anxiety disorders is not true?

    A. Adult panic attacks may have their origin in separation anxiety.
    B. Anxiety is the experience when repressed impulses break through into consciousness in distorted form.
    C. The effectiveness of analysis in treating anxiety disorders is consistent with the theoretical formulation.
    D. Anxiety may be a signal that the ego is in a dangerous situation.
    E. There is a biological predisposition to anxiety disorders.

14.7 Which of the following is not a usual differential made in the diagnosis of social phobia?

    A. paranoia
    B. avoidant personality disorder
    C. agoraphobia
    D. inadequate personality
    E. depression

14.8   Which of the following is not a significant subgroup of the obsessive-compulsive disorder?

- **A.**   excessive concern with dirt and contamination
- **B.**   pathological counting and checking
- **C.**   purely excessive, ego dystonic rumination
- **D.**   excessive slowness of activity
- **E.**   excessive fears about financial concerns

14.9   Predictions of favorable outcome in the treatment of obsessive-compulsive disorders do not include:

- **A.**   early age of onset
- **B.**   absence of compulsions
- **C.**   good premorbid adjustment
- **D.**   mild or atypical symptom pattern
- **E.**   short duration of symptoms

14.10   Which of the following is not a symptom associated with post-traumatic stress disorder?

- **A.**   guilt feelings about survival
- **B.**   prolonged episodes of intense affect
- **C.**   rapid habituation to stimuli
- **D.**   reexperience of the traumatic event in painful memories
- **E.**   psychic numbing

DIRECTIONS: For each of the statements or questions below, one or more of the alternative answers is correct. Choose answer

- **A**   if only 1, 2, and 3 are correct
- **B**   if only 1 and 3 are correct
- **C**   if only 2 and 4 are correct
- **D**   if only 4 is correct
- **E**   if all are correct

14.11   The diagnosis of panic disorder is made when which of the following conditions is (are) met?

1. A patient experiences at least four panic attacks in a four-week period that are discrete and spontaneous.
2. A patient experiences at least two panic attacks in a four-week period that are discrete and spontaneous.
3. A patient experiences one attack followed by a month of persistent anticipatory anxiety.
4. A patient experiences one panic attack followed by two weeks of persistent anticipatory anxiety.

14.12   The diagnosis of generalized anxiety disorder is made when:

1. a patient experiences at least six months of chronic anxiety or worry
2. at least six physical symptoms including sybtypes of motor tension, autonomic hyperactivity, and vigilance and scanning are present
3. the symptoms are not secondary to another disorder
4. the quality of the anxiety is difficult to describe or is free floating

14.13   Depression and anxiety disorders share many symptoms. Which of the following statements are useful in the differential between these two disorders?

1. Anxious patients have trouble falling asleep, whereas depressed people show early morning awakenings.
2. Diurnal mood fluctuation is uncommon in anxiety disorders.
3. Depressed patients show disturbances in appetite whereas anxious patients do not.
4. Depressed patients show disturbances in concentration.

14.14   Which of the following are not medical disorders that can mimic the anxiety disorders?

1. hyperthyroidism
2. Crohn's disease (irritable bowel disorder)
3. hypothyroidism
4. essential hypertension

14.15   Which of the following medications has (have) not been found to be useful in the treatment of panic disorder?

1. imipramine
2. alprazolam
3. desipramine
4. propranolol

14.16   Behavioral treatment of panic disorder involves which components?

1. breathing retraining to eliminate hyperventilation
2. relaxation
3. cognitive restructuring
4. systematic desensitization

14.17   Phobic disorder consists of which subtypes?

1. agoraphobia
2. social phobia
3. simple phobia
4. separation phobia

14.18   Most studies involving the pharmacological treatment of post-traumatic stress disorder indicate the effectiveness of:

1. diazepam
2. neuroleptics
3. lithium
4. antidepressants

14.19   Important considerations in the differential diagnosis of obsessive-compulsive disorder include:

1. generalized anxiety disorders
2. schizophrenia
3. mania
4. phobic disorders

14.20   Which of the following phenomena have been implicated in the etiology of obsessive-compulsive disorder?

1. first appearance during adolesence or early adulthood
2. first appearance precipitated by unusual stressor
3. an association with encephalitis
4. an association with head injury

ANSWERS

14.1   The answer is **A**.

Anxiety is a symptom that is associated both with aspects of normal functioning and with many different psychiatric disorders. A chronic anxiety condition is characterized by chronic tension, excessive worry, frequent headaches, or recurrent anxiety attacks.

Panic attacks are qualitatively different from the chronic anxiety conditions. Panic disorders are different in that the patients who suffer from these conditions will experience a panic attack in response to sodium lactate infusions. These patients also show familial aggregation and tend to develop agoraphobia. In addition, unlike patients who suffer from chronic anxiety states, patients with panic disorders tend to respond favorably to treatment with antidepressant medications. Panic attacks may first occur without a history of developed fear reactions.

14.2   The answer is **D**.

The first panic attack to strike a patient may occur during any routine activity. However, there appear to be a few conditions that frequently are associated with the first appearance of a panic attack. These conditions include a life-threatening illness or accident, the loss of a close interpersonal relationship, or separation from family.

The first panic attacks may occur in the early stages of developing either hypothyroidism or hyperthyroidism. Panic attacks may also first occur during the immediate postpartum period. Many patients state that their first panic attack occurred while under the influence of mind-altering drugs, including LSD, marijuana, sedatives, cocaine, or sympathomimetic drugs such as amphetamines.

14.3   The answer is **C**.

Panic attacks may occur during a period of routine activity. Suddenly the patient will experience a sense of impending doom, overwhelming terror, or apprehension. Associated physical symptoms include heart palpitations, dyspnea, chest tightening or pain, choking or smothering sensations, dizziness, or feelings of unsteadiness. There may be feelings of derealization or depersonalization, paresthesia, hot and cold flashes, sweating, faintness, trembling and shaking, and a fear of dying, going crazy, or losing control.

It is rare for an attack to last as long as an hour. Most panic attacks last between 5 and 20 mintues. However, attacks may subside and recur in waves. Other patients report feeling agitated and fatigued for several hours following the attack. Other patients who report long-lasting panic attacks may actually be suffering from some other psychopathological condition such as agitated depression or obsessional tension states.

14.4   The answer is **B**.

Anxiety disorders other than panic disorder are usually diagnosed as generalized anxiety disorder. The *Diagnostic and Statistical Manual of Mental Disorders (Third Edition-Revised) (DSM-III-R)* lists several characteristics of the generalized anxiety disorder. These include unrealistic or excessive worry and anxiety about two or more life situations. If another *DSM-III-R* Axis I diagnosis is present, the excessive worry and anxiety must be unrelated to the diagnosis. The disturbance cannot occur as part of a mood disorder or psychotic disorder. At least 6 of 18 symptoms must be present. These symptoms are divided into the categories of motor tension (trembling, muscle tension, restlessness, or easy fatigability), autonomic hyperactivity (shortness of breath, palpitations, sweating or cold clammy hands, dry mouth, dizziness or light headedness, nausea or other abdominal distress, hot flashes or chills, difficulty swallowing or lump in the throat), vigilance and scanning (feeling on edge, exaggerated startle response, difficulty in concentration, trouble in falling or staying asleep, or irritability). There cannot be an organic factor responsible for the symptoms. Therefore, it can be seen that the symptoms of generalized anxiety disorder can be grouped into four categories: motor tension, autonomic hyperactivity, apprehensive expectation, and vigilance and scanning.

14.5   The answer is **E**.

Panic disorder has been the subject of several different biological theorizations as has, to a lesser extent, the generalized anxiety disorder. One of the theories is that of increases in catecholamines, especially epinephrine. There are increased levels of catecholamines in the urine of patients with anxiety reactions and increases in the plasma levels of catecholamines of normal subjects exposed to stress. The beta-adrenergic theory is supported by the effectiveness of beta-blockers such as propranolol that tend to have a favorable impact on panic attacks. However, it is not clear whether administration of catecholamines can induce anxiety attacks.

Another biological theory involves the locus coeruleus. More than 50 percent of the noradrenergic fibers in the central nervous system are contained in the locus coeruleus. Electrical stimulation of the locus coeruleus can cause fear reactions in animals. Drugs that lower the firing of the locus coeruleus tend to inhibit anxiety reactions in humans. However, other experimental work indicates that the locus coeruleus is more highly associated with our response to novel stimuli rather than with anxiety.

Carbon dioxide sensitivity is yet another biological theory of panic disorder. Exposing panic disorder patients to a mixture of 5 percent carbon dioxide will precipitate a panic attack. Sodium lactate infusion will also cause panic attacks in many patients with this disorder, lending support to the lactate panicogenic theories. Finally, the genetic studies of panic disorder that indicate a higher prevalence in families of probands than in normal populations and the twin studies lend support to the biological theories.

14.6   The answer is C.

Psychoanalytic theory has offered many etiological conceptualizations of anxiety disorders and of the experience of anxiety. One of the aspects of this theory invokes castration anxiety. Other aspects relate adult anxiety to the separation anxiety experienced by children. Aside from the speculative theoretical conceptualizations, there is some empirical evidence that the same drugs that block panic attacks in adults may be effective in treating separation anxiety in children.

Freud also considered anxiety as a manifestation of incomplete or failed repression. When the repressed ideas become suffused with energy, they may break through to consciousness in a distorted form and be experienced as anxiety. Other psychoanalytic conceptualizations view anxiety as a sign that the ego is in a dangerous situation. Freud thought that there may be a biological predisposition to anxiety. A major caveat mitigating the validity of psychoanalytic conceptualizations is the failure of analytic methods to effectively treat anxiety or panic attacks.

14.7   The answer is D.

Social phobia is a persistent fear that one or more social situations resulting in scrutiny by others will result in humiliation for the patient. The fear of social situations is common to many different psychiatric disorders, and a careful differential diagnosis is necessary. For example, paranoid patients will avoid social situations, but this is because they fear that someone will do something untoward to them rather than that they themselves will do something embarrassing. Avoidant personality disorder patients will avoid social situations because of the fear that they will humiliate themselves, and these patients are difficult to differentiate from the social phobic patients.

Agoraphobic patients will avoid social situations, but this is because they fear that they will lose control and panic, thereby embarrassing themselves. Social withdrawal will occur in depression, but this is due to a lack of effort or motivation rather than to an actual fear of the social situation.

14.8   The answer is **E**.

The obsessive-compulsive disorders have as their essential feature the presence of recurrent and persistent troublesome thought patterns or the performance of idiosyncratic ritualistic behaviors or compulsions. There are several different subtypes of obsessive-compulsive disorders. One subtype involves patients who cannot bring themselves to throw anything away and who therefore tend to hoard even useless materials. Another group of patients have obsessions regarding dirt and contamination and spend much of their time washing and trying to avoid contact with (imagined) contaminated materials. Another group of patients spend much time obsessively counting and checking things. Yet another group exhibits obsessional thought patterns without exhibiting compulsive behavior. Finally, one group of patients with primary obsessional slowness spend many hours just performing everyday activities such as eating a single meal.

14.9   The answer is **A**.

The untreated course of obsessive-compulsive disorders reveals that between 24 and 33 percent of the patients show a fluctuating course. Between 11 and 14 percent will exhibit periodic remissions, and between 54 and 61 percent will have a constant or progressive course. In the past the prognosis of obsessive-compulsive disorders has been considered to be poor. Recent advances in the pharmacological and behavioral treatment of this disorder give new hope to patients with the disorder.

Prediction of favorable outcome in this disorder includes the presence of mild or atypical symptoms or a short duration of symptoms. Good premorbid adjustment and the absence of compulsions are also associated with a good prognosis. An early age of onset is associated with a poor prognosis.

14.10   The answer is **C**.

A post-traumatic stress disorder is thought to be associated with the experience of an event outside the usual range of human experience. This event is one that would be extremely distressing to almost anyone and includes witnessing the death or physical harm of another individual or the sudden destruction of one's home or community. The traumatic event is persistently reexperienced in distressing and intrusive memories, dreams, or flashbacks. There is a persistent avoidance of stimuli associated with the event or numbing of affective experience and a feeling of estrangement from others. There is also hypervigilance and an exaggerated startle response. Such individuals often experience guilt over having survived when others have perished. There are frequently episodes of extreme anger or increased irritability.

14.11   The answer is **B**.

Generally speaking, the diagnosis of panic disorder is made when a patient experiences at least four discrete, spontaneous panic attacks in a four-week period or one panic attack that is followed by a period of four weeks of persistent anticipatory anxiety. The diagnosis is made when an organic factor cannot be established as having initiated and maintained the panic attack. The panic attacks usually last for minutes or, more rarely, for a few hours. Initially the attacks are unexpected and do not occur immediately before or following exposure to a situation that usually causes anxiety. The attacks also cannot occur when the person is the focus of other people's attention. Later in the course of the illness, certain situations can become associated with having a panic attack. The attacks begin with a sense of impending doom. Sometimes the person does not experience the attacks as anxiety, but only as extreme discomfort. The average age at onset is in the late 20s.

14.12   The answer is **A**.

Generalized anxiety disorder is a residual category of anxious experience. This diagnosis is made when a patient has had at least six months of chronic anxiety or worry. In order for this diagnosis to be made, there must be present at least six symptoms from the general categories of motor tension, autonomic hyperactivity, and vigilance and scanning. The symptoms cannot be attributable to another disorder or to an organic factor. The characteristic feature of generalized anxiety disorder is unrealistic or excessive worry about two or more circumstances. Although there is some fluctuation possible in the level of tension, the patient is more often concerned about the circumstances than not, lasting for the entire period of the disorder. The diagnosis of generalized anxiety disorder is not given if the worry is about the symptoms of another disorder. However, the diagnosis can be given when another *DSM-III-R* Axis I diagnosis is present if the worry is not related to the other disorder.

14.13   The answer is **E**.

Individuals who are depressed can also show signs of anxiety. However, there are a few points of distinction that can be useful in making the differential diagnosis between the two disorders. Patients with a depressive disorder will show the vegetative signs of depression such as loss of appetite and early morning awakenings that are not present in anxiety disorders. Instead, anxiety disordered individuals have trouble initiating sleep. Diurnal mood fluctuations are common in depression but not in anxiety disorders. Anxious patients do not exhibit a decreased ability to enjoy things or to be cheered up. Finally, depressed individuals show a fairly consistent disturbance of concentration.

14.14   The answer is B.

Several organic medical disorders can mimic the symptoms of anxiety disorders. Hyperthyroidism and hypothyroidism can both result in feelings of anxiety, but these two medical disorders do not present with the other signs associated with the anxiety disorders. However, because of the similarity in affect, thyroid tests are necessary in all patients who complain of anxiety. Thyroid disorders can serve as the precipitant of panic attacks, and the panic attacks may outlast the thyroid disorder after it is successfully treated.

Hyperparathyroidism may also result in anxiety symptoms. It is therefore important to evaluate serum calcium levels in making a correct diagnosis. Other medical disorders mimicking anxiety disorders include pheochromocytoma and diseases of the vestibular nerve.

14.15   The answer is D.

Treatment of panic disorders relies on the use of pharmacological agents to block the occurrence of the panic attacks. There are several chemical agents that have been shown to be effective in reaching this goal. The most commonly used drugs for this purpose are the tricyclic antidepressants, usually imipramine, desipramine, and clomipramine. There have been no systematic studies of some of the other antidepressants, including nortriptyline and amitriptyline. Although monoamine oxidase inhibitors are effective in the treatment of panic disorders, they are usually reserved for those patients who do not respond to the tricyclics. Antidepressants can block the panic attacks but are not effective in treating the intervening anticipatory anxiety, for which a short course of benzodiazepines may be necessary.

The high-potency benzodiazepine alprazolam has also been used in the treatment of panic attacks. Furthermore, clonazepine appears to be promising in this regard. However, a drawback in the use of these drugs is the risk of withdrawal effects occurring during the tapering period. Beta-adrenergic drugs such as propranolol have been promoted by some as effective, but there are few scientific data to substantiate these claims. Clonidine has been found to be effective in the short run, but it appears to lose its effectiveness in a matter of weeks.

14.16   The answer is A.

Behavioral treatments have been very effective in treating phobic disorders, but have only recently been investigated in panic disorders. The components of a behavioral approach to panic disorders include retraining breathing patterns to eliminate hyperventilation, relaxation training, and cognitive restructuring to give a more benign interpretation to the symptoms. The patient is taught to change his or her cognitions from "My heart is racing; I'm having a heart attack" to "My heart is racing again, but this is a symptom of my panic disorder." Systematic desensitization is generally not used for this disorder.

14.17   The answer is A.

Phobic disorder is divided into three subcategories. The first subtype is agoraphobia. Agoraphobia may occur with or without panic attacks. In agoraphobia, there are three main themes: fear of leaving home, fear of being alone, and fear of being away from home in an inescapable situation or a situation where help cannot be obtained. Agoraphobic individuals fear using public transportation, being in crowds, or traveling a distance from home. Sometimes there is a trusted companion with whom the patient feels safe in traveling.

The second subtype of phobic disorder is social phobia. Here the patient fears being in a social situation and acting in such a way that would humiliate or embarrass her- or himself. These patients avoid social situations and situations where they would face the judgment of others. Common fears include those of public speaking, eating or writing, or using public lavatories.

The third category of phobic disorder is the simple phobia in which the patient fears specific objects, situations, or activities. There are three components to a simple phobia. One, there is an anticipatory anxiety brought on by the possibility of confronting the phobic object. Two, there is the central fear itself. Three, there is the avoidance behavior that the patient exhibits in order to minimize his or her anxiety.

14.18   The answer is D.

Although there have been no reports of controlled studies investigating the effectiveness of various pharmacological agents in the treatment of post-traumatic stress disorder (PTSD), there have been several reports of case studies and open clinical trials. One such report of open clinical trials reported that the use of beta-blockers (propranolol) was effective in reducing the symptoms of PTSD by self-report over a six-month period. A pilot study using clonidine also reported favorable effects.

Despite these initial reports of the effectiveness of adrenergic blocking agents, most of the reports involve the use of antidepressants. One report involved the use of imipramine and found it to be useful in reducing the symptoms of PTSD, a finding replicated in an independent case report. A retrospective study reported that a variety of antidepressants were effective in two-thirds of the cases examined. Phenelzine has also been reported to be moderately effective: however, a double-blind crossover study indicated that phenelzine may be no more effective than placebo. The use of neuroleptics and benzodiazepines in treating some of the specific symptoms of PTSD has been reported, but there has been no evidence of their efficacy in treating PTSD.

14.19   The answer is **C**.

The course of obsessive-compulsive disorder may resemble that of the psychotic disorders more than the neurotic disorders, but there are important considerations that can differentiate obsessive-compulsive disorder from other psychiatric disorders. For example, obsessions may resemble the delusions of thought disorders; however, closer evaluation indicates that whereas obsessions are resisted by the patient, the delusions are accepted and integrated into the patient's cognitive belief system. It is possible for both disorders to co-exist in the same patient.

Patients with obsessive-compulsive disorder may also have complicating depressions, and depressed patients may have complicating obsessions. However, obsessional patients tend to develop agitated depressions rather than retarded depressions. Both phobic patients and obsessive patients will exhibit avoidant behavior. One point of distinction is that phobic patients can usually manage to entirely avoid the phobic situation, but obsessive patients cannot avoid their obsessions.

14.20   The answer is **B**.

The usual age at onset for obsessive-compulsive disorders is in adolescence or early adulthood; however, it is possible for some cases to begin earlier than that. Usually, no precipitating event or stressor can be identified, and the disorder has an insidious onset. The course is often chronic and progressive. In those cases where patients report an abrupt onset, there may be a neurological etiology present. For example, obsessive-compulsive disorder has been reported following abnormal birth events, head injury, and encephalitis.

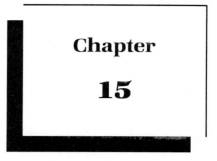

Chapter

15

Psychosomatic Disorders

DIRECTIONS: Each of the statements or questions is followed by five suggested responses or completions. Select the one that is the best choice or most complete answer in each case.

15.1 Who originally coined the classification coronary prone personality?

    A. Sigmund Freud
    B. Franz Alexander
    C. Flanders Dunbar
    D. Hans Selye
    E. Friedman and Rosenman

15.2 What percentage of patients who experience panic attacks have mitral valve prolapse?

    A. 20 percent
    B. 35 percent
    C. 50 percent
    D. 65 percent
    E. 80 percent

15.3 Which of the following psychological characteristics has not been associated with hypertension?

    A. depression
    B. confronting emotional conflicts
    C. angry coping style
    D. sadness
    E. anxiety

15.4 Which of the following immune functions are T-lymphocytes (T-cells) not primarily involved with?

    A. cancer cell surveillance
    B. delayed cutaneous hypersensitivity
    C. infectious agent control
    D. rejection of transplanted organ
    E. production of immunoglobulins

15.5 The individual who first postulated a general adaptation syndrome in response to stress is:

    A. Franz Alexander
    B. Hans Selye
    C. Flanders Dunbar
    D. George Engel
    E. William Osler

DIRECTIONS: For each of the statements below, one or more of the alternative answers is correct. Choose answer:

    A if only 1, 2, and 3 are correct
    B if only 1 and 3 are correct
    C if only 2 and 4 are correct
    D if only 4 is correct
    E if all are correct

15.6 Which of the following are traits that are most strongly correlated with coronary artery disease risks and mortality?

    1. competitiveness
    2. anger
    3. time pressure
    4. hostility

15.7   Hyperventilation is associated with which of the following?

    1. decreased serum CO_2
    2. focal neurological symptoms
    3. tetany
    4. increased sodium bicarbonate

15.8   Which of the following are associated with extrinsic asthma?

    1. a family history of allergy
    2. IgA antibodies
    3. triggered by allergens
    4. decreased vagal activity

15.9   Which of the following statements are true regarding patients with irritable bowel syndrome?

    1. Their slow-wave colonic activity decreases in response to stress.
    2. They generally have higher colonic motor activity.
    3. Colonic inflammation is associated with their diarrhea.
    4. Colonic hypermotility is seldom associated with pain.

15.10   Which of the following statements are true regarding the use of analgesic pain medications for the treatment of chronic pain?

    1. Analgesics tend to be underprescribed for biomedically caused chronic pain.
    2. Analgesics should be prescribed on a set schedule.
    3. The response to placebo medication is not useful in differentiating psychogenic from biomedical pain.
    4. Several nonsteroidal anti-inflammatory drugs increase the clearnace of lithium.

15.11   Factors that must be present simultaneously for a person to develop a psychosomatic disorder are:

    1. a biological predisposition to the biomedical disorder
    2. personality vulnerability
    3. a significant psychosocial stressor
    4. a specific family history of the biomedical disorder

15.12   The following factors have been positively correlated with basal, fasting serum gastrin levels in duodenal ulcer patients:

1. independence
2. achievement orientation
3. expressiveness
4. level of extroversion

15.13   Behavioral treatment of chronic pain conditions often involves:

1. the use of biofeedback and relaxation training
2. exposing neurotic conflicts that may underlie the condition
3. the reward of healthy, non-pain-related behaviors
4. the use of Gestalt therapy

DIRECTIONS: Each of the following questions consists of lettered headings followed by a list of numbered alternatives. Select the single lettered heading that is most closely associated with the appropriate numbered alternative. Each lettered heading may be chosen only once.

Psychosomatic disorder

A.   coronary heart disease
B.   rheumatoid arthritis
C.   asthma
D.   mitral valve prolapse
E.   peptic ulcer disease

Description

15.14   The primary physician should ensure that hypertension and hyperlipidemia are well controlled. Behavioral modification and stress monitoring may help decrease behavior traits associated with this disorder.

15.15   A selective beta-1 blocker such as atenolol is recommended. The anticholinergic side effects of some antidepressants may also be useful in the treatment of this disorder.

15.16   The use of histamine-2 blocking agents such as cimetidine may be useful in treating this disorder. In addition, antidepressants may be useful because of their histamine-blocking action.

15.17   Acute pain in this disorder is almost always accompanied by anxiety and therefore anxiolytics may be useful. Hypnosis or acupuncture may reduce anxiety in some patients.

15.18   Beta-blockers such as propranolol are sometimes used to block the peripheral manifestations of anxiety. Antidepressant medications may also be useful.

ANSWERS

15.1 The answer is **C**.

In her 1954 book *Emotions and Bodily Changes,* Flanders Dunbar described personality types that correlated with a number of medical illnesses. One such classification was "coronary prone personality."

15.2 The answer is **A**.

Recently, mitral valve prolapse (MVP) has been recognized as a cause of anxiety and panic symptoms. However, the exact connection between MVP and anxiety symptoms such as palpitations, dizziness, and weakness is not fully understood. Approximately 20 percent of patients who suffer from panic attacks suffer from MVP. MVP is usually benign but may result in arrhythmias and even in death. For this reasons, many individuals who are diagnosed as having MVP develop anxiety as well as symptoms of depression.

15.3 The answer is **B**.

A habitually angry coping style, including chronic suppressed anger, is a significant risk factor for essential hypertension. More specifically, there may be a tendency toward avoidance of emotional conflict in families with a hypertensive member. Acute depression has been found to cause arrhythmias and heart rate and blood pressure to increase at a rate comparable to changes seen with anxiety or anger. Sadness may cause blood pressure to be as high at rest as when exercising and may interfere with cardiovascular adjustments normally associated with exercise.

15.4 The answer is **E**.

The cellular immune system, of which T-cells are a component, protects against infectious agents; conducts surveillance within the body to control abnormal cells, probably including cancer cells; and controls delayed cutaneous hypersensitivity. T-cells must be suppressed to prevent rejection of transplanted tissues. The B-cells are responsible for the production of the circulating immunoglobulins, principally IgA, IgE, IgG, and IgM.

15.5 The answer is **B**.

In the 1960s and 1970s, Hans Selye postulated a general adaptation syndrome in response to stress. Selye stated that individuals experience a three-phase, sequential response to stress that includes an alarm response, sustained activation, and exhaustion if relief from the stress does not occur. Stress causes physiologic changes through both sympathetic and parasympathetic aspects of the autonomic nervous system. Selye also postulated that stress may lead to changes in hypothalamic–pituitary–adrenal cortical axis functioning.

15.6   The answer is C.

Certain character traits have been found to be associated with coronary heart disease, leading to the formulation of the "type A personality" as a descriptive diagnosis. Type A behaviors and attitudes include excessive consciousness of time deadlines, drive, ambition, competitiveness, aggressiveness, impatience, and hostility. This personality style leads to sustained stress and interpersonal difficulties and, through physiologic avenues, to coronary heart disease and myocardial infarction.

15.7   The answer is A.

Hyperventilation symptoms are often diverse and may mimic symptoms of many other disorders. Perioral tingling and "pins and needles" in the fingers and toes, or focal neurologic symptoms may develop. Carpopedal spasm and tetany may develop. The individual may become lightheaded and faint. Bizarre depersonalization or derealization may also occur. Emotional swings and inappropriate laughter may also be seen. The patient not being able to "catch his breath" as well as anxiety or tremulousness may also occur. A useful differential diagnostic strategy may be to have the patient hyperventilate in the physician's presence. If the symptoms are reproduced in this manner, this is strongly supportive of hyperventilation syndrome.

15.8   The answer is B.

Extrinsic asthma symptoms may be triggered by a wide variety of stimuli such as cold air, allergens, infections, and emotions. Extrinsic asthma has also been found to occur more in families that have strong allergic histories. Many patients with extrinsic asthma also form IgE antibodies.

15.9   The answer is C.

No specific pathological changes occur as a result of irritable bowel syndrome. There is no inflammation of the colon associated with diarrhea or constipation. The latter two conditions appear to be associated with changes in bowel motility. Patients with irritable bowel syndrome have higher colon motor activity than normals, and their slow-wave colonic activity increases in response to stress, whereas it decreases in controls. Patients with diarrhea who have hypomotility seldom complain of abdominal pain, whereas those who have accompanying pain usually have segments of hypermotility.

15.10   The answer is A.

Many analgesics are useful in decreasing pain. However, placebos decrease pain in at least one-third of individuals who are experiencing organically based pain. Therefore, response to placebo cannot be used to differentiate biomedical from psychogenic pain. If a biomedical disorder is underlying the pain, adequate analgesia should be assured. Some physicians underuse analgesia in treating pain disorders. This is probably due to an overestimation of the strength and half-lives of the drugs or to fears of addiction. To separate the association of increased perception of pain from receiving needed relief, analgesics should be given on a routine rather than as-needed basis.

15.11   The answer is A.

Three factors must be present simultaneously for a person to develop a psychosomatic disorder. First, the individual must have a biological predisposition to the particular disorder. This may be genetically determined, be secondary to trauma, or be due to environmental insults or damaging personal habits. Second, the individual must have a personality vulnerability. In other words, there must be a type or degree of stress that the individual's psychological defense mechanisms and personality structure cannot manage. Third, the individual must experience a significant psychosocial stress in his or her personality area.

15.12   The answer is A.

Duodenal ulcer disease tends to be responsive to emotional stimuli. Three psychological attributes have been positively correlated with basal, fasting serum gastrin levels in patients with this condition. These attributes are independence, achievement orientation, and expressiveness.

15.13   The answer is B.

Several behaviorally oriented approaches have been found to be useful in the treatment of chronic pain syndromes. Techniques such as biofeedback, relaxation training, and hypnosis may decrease the threshold for pain perception in some individuals. In addition, rewarding healthy, non-pain-related behaviors is also often helpful. Decreasing the secondary gain that the individual receives from the pain may also short-circuit escalation of the chronic pain cycle.

15.14 The answer is **A**.
15.15 The answer is **C**.
15.16 The answer is **E**.
15.17 The answer is **B**.
15.18 The answer is **D**.

A number of pharmacologic approaches may help reduce some of the risk factors of coronary heart disease. A primary physician should ensure that hypertension and hyperlipidemia are well controlled. Also, nicotine gum and other smoking cessation approaches should be vigorously recommended. Weight loss and appropriate exercise programs may also be helpful. A number of psychotherapy, behavior modification, and stress monitoring approaches may help decrease Type A traits, and there is evidence that these forms of treatment may be useful in coronary heart disease symptomatology as well as in preventing recurrent cardiac events.

Asthma may respond to treatment with several types of medications. A selective beta-1 blocker, such as atenolol, is recommended for asthmatic individuals or for other pulmonary patients for whom a beta-blocker may be indicated. Propranolol is both a beta-1 and beta-2 blocker and if beta-2 receptors are blocked, the ability to bronchodilate may be lost.

A major pharmacologic advance in the treatment of ulcer has been the development of histamine-2 blocking agents, such as cimetidine and ranitidine. In addition, controlled trials of some psychotropic medications, including antidepressants (due to their histamine-blocking effects) have also been shown to have healing effects on ulcer disease.

Many patients with early rheumatoid arthritis will demonstrate spontaneous improvement with little or no medication. Acute pain is almost always accompanied by anxiety, and on a short-term basis if the anxiety is marked, it may be lessened with anxiolytics, reducing the distress associated with the acute pain. Hypnosis or acupuncture may reduce anxiety in some patients.

Beta-blockers, such as propranolol or atenolol are sometimes useful in the treatment of mitral valve prolapse; propranolol may also block the peripheral manifestations of anxiety.

Chapter 16

Somatoform Disorders, Factitious Disorders, and Malingering

DIRECTIONS: Each of the statements or questions is followed by five suggested responses or completions. Select the one that is the best choice or most complete answer in each case.

16.1 Patterns of somatization are:

    A. usually related to autonomic nervous system function
    B. usually related to voluntary nervous system function
    C. usually related to cardiac function
    D. diverse
    E. idiosyncratic but narrowly defined for a single patient

16.2 Developmental considerations in the acquisition of somatization patterns include:

    A. difficulty in acquiring the capacity to verbalize emotional distress
    B. birth trauma
    C. fixation at the oral stage of analytic development
    D. fixation at the anal stage of analytic development
    E. poor peer relations during the latency stage

16.3 Under the *Diagnostic and Statistical Manual of Mental Disorders (Third Edition-Revised) (DSM-III-R)*, the diagnosis of conversion disorder requires:

    A. intentional production and manipulation of physical symptoms
    B. specification of the symbolic meaning of the symptoms
    C. family or subcultural norms of somatization patterns
    D. disappearance of symptoms under amytal interview
    E. lack of congruence between the symptom and culturally sanctioned response patterns

16.4 Conversion symptoms may function to do all of the following except:

    A. resolve early conflicts
    B. permit expression of a forbidden wish or impulse
    C. impose self-punishment
    D. remove oneself from an overwhelming life situation
    E. assume the sick role to allow gratification of dependency needs

16.5 Conversion disorders are:

    A. more common in men than in women
    B. more common in older individuals
    C. more common in rural populations
    D. more common in psychologically minded individuals
    E. more common in college-educated individuals

16.6 Probably the most important consideration in diagnosing a conversion disorder is:

    A. documentation of atypical symptom patterns
    B. ruling out neurological or medical disorders
    C. the use of the amytal interview
    D. history of "overuse" of medical services
    E. resistance of symptoms to customary treatment

16.7 Suggested treatment of conversion disorders includes:

    A. direct confrontation
    B. an initial standard psychosocial assessment
    C. use of major neuroleptics
    D. long-term hospitalization
    E. client-centered interview techniques

16.8   Suspicion of malingering is not increased by:

   A.   tampered medical records
   B.   knowledge of potential for financial compensation
   C.   overly dramatic complaints
   D.   well-defined symptoms
   E.   the fact that injuries appear to be self-induced

DIRECTIONS: For each of the statements or questions below, one or more of the alternative answers is correct. Choose answer:

   A   if only 1, 2, and 3 are correct
   B   if only 1 and 3 are correct
   C   if only 2 and 4 are correct
   D   if only 4 is correct
   E   if all are correct

16.9   Somatization disorder is:

   1. frequently seen in individuals with histrionic personality traits
   2. also known as Munchausen's syndrome
   3. associated with sociopathy in male relatives
   4. rarely associated with concurrent affective or anxiety disorders

16.10   The following disorders may be manifested clinically primarily by somatic complaints:

   1. anxiety disorders
   2. factitious disorders
   3. affective disorders (depression)
   4. somatoform disorders

16.11   The diagnosis of somatoform pain disorder requires:

   1. the ability of pathophysiological mechanisms to explain symptom patterns
   2. existence of symptoms for at least one month
   3. consistency of symptoms with known neuroanatomic distribution of pain receptors
   4. that the complaint not be secondary to other psychiatric disorders such as depression

16.12   In conversion disorders, favorable prognosis is associated with:

1. recent onset
2. good premorbid adjustment
3. clearly identifiable precipitating events
4. absence of severe associated psychopathology

16.13   Treatment of pain syndromes involves:

1. consideration of psychodynamic factors
2. little or no medication
3. use of behavioral techniques
4. reliance on neuroleptic medication

16.14   Epidemiologic studies of somatization disorder reveal:

1. increased prevalence when the family history is positive for the disorder
2. an associated increased rate of marital problems
3. an associated decreased level of work performance
4. an associated decreased rate of alcohol problems

16.15   The clinical presentation of somatization disorder includes:

1. negative history for affective disorder
2. flamboyant and dramatic symptoms
3. vaguely described complaints
4. history of multiple hospitalizations

16.16   The recommended psychotherapeutic treatment of somatization disorders includes:

1. ego supportive and empathic interactions
2. direct but gentle confrontation
3. fostering appropriate defenses and coping mechanisms
4. discounting physical symptoms

DIRECTIONS: Each of the following questions consists of lettered headings followed by a list of numbered alternatives. Select the single lettered heading that is most closely associated with the appropriate numbered alternative. Each lettered heading may be chosen only once.

A. Hypochondriasis
B. Conversion disorder
C. Somatization disorder
D. Somatoform pain disorder
E. Factitious disorder
F. Body dysmorphic disorder

16.17 includes complaints in excess of what would be expected from an underlying physical condition

16.18 is an unrealistic preoccupation with fear of having a disease

16.19 is characterized by the loss of, or an alteration in, physical functioning suggesting a physical disorder

16.20 is characterized by the presence of multiple somatic complaints that usually begin under the age of 30 years

16.21 is characterized by the exaggerated belief that the body is deformed

16.22 is characterized by the conscious, deliberate, and surreptitious feigning of physical or psychological symptoms

ANSWERS

16.1 The answer is **D**.

Somatization is defined as psychological distress expressed via physiological symptoms. In medical settings, somatization is a common manifestation of psychiatric problems. The pattern of somatization is diverse, although somatic complaints can be a manifestation of affective disorders, anxiety disorders, and psychophysiological disorders. Under *DSM-III-R*, somatization disorder is diagnosed when physical symptoms that usually suggest a physical disorder cannot be explained by organic findings or known physiological mechanisms and when these symptoms are strongly suspected of being linked to psychological factors or conflicts.

16.2   The answer is **A**.

Humans are born with the capacity to express affective responses with a variety of physical behaviors including facial expressions and preverbal vocalizations. The infant's caregivers respond to these physical behaviors with other behaviors that help set a pattern of communication. Later, when the infant learns to use symbolic language, the vocabulary of affective expression is greatly increased. Eventually, verbal expression comes to supplant somatic communication. However, if the infant has problems in learning to verbalize its affective feelings, it may become fixated at a somatic level of experiencing and communicating affect and psychological concerns. These individuals are theorized to be at risk for developing somatoform disorders.

16.3   The answer is **E**.

Under *DSM-III-R*, conversion disorders are defined as being characterized by a loss of, or an alteration in, physical functioning that suggests a physical disorder. Psychological factors are thought to be etiologically related to the onset of symptoms as exemplified by a temporal relation between a stressful event and the appearance of the symptoms. The individual with a conversion disorder is not consciously or intentionally producing the symptoms. An additional criterion is that the symptom cannot be congruent with a cultural response pattern and cannot be explained by a known physical disorder. It is not necessary to be able to specify the symbolic meaning of the symptoms, nor is it necessary for the symptoms to disappear under amytal interview techniques.

16.4   The answer is **A**.

Many theories seek to explain the development of conversion symptoms. Psychoanalytic theory states that conversion disorder symptoms represent a compromise between the unconscious need to express feelings and the fear of expressing these feelings. Behavioral theory states that the conversion symptom is an adaptation to a frustrating life experience. Celani postulates that conversion symptoms are attempts by the patient to express feelings of helplessness under the influence of cultural, social, and interpersonal variables. Some theorists state that conversion symptoms are a form of primitive communication similar to pantomime. These symptoms appear when direct verbal communication is not possible. Conversion symptoms have also been hypothesized as functioning to express forbidden wishes, to impose self-punishment, to remove oneself from a threatening situation, or to allow the patient to assume the sick role and allow dependent behavior.

16.5   The answer is **C**.

The prevalence of conversion disorders is unknown. The only epidemiological figures of incidence have been derived from studies of general hospital populations. In studies of general hospital psychiatric consultation services, estimates of between 5 and 13 percent have emerged. The diagnosis of conversion disorder occurs more frequently in women than in men, more frequently in patients under age 40, and more frequently in rural and unsophisticated populations.

16.6   The answer is **B**.

The diagnosis of conversion disorder is made more likely when there is an atypical pattern of symptoms, such as when patterns of sensory loss or paralysis do not follow known patterns of anatomical neurologic distribution. The amytal interview may also be useful, as may the resistance of symptoms to customary forms of treatment and a history of overuse of medical services. However, the most important factor in diagnosing a conversion disorder is in conducting a thorough evaluation for the presence of medical and neurological disease. Studies indicate that as many as 60 percent of individuals originally diagnosed as having a conversion disorder actually developed a physical problem or had died at a nine-year followup. Thirty percent of the individuals diagnosed as having conversion disorder in this study had initial symptoms that were related to their eventual medical diagnosis. The danger is in too quickly diagnosing a conversion disorder when an unusual medical disorder may instead be present.

16.7   The answer is **B**.

The treatment of conversion disorders has not been the subject of rigorous scientifc investigation. However, the research that has been conducted in combination with the accumulation of clinical experience suggests the course of successful treatment may be implemented using several guidelines. Treatment should begin with a thorough standard psychosocial assessment. This initial assessment optimally concentrates on uncovering the role of precipitating events, a description of past history of psychological trauma, and an evaluation of current associated psychopathology. The assessment interview and subsequent therapy need to be conducted carefully in order to avoid confrontation. Important information includes a detailed history of the family because a family history of interpersonal conflicts and communication deficits may be associated with the emergence of conversion disorder symptoms.

The use of confrontational techniques in the treatment of conversion disorders is likely to increase the defensiveness of the patient and therefore would be counterproductive. The therapist should instead listen to the somatic complaints of the patient without passing judgment on the validity of the complaints. The therapist can reassure the patient that the symptoms are likely to remit. New coping skills can be taught to the patient. Several forms of treatment have been reported as being successful in the treatment of conversion disorders. These successful forms of treatment include behavioral therapy, brief supportive therapy, hypnosis, psychoanalysis, faradic stimulation, and sodium amytal interview techniques. It should be noted that instances of spontaneous remission have also been reported. In some cases, the use of medication may be necessary in order to reduce anxiety or affective symptoms.

16.8   The answer is D.

Malingering involves the purposeful production of somatic symptoms motivated by external rewards. In these cases the clinician can identify a goal that the patient is apparently trying to reach by means of the symptoms. Usually when a patient is malingering, the symptoms are not well defined and may be vague. Other conditions also raise the suspicion of malingering, including an inconsistency between the history, the exam, and the diagnostic results and the presentation of the somatic complaints. The patient may be uncooperative during the diagnostic workup. A history of altered medical records, unexpected positive drug or toxin screen results, or repeated accidents and injuries, especially when these injuries appear to be self-induced, also raise the suspicion of malingering. These patients tend to overdramatize their complaints and may be resistant when a favorable prognosis is announced. The presence of possible motivations such as potential for financial compensation, requests for addictive drugs, or the ability of the symptom to have the patient removed from an unpleasant situation or aversive legal proceedings increases the level of suspicion. Finally the presence of antisocial personality traits can be associated with malingering.

16.9   The answer is B.

Somatization disorder is sometimes known as Briquet's syndrome in honor of the physician who first gave a detailed description of the disorder in 1859. A frequent personality pattern of individuals with somatization disorder includes many histrionic features, although elements of obsessional personality features may also be present. Epidemiological studies of somatization disorder indicate an increased prevalence of the disorder in first-degree relatives. Other associated factors include increased rate of marital difficulties, poor work performance, a higher percentage of teenage delinquency, alcohol problems, and sociopathy in first-degree male relatives.

16.10   The answer is E.

Somatic complaints may be the clinical manifestation of anxiety disorders, factitious disorders, affective disorders (especially depression), and somatoform disorders. Because of this wide variety of disorders, the presence of somatic complaints cannot be seen as being indicative of any given disorder. The development of somatization is related more to the failure to acquire adequate means of dealing with or communicating psychological distress than to the presence of a particular disorder.

16.11   The answer is D.

Under *DSM-III-R*, the diagnosis of somatoform pain disorder requires first that the patient's preoccupation with pain last at least six months. The second requirement for this diagnosis is that one of two conditions be met: either that appropriate evaluation uncovers no known organic pathology or pathophysiologic mechanism, or that if there is a related pathophysiologic mechanism, the complaint of pain or the resultant social and occupational impairment greatly exceeds what one would expect from the physical findings. The pain complaint should not be secondary to any other psychiatric condition such as an affective disorder. Usually psychological factors can be found to be related to the pain complaints, such as when the onset of pain follows some environmental stressor. However, this condition is not necessary for the diagnosis to be made.

16.12   The answer is E.

Most clinical reports indicate that spontaneous remission of conversion disorder symptoms may be common. Variables associated with favorable prognosis for conversion disorders include recent onset, clearly identifiable precipitating events, good premorbid adjustment, and the absence of severe psychopathology. It should be noted that not all prospective studies agree with the above clinical reports. One study followed 85 patients for between 7 and 11 years. Out of this sample, 82 percent had developed organic illnesses, schizophrenia, affective disorders, or chronic conversion symptoms, and four of these patients had committed suicide. Another study followed female patients for 20 years and found that nearly one-third developed a psychotic illness, primarily schizophrenia.

16.13   The answer is **B**.

There is an extremely wide variety of pain syndromes and, consequently, an extremely wide diversity of treatments for these disorders. Because there are so many etiologic agents involved in the appearance of pain syndromes, a multidisciplinary treatment approach is usually the best course. The role of psychodynamic factors needs to be investigated and appropriate psychotherapy can be initiated. The use of antidepressants, especially tricyclics, can be successful, particularly with chronic headache or facial pain.

Behavioral factors can play a very important role in the acquisition and maintenance of pain complaints. The role of pain complaints and pain-related behaviors in relation to eliciting helping behavior from other family members should be investigated. The role of family responses to pain behavior in reinforcing that behavior should also be evaluated. The family can be instructed in methods of changing their behavior and subsequently affecting the pain behaviors. Other behavioral techniques such as biofeedback or relaxation techniques can be implemented.

16.14   The answer is **A**.

Somatization disorder has received more systematic study than most other somatoform disorders. The St. Louis group at Washington University has made major contributions to our understanding of this disorder. It is from their work that we realized the familial role in the prevalence of somatization disorder. For example, there is a 20 percent prevalence of somatization disorder in first-degree relatives of individuals with this diagnosis. There also appears to be an increased rate of marital problems, poor work performance, teenage delinquencies, alcohol problems, and sociopathy in first-degree relatives of these individuals.

16.15   The answer is **C**.

Patients with somatization disorder often present with dramatic and flamboyant symptoms. These patients provide elaborately detailed descriptions of their symptoms, but their descriptions of history and the effects of previous treatments are vague and unhelpful. There is often a history of many previous hospitalizations and surgeries as well as a history of affective instability. Most of these patients are women, and they tend to marry abusive men and have unstable interpersonal relationships. Their personality patterns are primarily histrionic, but there may be elements of obsessional characteristics. There is also a pattern of frequent concurrent psychiatric disorders, including major affective disorder, phobic disorder, panic disorder, drug and alcohol abuse, and even schizophrenia.

16.16   The answer is **B**.

Psychotherapeutic approaches to the treatment of somatization disorder are generally supportive instead of interpretative or analytic. Confrontation, even when gently conducted, is likely to result in untoward effects for the patient. For many of these patients, the expression of their somatic complaints may be the only method they have for obtaining support from other individuals, and any attempts to remove these methods may be viewed as unempathetic or hostile. Instead the patient should be encouraged to develop new methods for obtaining support and coping with stress. The therapist can listen attentively when the symptoms are brought up without actually encouraging discussion of them. Gradually, other topics, such as interpersonal relations, can be introduced.

16.17   The answer is **D**.
16.18   The answer is **A**.
16.19   The answer is **B**.
16.20   The answer is **C**.
16.21   The answer is **F**.
16.22   The answer is **E**.

The diagnosis of somatoform pain disorder requires that there be a preoccupation with pain for a period of at least six months. The somatoform pain disorder is characterized by the presence of pain complaints, either when there is no organic pathophysiological reason or when the severity of the pain complaints and resultant restriction of activities are in excess of what would be expected on the basis of the physical findings. Usually psychological factors are thought to be involved in the appearance and maintenance of the pain complaints.

Hypochondriasis is best defined as the unrealistic fear of having a disease. The incidence of hypochondriasis has been estimated at between 3 and 13 percent of medical inpatients. Hypochondriacal complaints often accompany depressive episodes, and transient hypochondriasis is a common response to stressful life events. If an individual has been diagnosed with a serious disease such as cancer, minor aches and pains may be misinterpreted as serious symptoms. Many of these patients resist psychological interpretations of their problems and are seen by primary care physicians rather than psychiatrists.

Conversion disorders involve the loss or alteration of physical functioning in such a manner as to suggest a physical disorder. Manifestations of conversion disorders include paralysis, anesthesia, tunnel vision, spasm, weakness, and paraparesis. Before diagnosing a conversion disorder, it is important to first rule out neurological or medical illness.

Somatization disorder (Briquet's syndrome) is characterized by a history of the presence of multiple somatic complaints usually beginning under age 30 and persisting for many years. In order to give the diagnosis of somatization disorder, the patient must exhibit at least 13 symptoms involving gastrointestinal, reproductive, or cardiopulmonary systems, or pseudoneurological or pain symptoms. The disorder is more common among women than men.

Although it is considered part of the somatoform disorders, body dysmorphic disorder appears to have some features in common with delusional syndrome. Individuals with body dysmorphic disorder have an unrealistic belief that their bodies are deformed or, if there is an actual body defect, that the significance is grossly exaggerated. Although this disorder appears to have some features in common with delusional syndromes, in body dysmorphic disorder the belief cannot be as severely intense as it is in a delusional syndrome. That is, the patient must be able to admit that the defect has been exaggerated. Also the belief cannot appear in the presence of anorexia nervosa or transsexualism.

In factitious disorder, the patient deliberately and consciously uses subterfuge to fake physical or psychological symptoms. The factitious disorder differs from malingering in that for malingering a motivation can be discerned, whereas for factitious disorder the only motivation appears to be the chance to achieve the role of the patient. These patients submit willingly to even painful diagnostic or treatment procedures and often have multiple surgeries.

Chapter 17

The Dissociative Disorders

DIRECTIONS: Each of the statements or questions is followed by five suggested responses or completions. Select the one that is the best choice or most complete answer in each case.

17.1 The dissociative disorders are characterized by:
- A. dissociation or splitting of normal personality
- B. disturbances or alterations in memory, identity, or consciousness
- C. histrionic reactions to even minimal levels of stress
- D. "la belle indifference" reactions to symptoms of the disorder
- E. hypervigilance in social situations

17.2 Hilgard's research and theoretical conceptualizations support the notion that:
- A. unitary consciousness is necessary for normal functioning
- B. dissociative disorders have their roots in early childhood
- C. consciousness can be directed like a flashlight
- D. dissociation occurs only under extreme stress
- E. varieties of dissociation are inherent in normal mental function

17.3   Which of the following statements regarding the incidence of psychogenic amnesia is not true?

  A.   The incidence in the general population is around .03 percent.
  B.   The incidence in new admissions to a psychiatry service was found to be .26 percent.
  C.   Twenty percent of combat veterans are amnestic for their combat experiences.
  D.   The incidence rises during civilian disasters.
  E.   Soldiers exposed to prolonged marching and fighting under heavy fire may have a 35 percent rate of amnesia.

17.4   Which of the following statements regarding psychogenic amnesia is true?

  A.   It is characterized by recurrent amnestic episodes.
  B.   Often the patient will travel to another locale during the amnestic episode.
  C.   The essential feature is the sudden inability to remember important personal material.
  D.   Patients often assume another personality during the amnestic episode.
  E.   The diagnosis of psychogenic amnesia is easier to make in children than in adults.

17.5   Which of the following is not thought to be a precipitant of psychogenic amnesia?

  A.   a situation involving the threat of injury or death
  B.   the anticipated loss of an important object
  C.   an overwhelming and panic-inducing impulse
  D.   an alcoholic binge
  E.   narcissistic rage

17.6   Differences between psychogenic amnesia and organic memory disorders do not include which of the following?

  A.   Organic memory disorders are unlikely to have clearly demarcated beginnings and endings.
  B.   The memory disturbance in psychogenic amnesia has an onset related to a stressor.
  C.   Organic memory disorders are rarely followed by a full return of memory.
  D.   Cognitive functions are not disturbed in psychogenic amnesia.
  E.   Psychogenic amnesia is usually retrograde.

17.7   Which of the following statements regarding psychogenic fugue is not true?

A.   Psychogenic fugue usually occurs in the context of psychosocial stress.
B.   Psychogenic fugue states generally persist for months.
C.   The recovery from psychogenic fugue is usually rapid and sudden.
D.   Personal rejections, losses, failures, or financial pressures may precede a fugue state.
E.   Recurrences of psychogenic fugue are probably rare.

17.8   Multiple personality disorder is most often reported:

A.   in the wake of child abuse
B.   in lower socioeconomic status individuals
C.   in males
D.   in psychotic conditions
E.   in an isolated family member

17.9   Which of the following statements regarding multiple personality disorders is not true?

A.   The multiple personalities' awareness of each other varies.
B.   Approximately one-half of the contemporary cases have 10 or fewer personalities.
C.   Amnesia is always present.
D.   The personalities involved may be discrepant.
E.   It is a chronic post-traumatic dissociative disorder.

DIRECTIONS: For each of the statements or questions below, one or more of the alternative answers is correct. Choose answer:
A   if only 1, 2, and 3 are correct
B   if only 1 and 3 are correct
C   if only 2 and 4 are correct
D   if only 4 is correct
E   if all are correct

17.10   Varieties of psychogenic amnesia include:

1. localized
2. selective
3. generalized
4. continuous

17.11   Dissociative phenomena:

1. are always associated with psychopathology
2. cannot occur spontaneously
3. cannot be sought out
4. may be induced for therapeutic purposes

17.12   Signs that indicate the need for careful evaluation for multiple personality disorder include:

1. prior treatment failure
2. fluctuating symptoms and levels of function
3. time distortion or time lapses
4. the absence of concurrent psychiatric and somatic symptoms

17.13   The literature on the treatment of depersonalization disorder indicates that:

1. clozapine and phenazepam may be useful
2. electroconvulsive therapy is helpful in most cases
3. cognitive and behavioral approaches may be useful
4. short-term treatment is as efficacious as long term

17.14   Treatment of psychogenic fugue involves:

1. careful confrontation
2. the use of sodium amobarbital interviews
3. discouraging exploration of the other identity
4. pursuit of recovery of the missing memories

17.15   Possession states in multiple personality disorder can be classified as:

1. the somnabulic
2. the aggressive
3. the lucid
4. the passive

17.16   A predominant theory of the etiology of multiple personality disorder includes which factors?

1. a biological capacity to dissociate
2. experience of life events that overwhelm
3. the development of personalities as shaped by unique life events
4. an inability to heal hurts

DIRECTIONS: Each of the following questions consists of lettered headings followed by a list of numbered alternatives. Select the single lettered heading that is most closely associated with the appropriate numbered alternative. Each lettered heading may be chosen only once.

Dissociative disorder

A. Depersonalization disorder
B. Dissociative disorder not otherwise specified
C. Malingering
D. Psychogenic amnesia

Description

17.17 has memory impairment that centers around external incentives
17.18 usually occurs as a single episode
17.19 has a dissociative symptom as the predominant feature
17.20 refers to the feeling of being detached from one's mental processes or body

ANSWERS

17.1 The answer is **B**.

The dissociative disorders are characterized by disturbances or alterations in the usually integrative functions of memory, personal identity, or consciousness. These disorders include psychogenic amnesia, psychogenic fugue, multiple personality disorder, depersonalization disorder, and dissociative disorder not otherwise specified. They have little relation to histrionic disorders. "La belle indifference" may or may not be present. Likewise, hypervigilance has no systematic relation to the dissociative disorders. Split personalities have no specific technical definitions, although the term is sometimes used by laypersons to describe both schizophrenia and multiple personality disorder.

17.2   The answer is E.

Hilgard has proposed a neodissociation theory that is descended from Janet's original theorizations. Hilgard holds that both receptive and active mental functions can be regulated by overlapping control systems. These control systems may not always be accessible to conscious observation. One of his most famous concepts is the "hidden observer." The hidden observer is manifested when hypnotized individuals demonstrate the existence of an observing self that exists during the hypnotized state but is not accessible to conscious self-description until after the hypnotic state is terminated. Hilgard states that consciousness is not unitary and that varieties of dissociation are common in normal mental operations.

17.3   The answer is A.

Although there are no precise figures on the prevalence of the dissociative disorders in the general population, certain estimates have been made regarding the incidence in particular situations. For example, the incidence in new admissions to a psychiatric service has been reported as being around .26 percent. The incidence of dissociative disorders rises during episodes of extreme stress such as civilian disasters and during wartime. Reports indicate that as many as 20 percent of combat veterans are amnestic for their combat experience. Soldiers exposed to prolonged marching and fighting under heavy fire may have a 35 percent rate of amnesia for the experiences.

17.4   The answer is C.

The essential feature of psychogenic amnesia is the sudden inability to remember important personal material. Patients do not usually assume another identity and travel to another locale during the amnestic episode, as occurs in psychogenic fugues or multiple personality disorders. Psychogenic amnesia usually has a single episode in a given individual, although recurrences are possible. Recurrent amnestic episodes are more often associated with multiple personality disorder or temporal lobe epilepsy. Amnestic syndromes are rare in children. This may be partly due to the difficulty in assessing amnesia when normal development may involve the replacement of immature cognitive structures with more mature structures with a resultant discontinuity in mental operations.

17.5   The answer is D.

Psychogenic amnesia usually has a sudden beginning following a specific, severe psychosocial stressor. In some cases, the initiation is abrupt but may reflect the culmination of compounded stress. Precipitants of psychogenic amnesia include confrontation of situations involving the threat of injury or death, the actual or anticipated loss of an important object, overwhelming and panic-inducing impulses, mortifying shame, or narcissistic rage. Alcoholic binges may result in periods of blackout but are not associated with psychogenic amnesia. Instead, there is most likely a physiological reason for the loss of memory.

17.6   The answer is E.

Psychogenic amnesia and organic memory impairment may be differentiated on several bases. Organic memory disorders do not usually have a clearly indicated beginning and end, especially not endpoints related to psychosocial stressors. The memory impairment in organic memory disorders is more marked for recent events than for remote events and resolves slowly if at all. On the other hand, psychogenic amnesia is followed by a full return of memory. Organic memory impairment is usually accompanied by some degree of cognitive impairment.

When organic memory impairment is due to an intoxicant, there is rarely full recovery of the memory. The use of intoxicants can be documented in these cases. The alcohol-induced memory disorder is characterized by deficits in short-term recall in the presence of intact immediate memory. The memory impairment in psychogenic amnesia is related to a specific time period and cannot be characterized as a retrograde memory impairment.

17.7   The answer is B.

In the *Diagnostic and Statistical Manual of Mental Disorders (Third Edition-Revised)* definition of a psychogenic fugue state, the predominant disturbance is abrupt and unexpected travel away from home or usual place of work and activities with an inability to remember one's past. It is accompanied by an assumption of a new identity that is not due to multiple personality disorder or an organic mental disorder. It usually occurs in the context of psychosocial stress such as war or civilian disaster. Other precipitants may include personal rejections, losses, failures, marital and romantic problems, or financial troubles. It involves retrograde amnesia, and its course is usually brief, lasting days or hours. In rare cases, it may last for a period of a few months. The recovery is typically sudden and may occur upon awakening from sleep.

17.8   The answer is A.

Multiple personality disorder is seen as a post-traumatic dissociative disorder that occurs most frequently in the aftermath of child abuse.

Kluft feels that it may have its onset before the age of nine years, when the child is susceptible to hypnotizability and is in the Piagetian pre-operational stage. Between 75 and 90 percent of reported cases have involved females, although male cases may present to the legal system rather than to the mental health system. There are no reports of the relative incidence in different socioeconomic classes. The diagnosis tends to run in families. This familial trend may be the result of inherited biological capacities to dissociate or to the well-known transmission of child abuse patterns across generations. In order for multiple personality disorder to be diagnosed, a psychotic disorder must be ruled out.

17.9   The answer is C.

Multiple personality disorder is considered to be a chronic post-traumatic dissociative disorder. About 50 percent of contemporary cases of multiple personality disorder have 10 or fewer personalities. The transition from one personality to another is usually sudden but may occur slowly over the course of a few days. The different personalities may be discrepant and may even represent polar opposites. The multiple (alternate) personalities may have varying degrees of awareness regarding each others' existence. Over the lifetime of a patient, the degree of relative dominance of the different personalities may vary. Sometimes the personalities may only be aware of each other as dreams, but some personalities may interact with each other and even develop relationships with each other.

Amnesia is considered to be an important aspect of multiple personality disorder, but it is not always present. Even when amnesia is present, it may be difficult to document. Some individuals with multiple personality disorder deny that they have amnesia. These patients may confabulate narratives to cover the time periods when the other personalities take over. Other patients may remember the events that occur during the episodes as happening to the dominant personality. Still other patients may not report amnesia because they have been labeled crazy or were not believed when they previously reported no memory for events reported by others in their environment.

17.10   The answer is E.

The *DSM-III-R* diagnosis of psychogenic amnesia is given when the predominant disturbance is an episode in which the individual has a sudden inability to remember important personal information, and the loss of memory is too extensive to be explained by simple forgetfulness. The episode of amnesia cannot be due to a multiple personality disorder or to an organic memory disorder. There are several possible forms of psychogenic amnesia. One variant involves the loss of localized or circumscribed bits of memory. In some forms of psychogenic amnesia known as selective amnesia, only parts of the information are lost. It is also possible to have a generalized loss of information for the individual's life history. Some patients have intact skills for forming new memories, while other patients are continually impaired in their ability to form new memories.

17.11　The answer is **D**.

Contrary to popular opinion, dissociative phenomena are not always associated with forms of psychopathology. Dissociative phenomena may occur spontaneously, or they may be sought out by the individual. In some instances, dissociative phenomena may be induced for therapeutic reasons. Dissociative phenomena may share some underlying factors with hypnotizability. Some dissociative phenomena are common in everyday life. Examples of these forms of dissociative phenomena include self-absorption in thought to the extent that one is unaware of external events and fixation on the road while driving to the extent that one misses one's exit or suddenly becomes aware that one does not have any memory for the most recent few miles of driving. Some religious or spiritualistic practices also result in dissociative phenomena. The interpretation of dissociative phenomena is highly influenced by cultural variables. The trancelike states of ancient oracles and more modern instances of glossolalia are examples of dissociative phenomena that are not interpreted as psychopathology in their respective contexts.

17.12　The answer is **A**.

The failure to accurately diagnose multiple personality disorder may occur more commonly than we are aware. These patients may lack the awareness or the motivation to report the presence of the multiple personalities. A recent investigation found that there may be an average of almost seven years from the first appearance of symptoms to the time that the accurate diagnosis is made.

There are several signs in the presentation of patients that indicate the need for a more careful scrutiny for multiple personalities. These signs include a history of prior treatment failure and of three or more diagnoses on serial contacts with mental health professionals. The clinician should also be alerted by the presence of concurrent psychiatric and somatic symptoms and a history of fluctuating symptoms and levels of functioning. Other signs include reports of severe headaches, time distortions or time lapses, and reports of being told about behavior for which the patient has no memory. Sometimes individuals in the social environment report noticeable changes in the patient. Other signs involve the patient's reporting having found objects, behavioral products, or handwriting for which he or she is unable to account. Still another sign is when the patient uses the word "we" in the collective sense. Although it is possible to attempt to elicit other personalities via hypnosis or a sodium amobarbital interview, caution is recommended because such procedures may elicit a wide variety of phenomena.

17.13   The answer is **B**.

There is little literature on the treatment of depersonalization disorder. Although there is no medical treatment universally recognized as effective, some foreign reports indicate that the use of clozapine and phenazepam may be helpful. Electroconvulsive therapy does not appear to be useful even though it may help alleviate concomitant depression. Therapeutic hypnosis or long-term psychodynamic therapy may be useful, but a treatment course of more than five years may be necessary. Cognitive and behavioral approaches aimed at promoting active mastery may also be useful.

17.14   The answer is **C**.

The treatment of psychogenic fugue shares many features with the treatment of psychogenic amnesia. However, if the patient is still in a fugue state when seen, information regarding the baseline identity must first be obtained. Most of the literature regarding treatment of psychogenic fugue focuses on the recovery of memory and does not address whether issues related to the alternate personality should be explored. Hypnosis or sodium amobarbital interview techniques may be useful when coupled with psychotherapy. Although the usual focus is on recovering the missing memories, it may be wise to also work toward teaching the patient nondissociative methods of dealing with stressful experiences.

17.15   The answer is **B**.

Possession states are common phenomena in investigations of other cultures. In modern western culture, possession states are viewed as signs of multiple personality disorder, psychogenic fugue, or dissociative disorder not otherwise specified. Possession states can be divided into two general forms. In the first form, somnabulic possession states, the individual is not conscious of his or her usual self and does not have memory for the condition following the episode. In the second form, lucid possession states, the individual reports continual awareness of the usual self, but reports that he or she has no control over the emergence of the other personality.

17.16 The answer is **E**.

Multiple personality disorder may be the result of many different etiologies. Kluft has proposed a four-factor theory to account for the phenomenon. The first factor in the development of a multiple personality disorder is a biological capacity to dissociate, whether the dissociation is associated with hypnotism, epileptic phenomena, disordered neurological development, or state-dependent learning experiences. The second factor involves the experience of stressful life events that overwhelm the patient's coping responses. The patient then reverts to a dissociative strategy in order to deal with the stressful events. The third factor states that the quality of the different personalities is shaped by the learning experiences and developmental stage at the time of the emergence of the alternate personality. Finally, the fourth factor states that the people who develop multiple personality disorders are not able to heal their hurts.

17.17 The answer is **D**.
17.18 The answer is **C**.
17.19 The answer is **A**.
17.20 The answer is **B**.

Depersonalization is the experience of a feeling that one is detached from one's mental processes or body. One may feel like an observer of oneself, or that one is an automaton or is in a dream. Reality testing remains intact during the episode. Depersonalization may be experienced by a wide variety of normal individuals. It is only when the episodes of depersonalization are sufficient to impair social or occupational functioning and cannot be attributed to another disorder that they come to the attention of the psychiatrist. The disorder may first occur in childhood, but it usually has its onset in adolescence or early adulthood. It rarely has an onset after age 40. In psychiatric patients, the experience of depersonalization is the third most common type of complaint following depression and anxiety.

If an individual presents with the features that characterize the dissociative disorders, but does not meet the criteria for a particular disorder, the diagnosis of dissociative disorder not otherwise specified is given. Ganser's syndrome may be one form of this residual diagnosis, as may be derealization without depersonalization. Instances of this disorder may follow incidents of kidnapping or brainwashing.

There is always the possibility that an individual who appears to have a dissociative disorder may in fact be malingering. However, there are certain features of malingering that can be helpful in providing the correct diagnosis. The onset of symptoms in malingering can usually be clearly demarcated, but the precipitants are external incentives such as avoiding responsibility for criminal behavior. The duration of the symptoms is related to the utility of the response of other people to reports of the symptoms. Reported memory impairment usually centers around events related to the external incentives.

Psychogenic amnesia involves a single episode of loss of memory for important personal material. The onset is relatively clearly demarcated and is precipitated by severe psychosocial stress. Short-term memory remains unimpaired (except in the continuous form of the disorder). The deficits are generally related to anterograde memory. Recovery of memory is usually complete following successful treatment.

Chapter 18

Sexual Disorders

DIRECTIONS: Each of the statements or questions is followed by five suggested responses or completions. Select the one that is the best choice or most complete answer in each case.

18.1 The substance responsible for the embryologic differentiation of the testes is:

    A.   the H-Y antigen
    B.   the M-F antigen
    C.   the H-G antigen
    D.   the X-Y antigen
    E.   none of the above

18.2 The development of genitalia in utero depends on the presence or absence of what substance?

    A.   gamma-aminobutyric acid
    B.   testosterone
    C.   cholinesterase
    D.   estrogen
    E.   none of the above

18.3 Gender identity is usually established by what age?

    A. five years
    B. 12 years
    C. at birth
    D. three years
    E. 14 years

18.4 Which of the following statements is true regarding the capacity of gender identity to change?

    A. Gender identity is often changed with psychoanalytic therapy.
    B. Gender identity, once firmly established, is extremely resistant to change.
    C. Gender identity does not appear to be established until puberty.
    D. All possible biological factors involved in gender identity have been discovered.
    E. None of the above.

18.5 Which of the following statements is true regarding transsexualism?

    A. Almost all individuals who seek sex reassignment are transsexuals.
    B. Transsexualism is quite common in Europe.
    C. Transsexuals most commonly present requesting sex reassignment.
    D. Male transsexuals usually have a heterosexual orientation.
    E. Females are more likely to request sex reassignment than males.

DIRECTIONS: For each of the statements below, one or more of the alternative answers is correct. Choose answer:

    A if only 1, 2, and 3 are correct
    B if only 1 and 3 are correct
    C if only 2 and 4 are correct
    D if only 4 is correct
    E if all are correct

18.6 Suggested treatments for transsexuals include:

    1. supportive psychotherapy
    2. behavior therapy
    3. sex reassignment
    4. psychoanalysis

18.7   Behavioral treatments for paraphilias include:

   1. satiation
   2. assertiveness training
   3. covert sensitization
   4. flooding

18.8   Antiandrogenic medications are most helpful in treating paraphilias when the individual:

   1. participates in psychotherapy
   2. has a low sexual drive
   3. is self-motivated to pursue treatment
   4. has an antisocial personality disorder

18.9   Illnesses that may lead to sexual dysfunction are:

   1. multiple sclerosis
   2. hyperprolactinemia
   3. diabetes mellitus
   4. liver disease

18.10   Psychodynamic treatment of transsexuals should involve:

   1. limit setting
   2. ego support
   3. short-term goal setting
   4. therapist passivity

18.11   Children with gender identity disorder of childhood:

   1. are uncomfortable with their genitals
   2. identify with opposite-sex role models
   3. play at being the opposite sex
   4. have a high incidence of continued manifestations as adults

18.12   Individuals with paraphilias:

   1. are predominantly men
   2. usually have multiple paraphilias
   3. usually have onset of the paraphilias before age 18
   4. are usually disturbed by their disorder

18.13   Inappropriate sexual behavior can occur in those with:

1. antisocial personality disorder
2. dementia
3. psychosis
4. mental retardation

DIRECTIONS: Each of the following questions consists of lettered headings followed by a list of numbered alternatives. Select the single lettered heading that is most closely associated with the appropriate numbered alternative. Each lettered heading may be chosen only once.

Sexual disorder

A.   Transsexualism
B.   Paraphilias
C.   Hypoactive sexual desire disorder
D.   Sexual aversion disorder
E.   Premature ejaculation
F.   Vaginismus

Description

18.14   is characterized by involuntary spasm of the musculature of the female genitalia
18.15   refers to the self-perception of being the opposite sex despite anatomical characteristics of a given sex
18.16   is the disorder in which individuals generally report an absence of sexual fantasies
18.17   is characterized by repetitive or preferred sexual fantasies or acts that involve nonhuman objects
18.18   is characterized by an irrational fear of sex with subsequent avoidance of sexual contact
18.19   is treated primarily by the start–stop technique

ANSWERS

18.1 The answer is **A**.

The genetic sex of the individual is determined at conception, but development from that point on is influenced by many factors. For the first six weeks of gestation, the gonads are undifferentiated. If the Y chromosome is present in the embryo, the gonads will differentiate into testes. A substance referred to as the H-Y antigen is responsible for this transformation. If the Y chromosome or H-Y antigen is not present in the developing embryo, the gonads will develop into ovaries.

18.2 The answer is **B**.

Like the gonads, the internal and external genital structures are undifferentiated at first in the fetus. If the gonads differentiate into testes, fetal androgen–testosterone is secreted, and these structures develop into male genitalia (epididymis, vas deferens, ejaculatory ducts, penis, and scrotum). In the absence of fetal androgen, these structures develop into female genitalia (fallopian tubes, uterus, vagina, and clitoris). It is important to note that the development of genitalia in utero depends on the presence or absence of fetal androgen, from whatever source. Thus if fetal androgen is present (for example, in adrenal hyperplasia), male genitalia will develop, even in the presence of ovaries, and the child will be born with either ambiguous or male genitalia. Likewise, if fetal androgen is missing (for example, enzyme deficiency) or androgen receptors are defective (for example, testicular feminization), female genitalia will develop even though the individual has the Y chromosome and testes.

18.3 The answer is **D**.

Gender identity appears to develop in the early years of life and is generally established by age 3. Gender identity seems to depend on the manner in which the individual is reared, regardless of biologic factors. Evidence for this comes from studies of children born with genitalia that are ambiguous or opposite from their genetic sex. These children have been found to develop a gender identity consistent with the gender assigned to them at birth as long as their parents are unambiguous about the child's sex and surgical and hormonal corrections are made.

18.4 The answer is **B**.

Gender identity, once firmly established, is extremely resistant to change. For example, if a genetic female is reared as a boy (for example, because of exposure to fetal androgen), but suddenly develops breasts

and other female secondary sexual characteristics during puberty, his
gender identity will remain male and he will most likely desire correction
of the changes. However, if a child's physical appearance is ambiguous
or if the caregivers are inconsistent in their view of the child as male or
female, gender identity may not develop strongly, leading to possible
change in gender identity at a later time in life.

18.5   The answer is **C.**

Transsexuals most commonly present requesting sex reassignment—change in their physical appearance (usually by hormonal or
surgical means) to correspond with their self-perceived gender. However, it is important to remember that not all who seek sex reassignment
are transsexual: Cross-gender wishes may occur in transvestism, effem-
inate homosexuality, psychosis, and other psychiatric disorders. Therefore, it is important to carefully evaluate the patient and consider alternate
treatments before recommending sex reassignment.

18.6   The answer is **A.**

Because most gender-dysphoric individuals present with adamant
requests for sex reassignment, it is extremely difficult to engage these
patients in treatment with anything other than surgical sex reassignment
as the goal.

Supportive psychotherapy can serve various purposes in the transsexual individual. First, there have been reports of reversal of patients'
disordered gender identity in a few cases. Second, a trial of psychotherapy is often useful in cases in which the diagnosis is unclear. Third,
dealing with patients' fear of homosexuality can alleviate the wish for
surgical reassignment. Fourth, psychotherapy is important in the process of sex reassignment. Finally, therapy is often helpful in the postsurgical adjustment of transsexuals.

Psychoanalysis is generally not indicated in the treatment of transsexuals because of their poor ego functioning. Dynamic psychotherapy
may be useful but must involve the use of parameters often applied to
borderline patients: structured, with limit setting, ego support, and short-
term goals. Behavior therapy has been used with success in several cases
using videotapes and modeling.

18.7   The answer is **A.**

A variety of behavioral therapies have been used to treat paraphilias.
Various aversive conditioning methods such as electric shocks, apo-
morphine (to induce nausea), and covert sensitization have been used
to decrease deviant sexual behavior. Satiation is a technique in which

the individual uses his or her deviant fantasies postorgasm in a repetitive manner to the point of satiaty with the deviant stimuli, in essence making the fantasies boring.

Recent treatments have used a multicomponent approach. Covert sensitization and satiation are used to decrease inappropriate sexual arousal while cognitive therapy is used to change the paraphiliacs' inappropriate beliefs concerning sexual behavior. Social and assertive skills training are used to enable these individuals to relate to adult partners in an appropriate manner.

18.8   The answer is **B**.

Antiandrogenic medications have been widely used to treat sex offenders throughout the world since the 1960s. They have been used less extensively in the United States because of ethical and legal considerations, that is, the ability of the individual facing a prison term to give informed consent. They do not appear to influence the direction of sexual drive toward appropriate adult partners; rather they act to decrease libido and thus break the individual's pattern of compulsive deviant sexual behavior. These medications work best in those paraphiliacs with a high sexual desire or with antisocial personality.

18.9   The answer is **E**.

Sexual arousal requires intact neural and vascular connection to the genitals along with normal endocrine functioning. Any illness that interferes with these systems can lead to sexual dysfunction: neurologic diseases (for example, multiple sclerosis, lumbar or sectorial spinal cord trauma, or herniated disk), thrombosis of the veins or arteries of the penis, diabetes mellitus, endocrine disorders (for example, hyperprolactinemia), and liver disease.

18.10   The answer is **A**.

Dynamic psychotherapy may be used but must involve the use of parameters applied to borderline patients: structured, with limit setting, ego support, and short-term goals.

18.11   The answer is **E**.

Individuals diagnosed as having gender identity disorder of childhood express a desire to become a member of the opposite sex. Boys wish to have a vagina and may play at breast feeding. Girls wish to have a penis and may simulate a penis with various objects or stand to urinate. Both sexes identify with role models of the opposite sex (for example, a boy insisting that he be Supergirl in a game). Retrospective studies of transsexuals have shown a high incidence of childhood cross-gender behavior. Follow-up of gender-disordered children has shown a high incidence of continued manifestations in adulthood, with a higher incidence of homosexual or bisexual behavior and fantasies than in a control group.

18.12   The answer is A.

The vast majority of individuals with paraphilic disorders are men. For example, among reported cases of sexual abuse, over 90 percent of offenders are men. It has also been traditionally held that paraphiliacs engage in only one type of deviant sexual behavior. However, recent studies have suggested that these individuals often have multiple paraphilias. It is also important to note that over 50 percent of these individuals develop the onset of their paraphilic arousal prior to age 18.

18.13   The answer is E.

Inappropriate sexual behavior is not always the result of paraphilia. A psychotic patient may cross-dress because of a delusional belief that God wishes him to hide his true sex. A manic patient may expose himself to women because of his hypersexuality and belief that he will be able to "pick them up." A patient with dementia can behave in a sexually inappropriate manner because of her cognitive impairment. An individual with mental retardation may engage in sexually inappropriate behavior because of cognitive impairment, poor impulse control, and lack of sexual knowledge. Antisocial personalities can also commit deviant sexual acts; this is usually the result of their overall disregard for social norms and sanctions.

18.14   The answer is F.
18.15   The answer is A.
18.16   The answer is C.
18.17   The answer is B.
18.18   The answer is D.
18.19   The answer is E.

Vaginismus is characterized by involuntary spasm of the musculature of the outer one-third of the vagina so that penile penetration is prevented. This problem can only be diagnosed with certainty by a gynecologic examination. Some women who are anxious about sex may experience some pain during penetration, but these women do not have vaginismus.

Transsexualism is a disorder of gender identity. An individual, despite having the anatomical characteristics of a given sex, has the self-perception of being the opposite sex. This disorder is rare, with estimates of 30,000 cases worldwide.

Hypoactive sexual desire disorder is characterized by pervasive or persistent inhibition of sexual desire. Generally, a patient with such a presenting problem reports an absence of sexual fantasies and a lack of desire or interest in engaging in sexual activities.

The paraphilic disorders are characterized by repetitive or preferred sexual fantasies or acts that involve nonhuman objects. Examples are fetishism, transvestism, pedophilia, and zoophilia.

Sexual aversion disorder is characterized by an irrational fear of or aversion toward sex with subsequent avoidance of sexual contact. It is important to differentiate this disorder from hypoactive sexual desire disorder.

Premature ejaculation is characterized by persistent and recurrent absence of voluntary control over ejaculation, with the result that the individual ejaculates before he wishes to do so. The treatment of premature ejaculation involves training the individual to tolerate high levels of excitement without ejaculating and reducing anxiety associated with sexual arousal. One successful intervention is the start–stop technique. This technique involves having the patient lie on his back while his partner strokes his penis. When the patient feels that he is about to ejaculate, he signals his partner to stop stimulation. The patient should start–stop at least four times prior to ejaculation.

Chapter 19

Adjustment Disorders and Impulse Disorders Not Otherwise Classified

DIRECTIONS: Each of the statements or questions is followed by five suggested responses or completions. Select the one that is the best choice or most complete answer in each case.

19.1 One of the major catalysts for the development of a standard diagnostic system for adjustment disorders was:

- **A.** World War I
- **B.** the Vietnam conflict
- **C.** World War II
- **D.** the American Civil War
- **E.** the Korean conflict

19.2   Which of the following statements is true regarding the use of the BICEPS principles (brevity, immediacy, centrality, expectance, proximity, and simplicity) in the treatment of adjustment disorders associated with combat?

    A.   The therapeutic focus should be on underlying neurotic conflict.

    B.   Delaying treatment for more than 72 hours following the stressor is likely to enhance therapeutic response.

    C.   The therapeutic approach should focus on the discussion of present events.

    D.   The soldier should be treated as a "patient" to clearly define the individual as being psychologically unstable.

    E.   None of the above.

19.3   Of the adjustment disorders defined in the *Diagnostic and Statistical Manual of Mental Disorders (Third Edition-Revised) (DSM-III-R)*, which has been found to have the poorest outcome?

    A.   adjustment disorder with anxious mood

    B.   adjustment disorder with mixed emotional features

    C.   adjustment disorder with depressed mood

    D.   adjustment disorder with disturbance of conduct

    E.   adjustment disorder with work (or academic) inhibition

19.4   Which of the following is true regarding adjustment disorders, as defined by *DSM-III-R*?

    A.   The prognosis for these disorders may not be as benign as was originally suspected.

    B.   Adjustment disorders are rare phenomena.

    C.   Adjustment disorders usually do not resolve within six months following the removal of the stressor.

    D.   Adjustment disorders may occur without any discernible stressor.

    E.   None of the above.

19.5   Which of the following are true regarding the use of behavioral treatments of compulsive gambling?

    A.   Behavioral treatments have been found to be overwhelmingly effective.

    B.   There has been a trend away from single procedures to the use of a multimodal approach.

    C.   Aversive treatments have been more effective than other techniques.

    D.   Systematic desensitization has been found to be highly effective.

    E.   None of the above.

19.6   Which of the following is not included as a *DSM-III-R* diagnostic criterion for kleptomania?

    A.   an increasing sense of tension immediately before committing the theft

    B.   experiencing pleasure or relief at the time of committing the theft

    C.   The theft is not committed due to a conduct disorder or antisocial personality disorder.

    D.   The stolen items are taken for personal use or monetary gain.

    E.   Stealing is not secondary to a manic episode.

DIRECTIONS: For each of the statements below, one or more of the alternative answers is correct. Choose answer:

    A   if only 1, 2, and 3 are correct
    B   if only 1 and 3 are correct
    C   if only 2 and 4 are correct
    D   if only 4 is correct
    E   if all are correct

19.7   As classified in *DSM-III-R*, adjustment disorder and impulse control disorders not elsewhere classified share the following features:

    1. Both disorders are quite common.
    2. Both disorders are often triggered by stressors.
    3. Both categories of psychiatric disorders respond to the same treatment strategies.
    4. Both the diagnostic criteria and the individual disorders contained in these two classifications have changed as our understanding of them has increased.

19.8　The following factors have been found to play an important role in determining who will experience an adjustment disorder:

1. intensity of the stressor
2. the quality of the support system
3. the vulnerability of the individual
4. severity of the stressor

19.9　The following are thought to be essential features common to all impulse control disorders not elsewhere classified:

1. There is a failure to resist an impulse, drive, or temptation to perform the act.
2. There is an increasing sense of tension or arousal before the act is committed.
3. The patient experiences pleasure, gratification, or relief at the time of committing the act.
4. The act does not often lead to personal danger or to danger to others.

19.10　Treatment approaches to pyromania have included:

1. psychoanalytically oriented psychotherapy
2. structured fantasy with positive reinforcement
3. stimulus satiation
4. positive reinforcement with the threat of punishment

19.11　Which of the following are true regarding compulsive gamblers?

1. The overwhelming majority are men.
2. Compulsive gamblers often have parents who suffer from the disorder.
3. Compulsive gamblers are often described as being competitive and optimistic.
4. Compulsive gamblers and alcoholics often have similar premorbid personality structures.

19.12　Which of the following statements are true regarding trichotillomania?

1. This disorder is most common in children.
2. This disorder is more common in men than in women.
3. This disorder is often associated with nail biting, hair biting, or automutilation.
4. Most cases of this disorder in children do not resolve without psychiatric treatment.

DIRECTIONS: Each of the following questions consists of lettered headings followed by a list of numbered alternatives. Select the single lettered heading that is most closely associated with the appropriate numbered alternative. Each lettered heading may be chosen only once.

Adjustment disorder

A. Adjustment disorder with mixed disturbance of emotions and conduct
B. Adjustment disorder with mixed emotional features
C. Adjustment disorder not elsewhere classified
D. Adjustment disorder with physical complaint
E. Adjustment disorder with depressed mood

Description

19.13 is characterized predominantly by tearfulness, hopelessness, and dysphoria
19.14 is characterized predominantly by a combination of affective symptoms and behavior control difficulties
19.15 represents a residual diagnosis within the diagnostic category
19.16 is new in *DSM-III-R* and may be confused with somatoform disorder
19.17 is characterized predominantly by a combination of symptoms of anxiety and depression

ANSWERS

19.1 The answer is **C.**

One of the major catalysts for the development of a standard diagnostic system was World War II. Psychiatrists with military experience returned to the United States having witnessed numerous psychiatric responses caused by combat stress. This, combined with general frustration in the field regarding the lack of consistent nomenclature within psychiatry, led to the creation of the standardized diagnostic system, the *Diagnostic and Statistical Manual of Mental Disorders (First Edition)*, in 1952.

19.2   The answer is C.

In 1929, Salmon and Fenton articulated the basic principles of crisis intervention important in the treatment of psychiatric sequelae of combat related experiences. The treatment principles were brevity, immediacy, centrality, expectance, proximity, and simplicity (BICEPS). The treatment approach is brief, usually 72 hours or less. Immediate recognition and treatment of stress-related symptoms are crucial. Delay in treatment usually results in an increase in symptom severity. Treatment occurs in a central area, where appropriate triage can occur. Soldiers are not treated as patients, because the sick role can lead to a continued avoidance of the stressor. In addition, the treatment team has the expectation that the soldier will return to useful function. Bonding with and support from the combat unit are essential for the psychological stabilization of the soldier. The therapeutic approach is uncomplicated and the focus is on the discussion of immediate events rather than on underlying neurotic or personality issues.

19.3   The answer is D.

Studies of adolescents receiving an adjustment disorder diagnosis yield more pessimistic results with regard to prognosis than do comparable studies with adult populations. For example, Masterson found that 62 percent of an adolescent population who had received an adjustment disorder diagnosis had either a moderate or severe impairment rating at five-year follow-up. Along similar lines, Andreasen et al. found that only 44 percent of an adolescent population were psychiatrically well at five-year follow-up. In general, research in the area suggests that regardless of age of patient, adjustment disorders with disturbance of conduct have a poorer outcome.

19.4   The answer is A.

Although there are currently no reliable studies on the epidemiology of adjustment disorders, these disorders are probably quite common. Estimates of incidence range from 4.8 percent of psychiatric conditions to approximately 19 percent. Further research into the epidemiology and prognosis of adjustment disorders is clearly needed in this area, but existing research suggests that the prognosis for adjustment disorders may not be as benign as was originally suspected.

19.5   The answer is **B**.

Behavioral treatments, particularly aversive therapy, have been used to treat compulsive gamblers. However, a review of the literature on aversive treatments reveals disappointing results. For example, McConaghy compared aversive therapy with imaginal desensitization and found the latter to be more effective. In addition, there has been a general trend away from the use of single limited procedures such as aversion therapy toward a multimodal approach to therapy.

19.6   The answer is **D**.

The *DSM-III-R* diagnostic criteria for kleptomania are as follows: failure to resist impulses to steal objects; objects are not stolen for personal use or for their monetary value; an increasing sense of tension immediately before committing the theft; experiencing pleasure or relief at the time of committing the theft; the theft is not committed to express anger or revenge; and the theft is not due to antisocial personality disorder. Besides kleptomania, the differential diagnosis for thievery includes ordinary stealing, antisocial personality disorder, conduct disorder, manic episode, and malingering. Individuals with organic mental disorder, schizophrenia, or depression may also be referred by the court for psychiatric evaluation following an alleged theft.

19.7   The answer is **C**.

Although adjustment disorders and impulse control disorders not elsewhere classified differ in frequency (adjustment disorders are quite common whereas impulse control disorders not elsewhere classified are relatively rare), the diagnoses in these categories share certain features. First, adjustment disorders are precipitated by a psychological stressor, and impulse control disorders are often modulated directly by the severity of the psychological stressor. In addition, both the diagnostic criteria and the individual disorders in these two classifications have changed as research has broadened our understanding of them.

19.8   The answer is **E**.

There are several factors that appear to play an important role in the determination of who will experience an adjustment disorder following a stressful event. These factors include the severity or intensity of the stressor, the quality of the support system available to the individual, and the vulnerability of the individual to development of an adjustment disorder. The direct relationship between the intensity of the stressor and the development of psychiatric sequelae has been well documented, especially by military psychiatrists. The quality of the support system is important in both the development of adjustment disorders and in their outcome. For instance, it is well known within military psychiatry that the higher the "esprit de corps" of the unit, the lower the number of psychiatric casualties. The vulnerability of the individual to development of an adjustment disorder has also been recognized as an important factor and may have constitutional as well as psychological underpinnings.

19.9   The answer is A.

The essential features common to all impulse control disorders not elsewhere classified are 1) a failure to resist an impulse, drive, or temptation to perform some act that is harmful to the person or others; 2) an increasing sense of tension or arousal before committing the act; 3) the experience of pleasure, gratification, or relief at the time of committing the act. The act is ego syntonic in that it is consonant with the immediate conscious wish of the individual. Immediately following the act there may or may not be genuine regret, self-regret, or guilt.

19.10   The answer is E.

Although most writers on the treatment of pyromania approach this diagnostic group from a psychoanalytic perspective, many behaviorally oriented researchers have used aversive therapy to treat firesetters. Still others have used positive reinforcement with threats of punishment, stimulus satiation, and operant structured fantasies with positive reinforcement.

19.11   The answer is E.

It is estimated that one percent of the adult male population are compulsive gamblers, and *DSM-III-R* places the prevalence at two to three percent of the adult population. It is likely that equal numbers of women and men gamble, but the vast majority of compulsive gamblers are men. In addition, pathologic gambling is more common in the fathers of men with the disorder and in the mothers of women with the disorder. Predisposing factors listed in *DSM-III-R* include inappropriate or inconsistent parental discipline, exposure to gambling as an adolescent, a family who places a high value on material symbols, and a family who places a low emphasis on savings, budgeting, and future financial planning.

19.12   The answer is B.

Trichotillomania (the pulling out of one's own hair) is mostly found in children and young adults. In a 1986 study, Oranje found the female-to-male ratio of this disorder to be 2.5 to 1. He also found that 25 percent of the children with this disorder had associated onychophagy (nail biting), trichophagy (hair biting), or automutilation. Most cases of trichotillomania in young children resolve spontaneously. However, the course and prognosis of trichotillomania in adults are unknown.

19.13 The answer is **E**.
19.14 The answer is **A**.
19.15 The answer is **C**.
19.16 The answer is **D**.
19.17 The answer is **B**.

The predominant symptoms associated with adjustment disorder with depressed mood are those of a minor depression. For example, the symptoms might be depressed feelings, tearfulness, and feelings of hopelessness.

The diagnosis of adjustment disorder with mixed disturbance of emotions and conduct is made when the disturbance combines affective and behavioral features of adjustment disorder with mixed emotional features (anxiety and depression) and adjustment disorder with disturbance of conduct characterized by violation of societal expectations or norms.

Adjustment disorder not elsewhere classified is a residual diagnosis within the diagnostic category. This diagnosis can be used when a maladaptive reaction that is not classified under other adjustment disorders occurs in response to stress.

Adjustment disorder with physical complaint is a new diagnostic category in *DSM-III-R*. It was added because the criteria for all of the somatoform disorders require a duration of at least six months. The clinical symptoms include headache, backache, fatigue, or other aches and pains.

A diagnosis of adjustment disorder with mixed emotional features is given when the predominant complaints are a combination of depressive symptoms and anxiety or other emotions.

Chapter 20

Personality Disorders

DIRECTIONS: Each of the statements or questions is followed by five suggested responses or completions. Select the one that is the best choice or most complete answer in each case.

20.1 Which one of the following statements regarding personality disorders is not true?

- **A.** Personality disorders are patterns of inflexible and maladaptive traits.
- **B.** Personality disorders significantly impair the ability of the patient to adjust to and accommodate stress.
- **C.** Personality disorders are, by definition, time limited.
- **D.** Personality disorders cause significant impairment in social or occupational functioning.
- **E.** Personality disorders are maladaptive ways of thinking, feeling, and behaving.

20.2   What has been the most common method of classifying personality disorders in psychiatry?

  A.   a dimensional personality classification on the basis of responses of self-report instruments
  B.   a categorical model based on laboratory research
  C.   an empirically derived system based on differences in observed patterns of interaction with other individuals
  D.   a categorical model based on theoretical formulation and clinical observations
  E.   empirically derived and statistically validated clusters of types

20.3   Common assessment methods for the diagnosis of personality disorders do not include:

  A.   laboratory test results
  B.   clinical interview
  C.   semistructured interviews
  D.   self-report inventories
  E.   projective assessment methods

20.4   Which of the following treatment approaches focuses on personality structure?

  A.   chemotherapy
  B.   systems
  C.   cognitive
  D.   rational–emotive therapy
  E.   psychodynamic

20.5   Which of the following statements regarding the schizotypal personality disorder is not true?

  A.   Schizotypal personality disorder was a new addition to the *Diagnostic and Statistical Manual of Mental Disorders (Third Edition) (DSM-III)*.
  B.   It is a pattern of odd behavior, speech, thinking, and perception.
  C.   The schizotypal patient is typically withdrawn and avoidant.
  D.   Nearly all schizotypal patients have a family history of schizophrenia.
  E.   Recent research has focused on biological markers of schizotypal personality disorders.

20.6 Why are schizoid patients unlikely to be seen in psychotherapy?

    A. They are usually given pharmacotherapy only.

    B. Due to downward drift, few of these patients possess the resources to pay for therapy.

    C. They have little motivation for change and lack the ability to establish rapport with a therapist.

    D. The expression of anger typical of these patients precludes intimate interpersonal relations such as found in psychotherapy.

    E. Generally, their adjustment problems are not severe enough to warrant therapy.

20.7 Research on paranoid personality disorder suggests that it may have a biogenetic association with:

    A. major affective disorder

    B. schizophrenia

    C. avoidant personality disorder

    D. borderline personality disorder

    E. inadequate personality disorder

20.8 Which of the following is not a characteristic of narcissistic personality disorder?

    A. insensitivity to the evaluation of others

    B. expressions of grandiosity

    C. low empathy

    D. preoccupation with fame and wealth

    E. shallowness

DIRECTIONS: For each of the statements or questions below, one or more of the alternative answers is correct. Choose answer:

    A if only 1, 2, and 3 are correct

    B if only 1 and 3 are correct

    C if only 2 and 4 are correct

    D if only 4 is correct

    E if all are correct

20.9   Which of the following has been proposed as an explanation for the low base rate of schizoid personality disorder?

1. a low actual rate of the disorder
2. a low rate of presentation to mental health professionals
3. annexation of the symptoms by the avoidant and schizotypal personality disorders
4. the monothetic diagnostic criteria in *DSM-III*

20.10   Which of the following personality disorders have been criticized for being sex biased?

1. self-defeating personality disorder
2. histrionic personality disorder
3. dependent personality disorder
4. schizotypal personality disorder

20.11   Antisocial personality disorder is a pattern of:

1. disregard for social norms
2. social withdrawal
3. failure to conform to the law
4. suffocatingly close interpersonal relationships

20.12   Borderline personality disorder is characterized by:

1. a pattern of superficial interpersonal relationships
2. affective instability
3. rigid personal values
4. self-destructive behaviors

20.13   Type A personality style shares characteristics with which personality disorders?

1. avoidant
2. narcissistic
3. paranoid
4. obsessive-compulsive

20.14   Research has indicated which pattern(s) of covariation of avoidant personality disorder?

1. large covariation with schizoid personality disorder
2. little covariation with schizoid personality disorder
3. little covariation with borderline personality disorder
4. large covariation with dependent personality disorder

20.15 Which of the following therapy approaches have been found to be useful with avoidant personality disorder?

1. insight therapy
2. client-centered therapy
3. cognitive techniques
4. neuroleptic pharmacology

20.16 Which of the following can be considered characteristic of dependent personality disorder?

1. an extreme desire to be alone
2. a tendency to make impulsive and ineffective decisions
3. rigidity of thought resulting in stubbornly resisting the suggestions of others
4. failure to demonstrate assertive behavior

DIRECTIONS: Each of the following questions consists of lettered headings followed by a list of numbered alternatives. Select the single lettered heading that is most closely associated with the appropriate numbered alternative. Each lettered heading may be chosen only once.

Personality disorder

A. Self-defeating personality disorder
B. Obsessive-compulsive personality disorder
C. Passive-aggressive personality disorder
D. Sadistic personality disorder

Description

20.17 involves indirect resistance to authority
20.18 is characterized by behavior demeaning to others
20.19 includes disinterest or boredom with success
20.20 is characterized by behavioral rigidity

ANSWERS

20.1   The answer is **C**.

Personality disorders can be thought of as relatively enduring patterns of inflexible and maladaptive behavioral traits. Personality disorders result in markedly impaired social and occupational functioning. They can also be thought of as maladaptive ways of thinking, feeling, and behaving that significantly impair the ability of the person to adjust to and accommodate to stress. By definition, these disorders are not time limited.

20.2   The answer is **D**.

Psychology and psychiatry have two different traditions of classifying personality disorders. Psychiatry's most common method of classification involves a categorical model based on theoretical formulation and clinical experience. Here the definition of a personality disorder posits the definition of an ideal type that is usually an exaggeration of the manifestations seen in clinical practice. This ideal type is an exemplar against which actual clinical presentations are compared for similarity.

In psychology the most common method of classifying personality disorders involves categorizing patients on a dimensional basis secondary to the responses of the patient to a self-report inventory. This method is consistent with the psychometric tradition of psychology. Some of the more common dimensions include Cattell's 16 source traits; Eysenck's neuroticism, introversion–extroversion, and psychoticism traits; Murray's basic human needs; Millon's biosocial taxonomy; and Leary's interpersonal circumplex.

20.3   The answer is **A**.

The most common method of diagnosing personality disorders has traditionally been the clinical interview. The semistructured interview is also used, and may be preferred by some because the standardized method of asking predetermined questions may increase reliability. Other methods include self-report inventories and projectives, although the utility of projectives may be limited to the diagnosis of borderline personality disorders. In general, laboratory testing has not been found to be useful.

20.4   The answer is **E**.

The traditional treatment approach to personality disorders used by psychiatrists has been psychodynamic therapy. Psychodynamic therapy focuses on restructuring the personality. Interpersonal therapies such as systems and family therapies are applicable to treatment of personality disorders because their focus on interpersonal behavior attacks the symptoms that tend to be salient in personality disorders. Behavioral and cognitive therapies are also useful and tend to be symptom focused. Chemotherapy can be helpful in targeting certain symptoms of personality disorders such as the affective features of borderline personality disorder, the cognitive–perceptual dysfunctions in schizotypal personality disorder, and the anxiety in avoidant personality disorder.

20.5   The answer is **D**.

Schizotypal personality disorder was a new diagnosis in the *DSM-III*. It is characterized by a pattern of peculiar and odd behavior, speech, thinking, and perception. Usually these patients are withdrawn and avoidant. They may have mild parnoid tendencies and inappropriate or constricted affect. Current conceptualizations of the schizotypal personality disorder view it as a phenotypic variant of a schizophrenic genotype, even though many schizotypal personality disorder patients are negative for a family history of schizophrenia. Current research is pursuing the identification of a biological marker for the schizotypal personality disorder.

20.6   The answer is **C**.

Patients with schizoid personality disorder are unlikely to be seen in therapy, mainly because they lack the motivation for change, have little insight, and lack the ability to establish a rapport with the therapist. In fact, if one of these patients does become involved in therapy, it is likely that what is being treated is a misdiagnosed case of avoidant personality disorder. Despite the aloofness of the schizoid patient, attempts by the therapist to provide warmth and genuine caring may be successful in finally reaching the patient. Behavioral shaping of social behavior can be helpful in the treatment of these individuals. One unfortunate aspect of the patient with schizoid personality disorder is that the symptoms that cause the discomfort may also make therapy extremely difficult.

20.7   The answer is **B**.

Recent research on the paranoid personality disorder indicates that it may share a biogenetic association with schizophrenia and other paranoid disorders. There may be a continuous spectrum of schizophrenic disorders where paranoid personality disorder is a characterologic manifestation of a genetic predisposition. Certain theorists have suggested a learning–behavioral model of the acquisition of paranoid personality disorder. In this conceptualization, a process of learned suspiciousness leads to withdrawal and ruminative suspiciousness which is reinforced by the critical and avoidant responses of others in the social environment. The inadequate personality disorder is a diagnosis from the *DSM-II* that was not retained in the *DSM-III*.

20.8   The answer is **A**.

Narcissistic personality disorder is characterized by expressions of grandiosity, entitlement, exploitation, shallowness, and low empathy. These individuals are preoccupied with fame, fortune, and magnificent accomplishments and achievements. They tend to be oversensitive to the criticisms of others and react to even mild criticism with shame, rage, humiliation, or expressions of grossly indifferent denial that the opinions of others matter. Patients with narcissistic personality disorder tend to be arrogant and conceited, but at the same time are envious of others. They also require constant attention and admiration.

20.9   The answer is **E**.

The schizoid personality disorder is practically ubiquitous in most taxonomies. However, there are questions raised as to whether to keep this diagnosis in the *DSM* because of the rarity of its actual diagnosis. There are several proposed reasons why the schizoid personality disorder may be rarely diagnosed. One reason is that it may actually have a low rate of occurrence. Another proposed reason involves the requirement of *DSM-III* that all such patients show certain of the associated symptoms. This problem may have been alleviated by the *DSM-III-R*, which does not require that all patients with this diagnosis be void of any warm feelings. Another reason may be that these patients rarely present in mental health settings. Perhaps the most pertinent reason is that many patients previously diagnosed as schizoid are now likely to be diagnosed as avoidant or schizotypal personality disorders.

20.10   The answer is **A**.

The diagnostic criteria for personality disorders are meant to be objective and impartial. However, there have been criticisms regarding the criteria of some of the categories of personality disorders. The best known example involves the criteria for histrionic personality disorder. Some theorists have suggested that the histrionic personality disorder may be the feminine phenotypic manifestation of an underlying genotype whose masculine version is antisocial personality disorder. Both of these disorders are thought to have a disinhibition. In the female this disinhibition may be reflected through sexual seductiveness, affective lability, and manipulation of others. In the male the disinhibition may be reflected by impulsivity, aggressive behavior, drug abuse, and numerous shallow sexual relationships. Some theorists have suggested that the histrionic personality disorder may be a caricature of feminine stereotypes.

Likewise the criteria for self-defeating personality disorder have been criticized as being biased against women. The original title of this disorder was masochistic personality disorder. However, that name was changed because of the historical notion of masochism as a primarily feminine trait. There is some concern that the diagnosis of self-defeating personality will lead clinicians to blame the victim in spouse abuse situations. Certainly, there is potential to misuse this diagnosis, and application of the diagnosis should be carefully evaluated.

The diagnosis of dependent personality disorder is more frequently given to women than to men. It has been proposed that this differential of diagnosis is due to masculine ideas regarding what is healthy behavior as well as the use of stereotypic feminine behavior in the criteria of *DSM-III*. Yet another reason may be that clinicians, who are predominantly male, may not recognize masculine dependent behavior.

20.11   The answer is B.

The hallmark of antisocial personality disorder is behavior that is in disregard for the usual norms of social behavior, rather than the avoidance of social contact. In fact, the patient with antisocial personality disorder may be quite "social" and superficially charming. However, the patient with antisocial personality disorder exhibits a constellation of behaviors that are socially irresponsible and exploitative of others. These individuals do not show signs of guilt over their behaviors. They fail to conform their behavior to the law as well as to social mores. As might be expected, they do not tend to form stable relationships. They have unstable work histories. If they are parents, these individuals do not function as responsible caregivers, and their charges often have to rely on neighbors or other individuals for food or shelter. They tend to have a series of shallow sexual relationships.

20.12   The answer is C.

The borderline personality disorder is characterized by an inefficiency in interpersonal and occupational functioning due to dysfunctional relationships and problems of identity. There is usually a series of intense and chaotic relationships, rapidly changing affective states, and fluctuations between extremes of attitudes regarding other people. The borderline may fluctuate between idealization of another person and vilification of that same individual. Their life histories usually reflect a pattern of self-destructive behavior, and they appear to have little insight into the effect of such behavior on themselves. Patients with borderline personality disorder often lack a clear sense of identity or life plan. Their life values are also indeterminate.

The diagnostic criteria for borderline personality disorder require a pervasive pattern of unstable mood, interpersonal relations, and self-image beginning in early adulthood and manifested in a variety of contexts. The criteria also require that at least five of the following eight categories of symptoms be present: 1) unstable and intense relations characterized by alternation between idealization and devaluation of the other person; 2) impulsiveness in at least two areas that are self damaging (for example, sex, finances, shoplifting); 3) affective instability, with affective states lasting a few hours to a few days; 4) inappropriate, intense anger; 5) recurrent suicidal gestures or self-mutilatory behavior; 6) marked and persistent identity disturbance; 7) chronic feelings of boredom or emptiness; and 8) frantic efforts to avoid real or imagined abandonment.

20.13   The answer is D.

The Type A behavioral style is marked by intense ambition, a sense of time urgency, and competitiveness. These individuals are easily aroused to anger and hostility. There is a large association with early cardiovascular disorders. It can be seen that there is some overlap between the concept of Type A behavior and the concept of the obsessive-compulsive personality disorder.

The obsessive-compulsive personality disorder is characterized by behavioral rigidity and affective constriction. These individuals are perfectionistic, overly disciplined, and formalistic. Although they tend to intellectualize and attend to small details, their output is marred by circumstantiality. They have ruminative doubts about their ability and are plagued by indecisiveness. Their rigid style tends to interfere with their efficiency and productivity.

20.14   The answer is C.

Originally it was thought that there would be problems in differentiating the schizoid personality disorder from the avoidant personality disorder. That is because both disorders have social withdrawal as an important characteristic. However the reasons for this common characteristic vary across the two disorders. The schizoid personality disorder patient withdraws because of a lack of interest; the avoidant personality disorder patient withdraws because of insecurity and anxiety surrounding social interaction. It should be noted that the patient with avoidant personality disorder usually has a strong desire to form interpersonal relations, but is unable to do so.

More recent research has indicated that there is little covariation of the schizoid personality disorder with the avoidant personality disorder. However, there appears to be substantial overlap between the avoidant personality disorder and the dependent personality disorder. Both of these disorders share insecurity in personal relations, a strong desire for interpersonal relationships, and low self-esteem.

20.15 The answer is **B**.

Both cognitive approaches and insight-oriented therapy are useful in the treatment of the patient with an avoidant personality disorder. These patients have extremely high standards for themselves amd tend to feel that other individuals apply the same standards to the patient. Acknowledging the unrealistic nature of these thoughts and feelings is helpful in removing them. Cognitive techniques can be aimed at challenging the assumptions of inadequacy and threat. Assertiveness training, social skills training, and systematic desensitization may all be helpful in removing the symptoms of shyness and social introversion.

20.16 The answer is **D**.

Far from having a strong desire to be alone, the patient with a dependent personality disorder tends to rely excessively on another individual for emotional support, even to the extent that these patients will let others make important decisions for them. They tend to feel helpless when left alone. They act submissively, will subordinate their needs and desires to those of other individuals, and will tolerate mistreatment from others in order to remain in their company. They will demean themselves in order to gain acceptance. These patients will fail to behave appropriately in those situations that require assertive behavior.

These patients have difficulty initiating projects on their own. They are easily hurt by criticism, even if the criticism is offered in a humorous vein. They will agree with the prevailing opinion rather than state their own opinion and, in their minds, risk rejection. They tend to be preoccupied with fears of being abandoned.

20.17 The answer is **C**.
20.18 The answer is **D**.
20.19 The answer is **A**.
20.20 The answer is **B**.

Self-defeating personality disorder is characterized by chronic pessimism, a submissive and acquiescent attitude, and a resignation to failure, suffering, defeat, and exploitation. Self-defeating individuals tend to be bored with or disinterested in success and in developing supportive relationships. They believe that their misfortunes are deserved, justified, expected, and unavoidable. They tend to place themselves in situations and relationships that may be harmful, painful, disappointing, or abusive. They are difficult to treat because they expect treatment to fail and will behave in such a way as to contribute to that failure.

Obsessive-compulsive personality disorder patients tend to show a combination of extreme orderliness, parsimoniousness, and obstinacy. These individuals tend to be behaviorally rigid and perfectionistic. They are effectively constricted, overly disciplined, and formalistic. Their work and interpersonal behavior patterns are marked by intellectualization, circumstantiality, and attention to small detail. They devote themselves to their work, often neglecting family and friends. Other people are likely to view these individuals as formal, stiff, domineering, and stubborn. They are often plagued by indecisiveness as they search for the perfectly right answer.

Patients with passive–aggressive personality disorder tend to be passively and indirectly resistant to authority, demands, obligations, and responsibilities. They tend to respond to requests for compliance with dawdling, procrastinating, and forgetting engagements. Others see these patients as irritable, whining, argumentative, and discontented. They do not express their negative emotions directly, but instead express them through resistant and negativistic behavior. When asked to do something, they may respond slowly or with sloppy work methods. They have unreasonable criticism of people in authority and often complain that others' demands are excessive.

The sadistic personality disorder is a new addition to the *DSM-III-R*. It is marked by the tendency to be demeaning to others, aggressive, and exploitative. There may be evidence of physical cruelty and violent behavior. Persons with this disorder engage in both public and private humiliation of other individuals. Their cruel behavior cannot be understood as being instrumental or in the pursuit of some goal. Instead they seem to derive pleasure from the humiliation and pain of other people. They are usually domineering and controlling in relationships. They seem to be fascinated by symbols of aggression.

Chapter 21

Disorders Usually First Evident in Infancy, Childhood, or Adolescence

DIRECTIONS: Each of the statements or questions is followed by five suggested responses or completions. Select the one that is the best choice or most complete answer in each one.

21.1 Attention-deficit hyperactivity disorder (ADHD):
- **A.** rarely leads to antisocial personality disorder in adulthood
- **B.** may be a presentation of fetal alcohol syndrome or lead poisoning
- **C.** is associated with conduct disorder in less than half of ADHD cases
- **D.** generally responds poorly to antidepressant medications
- **E.** is rarely seen in Tourette's disorder

21.2 Conduct disorder:
- **A.** can be a presentation of mood disorder in children
- **B.** responds poorly to limit setting
- **C.** appears rarely with developmental reading disorder
- **D.** is defined by criminal behavior
- **E.** none of the above

21.3 Separation anxiety disorder is associated with:

    A. school absenteeism in rare cases
    B. a low rate of anxiety or mood disorder in the parents
    C. successful antidepressant treatment in some cases
    D. good adult outcome in virtually all cases
    E. developmental reading disorder

21.4 Tourette's disorder:

    A. has a waxing and waning presentation in rare cases
    B. is always associated with coprolalia
    C. cannot be seen in association with ADHD
    D. is associated with high rates of adult unemployment
    E. none of the above

21.5 Mental retardation:

    A. appears equally prevalent in all socioeconomic classes
    B. is often due to Fragile X Chromosome syndrome in females
    C. is often associated with treatable concomitant psychopathology.
    D. is defined as having an IQ below 70
    E. is often reversible

21.6 Autistic disorder:

    A. is typically the result of faulty parenting
    B. rarely occurs with seizure disorders
    C. does not respond to treatment interventions
    D. might be associated with antibodies to serotonin receptors
    E. none of the above

21.7 Language and speech disorders:

    A. occasionally appear with concomitant Axis I diagnoses in childhood
    B. are generally transient disorders of childhood
    C. can result from mild persistent hearing loss in some cases
    D. can be appropriately treated without prior general medical evaluation
    E. none of the above

21.8   Standardized assessment instruments generally:

A.   show few discrepancies between child and parent reports of psychopathology
B.   show parents are invariably more reliable reporters of psycho-pathology than children
C.   are less systematic and complete than routine clinical evalua-tions
D.   suggest that parents and children offer useful but different observations
E.   have not been found to be useful in the assessment of child psychopathology

DIRECTIONS: For each of the statements below, one or more of the alternative answers is correct. Choose answer:
A   if only 1, 2, and 3 are correct
B   if only 1 and 3 are correct
C   if only 2 and 4 are correct
D   if only 4 is correct
E   if all are correct

21.9   Which of the following are characteristics of oppositional defiant disorder?

1. disrespect for the personal rights of other people
2. argumentative and disobedient behavior
3. infrequent association with ADHD
4. a self-defeating stand in arguments

21.10   Which of the following are characteristics of overanxious disorder?

1. anxiety, worrying, and tension
2. perfectionistic style
3. habit disturbances
4. multiple somatic complaints

21.11 Which of the following are true regarding ADHD?

1. Motoric hyperactivity, inattention, and emotional lability are common.
2. Hyperactive children demonstrate a much higher level of motoric activity than do normal children in settings such as gym and recess.
3. Children with ADHD tend to be impulsive, with the level of impulsivity increasing with emotional and sensory stimulation.
4. "Overflow" into impulsivity is usually more evident at home than in the classroom.

DIRECTIONS: Each of the following questions consists of lettered headings followed by a list of numbered alternatives. Select the single lettered heading that is most closely associated with the appropriate numbered alternative. Each lettered heading may be chosen only once.

Childhood disorder

A. Functional encopresis
B. Cluttering
C. Reactive attachment disorder
D. Stereotypy

Description

21.12 is a disorder of speech dysfluency involving excessive rate and rhythm, resulting in the condensation of sounds and the collapsing of words

21.13 is an elimination disorder involving fecal soiling after age 4

21.14 is characterized by abnormal interpersonal behavior and emotional excitability following emotional abuse by a caretaker

21.15 involves repetitive and purposeless motor behavior that causes functional interference or injury to the child

ANSWERS

21.1   The answer is **B**.

There are a variety of neuromedical etiologies of ADHD. These include brain damage, neurological disorder, low birth weight, and exposure to neurotoxins. Intrauterine exposure to toxic substances, including alcohol or lead, can have significant effects of behavior. Symptoms associated with fetal alcohol syndrome often include hyperactivity, impulsivity, and inattention as well as physical anomalies.

Conduct disorder is seen in 70 percent of children with ADHD. Aggressivity, behavioral disorders, and subsequent antisocial personality disorder are commonly seen in association with ADHD. Children formally diagnosed as "attention deficit disorder without hyperactivity" only occasionally have conduct disorder.

There is an overrepresentation of ADHD in Tourette's disorder (20 to 60 percent of male Tourette's patients have ADHD). Obsessive-compulsive disorder is also probably overrepresented in children with ADHD.

With regard to treatment, approximately, 75 percent of children with ADHD respond to psychostimulants or antidepressants.

21.2   The answer is **A**.

Conduct disorder is the most common diagnosis of children and adolescents in both clinic and hospital settings. The syndrome is not a single medical entity but rather the final pathway for a variety of forms of misbehavior. Conduct disorders can result from biopsychiatric disease (mood disorders, psychosis), organic impairment, or personality disorders.

Academic underachievement is typical in association with conduct disorders and can be related to disorders such as developmental reading disorder and expressive language disorder.

With regard to the treatment of conduct disorder, it is important that a containment structure is established and limits are set to provide safety to both the child and others. Creating or reinforcing these limits can involve parent counseling, psychiatric treatment of parents, increased supervision at home, or the use of legal measures.

21.3   The answer is **C**.

In separation anxiety disorder, cognitive, affective, somatic, and behavioral symptoms of anxiety appear in response to genuine or fantasied separation from attachment figures. This disorder is thought to be one of the major sources of school absenteeism. Separation anxiety disorder appears to run in families and over half of children with separation disorder have parents with mood or anxiety disorders.

Although the use of antidepressant medications in children with separation anxiety disorder is common, there have been no large-scale studies of the effectiveness of antidepressant drugs with this population. However, antidepressants are probably effective in treating school absenteeism when the underlying etiology is separation anxiety disorder.

Follow-up studies of separation anxiety disorder are currently not available, but it is presumed that there is a high risk for the development of mood or anxiety disorders in this diagnostic group.

21.4 The answer is **D**.

Tourette's disorder is a lifelong disease entailing vocal and multiple motor tics. There is a typical course of waxing and waning symptoms over time, with much variation in symptom severity. Classical coprolalia (obscene language) is observed in 60 percent of patients with this disorder with an initial appearance in early adolescence. Copropraxia (complex obscene gestures) may appear later, as coprolalia resolves.

Attention-deficit hyperactivity disorder and conduct disorder are often associated with Tourette's disorder. Obsessive-compulsive disorder is also commonly observed in conjunction with Tourette's disorder. With regard to occupational attainment in Tourette's patients, up to 50 percent of adult Tourette's patients are unemployed.

21.5 The answer is **C**.

The definition of mental retardation encompasses three features: a) subaverage intelligence (IQ of 70 or below), b) impaired adaptive functioning, and c) childhood onset. Mental retardation is often associated with treatable accompanying psychopathology and there is a two- to fourfold increase of psychiatric disorders in mentally retarded individuals, compared with the "normal" population. Diagnoses such as ADHD, pica, stereotypy/habit disorder, cluttering, and stuttering often accompany mental retardation. However, mentally retarded patients receive less treatment for their concomitant psychopathology than do other groups, because of low expectations, economic limitations, and difficulties in managing complex organizational systems. With regard to the epidemiology of mental retardation, severe and profound mental retardation are distributed evenly across all socioeconomic classes, but mild retardation is much more common in lower socioeconomic classes.

Fragile X Chromosome syndrome is a newly described and common disorder, which is the second most common genetic cause of moderate and severe mental retardation. It accounts for 40 percent of male predominance in moderate and severe mental retardation.

21.6 The answer is **D**.

Autistic disorder presents with a wide spectrum of symptoms and varying severity. The classical form of this disease was described by Kanner as a disorder characterized by infantile onset, profoundly disturbed social relations, communication disruption, motor abnormalities, affective disturbance, massive cognitive impairments, multiple behavioral oddities, distorted perceptions, and bizarre thoughts. This disorder is thought to be genetically and biologically mediated; there is no evidence that psychological factors or parenting abnormalities cause this disorder. Neurochemical assays suggest a decrease in urinary catecholamines and an increase in dopamine metabolite (HVA) in cerebrospinal fluid. There is also an elevation in blood serotonin, which appears to be a stable trait that remains present for decades. However, the elevated blood serotonin level does not appear to correlate with specific clinical features.

With regard to the treatment of autism, the availability of educational and supportive services has a marked beneficial impact. For less severe cases, some adaptive skills can be learned. Social skills training (in mild cases) may permit blending into ordinary social life.

21.7 The answer is **C**.

Communication problems are usually chronic disorders observed in approximately 7 to 12 percent of the general population, and are common in individuals who have psychiatric disorders, hearing disorders, or mental retardation (about 50 percent of children with language and speech disorders have concomitant Axis I diagnoses and another 20 percent show a subsequent appearance of developmental disorders). Hearing loss plays a large role in the etiology of language and speech disorders, presumably because hearing is crucial for the development of speech and language. Evaluation of communication disorders should include language and speech assessment as well as medical, psychiatric, social, and developmental work-up.

21.8 The answer is **D**.

Structured and semistructured interview protocols, checklists, questionnaires, and rating scales have been developed for the evaluation and follow-up of many childhood psychiatric disorders and may often be useful as a supplement to the clinical evaluation of children. However, standardized instruments can yield findings that are often different from clinical evaluations and are more systematic and complete than clinicians in scanning for certain disorders. Children and parents each contribute useful but different observations. In general, children are more effective in reporting mood symptoms, and parents are more effective in reporting behavioral symptoms. However, features of conduct disorder may be reported at higher rates either by children or by parents, depending on the clinical situation.

21.9   The answer is **B**.

Children with oppositional defiant disorder show argumentative and disobedient behavior but, unlike children with conduct disorder, respect the personal rights of others. A crucial feature of the oppositional struggling seen in this disorder is the self-defeating stand that these children take in arguments. For instance, they may be willing to lose something they want (such as a toy), rather than lose the struggle.

21.10   The answer is **E**.

In addition to anxiety, worry, and tension, children with overanxious disorder often appear shy, self-doubting, and self-deprecating. Some of these children appear hypermature and overly serious, sometimes having the behavioral mannerisms of older children. Perfectionism and excessive compliance to authority with superficial pride and confidence are also common characteristics. These children often have concomitant habit disturbances such as nail biting, hair pulling, thumb sucking, and enuresis. Multiple somatic complaints and excessive attention seeking behaviors are also common.

21.11   The answer is **B**.

Major symptoms of ADHD include motoric hyperactivity, impulsivity, inattention, and emotional lability. The naturalistic observations of children with this disorder show that motor activity is high across various environmental settings and is most different from normal children in structured classroom situations. Children with ADHD tend to be impulsive in all settings, and the degree of impulsivity varies across settings, increasing with sensory or emotional stimulation. "Overflow" into impulsivity is particularly clear in the classroom.

21.12   The answer is **B**.
21.13   The answer is **A**.
21.14   The answer is **C**.
21.15   The answer is **D**.

Cluttering is a form of speech dysfluency disorder that involves excessive rate and irregular rhythm of speech, resulting in the condensation of sounds and the collapsing of words. Speech is slurred and is not distinct. The rate of speech is rapid and fluctuating. In addition to articulation problems, there are also often organizational and syntactic difficulties reflected by repetitious form and missing or extraneous linguistic elements. This disorder influences not only speech but also reading and writing.

Functional encopresis is an elimination disorder that includes fecal soiling of clothes, voiding in bed, and excretion onto the floor. This disorder occurs after age 4, by which time full bowel control is developmentally expected. Functional encopresis during the daytime is much more common than nocturnal encopresis. Stomachaches, large stools, and chronic constipation are commonly seen. Since medical causes for encopresis need to be excluded prior to labeling the problem as "functional," medical evaluation is a necessity.

This disorder is defined as abnormal interpersonal behavior following physical or emotional abuse by a caretaker and is characterized by a variety of behavioral, cognitive, and affective presentations. In children, odd social responsiveness, weak interpersonal attachment, apathy, or inappropriate excitability are common. However, any failure of normal development may be labeled as reactive attachment disorder providing it is clearly preceded by failure in ordinary care of the child. Infants with this disorder appear lethargic and show little body movement or activity. Sleep is excessive and disrupted. Weight gain is slow. The infants often resist being held and there is often little interest in the environment. In older children, this disorder often presents with socialization defects.

Examples of stereotypies and habits include head banging, body rocking, hand flapping, whirling, stereotyped laughing, thumb sucking, hair fingering, face touching, eye poking, object biting or self-biting, self-scratching, self-hitting, teeth grinding, and breath holding. It is common for several stereotypies to co-occur, and different stereotypies may become more prominent at different times. Frequency of stereotypies may increase during periods of tension, frustration, boredom, isolation, or just before bedtime. Two of the most common stereotypies are head banging and body rocking.

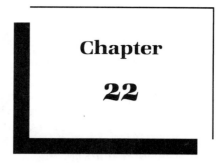

Chapter

22

Sleep Disorders

DIRECTIONS: Each of the statement or questions is followed by five suggested responses or completions. Select the one that is the best choice or most complete answer in each case.

22.1 Typically, cycles of rapid eye movement (REM) and non-rapid eye movement (NREM) sleep last:

- **A.** approximately 60 minutes
- **B.** between 25 and 60 minutes
- **C.** approximately 90 minutes
- **D.** between 75 and 95 minutes
- **E.** between 70 and 100 minutes

22.2 As sleep becomes deeper in a sleep session:

- **A.** the overall incidence of slow waves in the electroencephalogram (EEG) increases
- **B.** the overall incidence of slow waves in the EEG remains constant
- **C.** the overall proportion of slow-wave activity approaches 20 percent
- **D.** the overall incidence of slow waves decreases
- **E.** the overall proportion of slow waves plateaus at 35 percent

22.3 Stage 2 sleep is characterized by:

   A. the reduction of slow-wave activity
   B. relatively regular conjugate eye movement
   C. the appearance of spindles and K-complexes in the EEG
   D. desynchronous EEG activity
   E. preponderance of alpha rhythm activity in the EEG

22.4 Which of the following statements regarding REM sleep is not true?

   A. REM sleep is characterized by the loss of thermoregulation.
   B. Brain oxygen consumption rises during REM sleep.
   C. Penile erections typically occur during REM sleep.
   D. Skeletal muscle tone is greater in REM than in NREM sleep.
   E. Heart rate is more variable during REM sleep than during wakefulness.

22.5 The effects of prolonged REM sleep deprivation are:

   A. unknown
   B. fatal
   C. decreased cognitive efficiency
   D. related to a disruption of normal mood
   E. primarily related to the rebound effect

22.6 The effects of aging on sleep do not include:

   A. decreases in the ability to achieve long uninterrupted periods of sleep
   B. inability to achieve depth of sleep
   C. increases in daytime sleeping
   D. a shift of REM sleep into earlier parts of the sleep session
   E. a more concentrated distribution of REM sleep

22.7 The incidence of sleep disorders in the general population is estimated to be:

   A. greater in males than in females
   B. around one percent
   C. between 16 and 17 percent
   D. between 10 and 12 percent
   E. somewhat greater than 20 percent

22.8   The sleep patterns associated with depressive disorders include:

   A.   lack of the REM rebound effect
   B.   an abbreviated first NREM period
   C.   smaller proportion of Stage 2 relative to Stage 3 sleep
   D.   shortened overall REM incidence
   E.   greater proportion of Stage 2 relative to Stage 3 sleep

DIRECTIONS: For each of the statements or questions below, one or more of the alternative answers is correct. Choose answer:

   A   if only 1, 2, and 3 are correct
   B   if only 1 and 3 are correct
   C   if only 2 and 4 are correct
   D   if only 4 is correct
   E   if all are correct

22.9   The most common sleep/wake complaint(s) is (are):

   1. insomnia
   2. sleep apnea
   3. excessive daytime sleepiness
   4. delayed sleep phase syndrome

22.10   In contrast to the *Diagnostic and Statistical Manual of Mental Disorders (Third Edition-Revised) (DSM-III-R)*, the Association of Sleep Disorders Center groups sleep disorders into which of the following categories?

   1. disorders of initiating and maintaining sleep
   2. disorders of excessive sleepiness
   3. disorders of the sleep/wake cycle
   4. parasomnias

22.11   Which of the following statements regarding narcolepsy/cataplexy are not true?

   1. There are approximately 20,000 narcoleptics in the United States.
   2. Narcolepsy is a time-limited disorder.
   3. Narcolepsy is associated with cataplexy in 20 to 30 percent of the cases.
   4. The rapid descent from wakefulness into REM sleep is an essential characteristic of narcolepsy.

22.12   Which of the following statements regarding parasomnias is true?

1. The most common parasomnias of childhood are myoclonus, early morning awakenings, and night terrors.
2. Parasomnias are more common in young boys than in young girls.
3. Parasomnias are no more common in proband families than in the general population.
4. Parasomnias are benign.

22.13   Routine interventions for sleep disorders include:

1. attention to sleep/wake hygiene
2. psychoactive drug detoxification
3. stimulus control
4. use of sedative hypnotic drugs

22.14   The *DSM-III-R* includes which categories in its classification of sleep disorders?

1. disorders of initiating and maintaining sleep
2. dyssomnias
3. disorders of excessive daytime sleepiness
4. parasomnias

22.15   Which of the following statements regarding myoclonic sleep disorder are true?

1. Approximately 5 percent of patients with chronic insomnia suffer from myoclonic sleep disorder.
2. When recorded in the laboratory, many of these patients show paradoxically deep sleep EEGs.
3. Observations by bed partners are not useful in the assessment of this disorder.
4. Propoxyphene may hold promise for treatment of this disorder.

DIRECTIONS: Each of the following questions consists of lettered headings followed by a list of numbered alternatives. Select the single lettered heading that is most closely associated with the appropriate numbered alternative. Each lettered heading may be chosen only once.

Sleep disorder diagnoses

A. severe obstructive sleep apnea syndrome
B. narcolepsy–cataplexy
C. delayed sleep phase syndrome
D. conditioned or learned insomnia
E. insomnia associated with central nervous system depressant dependency

Suggested treatments

22.16 methylphenidate, imipramine
22.17 detoxification
22.18 modified, chronic tracheotomy
22.19 stimulus control
22.20 chronotherapy

ANSWERS

22.1 The answer is **E.**

There are three basic states in the operation of a healthy functioning human central nervous system. These three states are waking and the two sleep states of rapid eye movement (REM) and non-rapid eye movement (NREM). The sleep and wake states show a lifelong pattern of cycles lasting slightly more than 24 hours. The two sleep states show a cycle lasting between 70 and 100 minutes. REM sleep states occupy approximately 20 to 25 percent of total sleep time, and NREM states occupy the remaining 75 to 80 percent of total sleep time.

22.2   The answer is **A**.

NREM sleep appears to occur in four stages. Stage 1 is drowsiness and is best conceptualized as the passage from wakefulness to sleep. Stage 2 occupies about 50 percent of total sleep time. Stages 3 and 4 are known as slow-wave sleep and are characterized by the presence of at least 20 percent slow-wave or delta activity in the EEG. Stage 4 is characterized by between 20 and 50 percent delta-wave activity. Therefore, it can be seen that as sleep becomes deeper in the sleep session, the overall proportion of slow-wave activity in the EEG tracing increases.

22.3   The answer is **C**.

Stage 2 sleep is identified by the presence of characteristic EEG activity known as sleep spindles and K-complexes. The arousal threshold of Stage 2 is less than that in Stages 3 and 4. Relatively regular conjugate eye movements occur in REM sleep, and in fact it is these eye movements that give REM sleep its name. The preponderance of alpha-wave activity characterizes wakefulness. Desynchronous EEG patterns also occur in REM sleep.

22.4   The answer is **D**.

Skeletal muscle tone is actually decreased in REM sleep compared with that in NREM sleep. Heart rate, respiration rate, and blood pressure all show greater variability during REM sleep than during NREM sleep or wakeful states. Brain oxygen consumption rises during REM sleep, and REM sleep also shows increases in the arousal threshold to inspired carbon dioxide. Brain oxygen consumption in NREM sleep is approximately equal to that in waking states. The arousal threshold increases in NREM sleep as the preponderance of slow-wave EEG activity increases. Penile erections and the presence of regular lateral eye movements are also found in REM sleep. The loss of thermoregulation characterizes REM sleep. Humans report having been dreaming following awakening 80 percent of the time when such awakenings occur during REM sleep.

22.5   The answer is **B**.

REM sleep appears to have an essential function in mammals. Prolonged REM deprivation is followed by death in rats. A hypermetabolic state precedes death in these cases. Some theorists have speculated that sleep is necessary for processes of energy regulation. Slow-wave sleep also appears to be important in the function of organisms. Sleep deprivation results in a slow-wave sleep rebound, but there is a diminished capacity for slow-wave sleep rebound in patients with affective disorders and schizophrenic disorders. There appears to be a correlation between the amount of slow-wave sleep rebound and improvement in mood following sleep deprivation in mood-disordered patients. There also appears to be an association between slow-wave sleep and anabolic steroid secretion.

The above observations have led some researchers to propose that there is some protective function of slow-wave sleep. For example, it may be possible that prolonged REM sleep deprivation results in the disinhibition of catabolic processes that overwhelm the anabolic processes of slow-wave sleep.

22.6   The answer is E.

Aging results in significant effects on sleep characteristics. Increased age is associated with decreased ability to attain long, uninterrupted periods of sleep and a decreased abililty to achieve deep sleep. There is an increase in the number of arousals during sleep as well as a decrease in slow-wave sleep associated with increased age. In healthy younger subjects, the greater preponderance of REM sleep occurs during the second half of sleep. As humans grow older, there is a shift of the proportion of REM sleep to the earlier sleep periods. As a result, the distribution of REM time becomes more evenly spread out over the total sleep period.

22.7   The answer is C.

It is estimated that between 16 and 17 percent of the population of the United States complain of a sleep problem at any given time. Approximately 15 percent of the population complain of sleep disturbance, usually insomnia, and the additional one to two percent complain of excessive sleepiness. There is a greater preponderance of sleep complaints in older individuals than in younger individuals. The more prevalent complaints in older individuals involve early morning awakenings and problems in maintaining sleep. The increase in sleep complaints and in use of sleeping medications that occurs with aging is more prevalent in females than in males. However, it may be that females are more likely to report sleep difficulties.

22.8   The answer is B.

Thirty-five percent of the patients seen in United States sleep centers are given psychiatric diagnoses. Several psychiatric diagnoses show associated impairment in sleep continuity and loss of slow-wave sleep. It is still unclear whether depressive disorders and schizophrenic disorders share common sleep disturbances. This is partly because although the sleep disturbances associated with depression have been fairly consistently documented, the data concerning schizophrenic disorders are less consistent.

Depressive disorders show a shortened first NREM period and a prolonged first REM period with increased density of rapid eye movements. The REM rebound effect is very robust in depressive disorders, with large increases in early REM sleep following REM sleep deprivation. Most patients with a depressive disorder (between 80 and 85 percent) show hyposomnia, with a maximum sleep efficiency of 85 percent. The other patients show hypersomnia, with sleep efficiency ratings of 95% or more.

22.9   The answer is **B**.

Insomnia and excessive daytime sleepiness are the two most common complaints among sleep disorders. Insomnia involves patient subjective complaints of restless, disturbed, or shortened sleep. In general, the sleep is experienced by the patient as nonrestorative. Excessive daytime sleepiness occurs when the patient complains of an inability to remain awake during the day. In these cases sleep occurs unintentionally and results in sleeping during inappropriate times.

The National Institutes of Health Consensus Conference on Insomnia recommends that the physician determine the correlates of the sleep disorder in order to help determine the etiology and plan the treatment. For example, the duration of the sleep complaint can help with the differential diagnosis because sleep complaints lasting less than two or three weeks are generally associated with transiently stressful periods in the patient's life. A sleep complaint that lasts longer than two or three weeks is most likely associated with a medical or psychiatric disorder.

22.10   The answer is **E**.

The ASDC classifies sleep disorders into four main groups: 1) disorders of initiating and maintaining sleep, 2) disorders of excessive sleepiness, 3) disorders of the sleep/wake cycle, and 4) parasomnias. The ASDC classification system is more detailed than the *DSM-III-R* system and relies more heavily on the use of laboratory testing to determine the etiology of the sleep disorder. The ASDC system also differentiates among the various physical causes of sleep disorders, but the *DSM-III-R* considers all of these disorders under the classification "hypersomnia related to a physical condition."

Patients with disorders of initiating and maintaining sleep (DIMS) tend to receive psychiatric diagnoses about 35 percent of the time, while the diagnosis of persistent psychophysiological DIMS is given another 15 percent of the time. Sleep-disordered breathing and periodic leg movements account for another 10 percent each. In 30 percent of the cases of DIMS, the disorder is related to a concurrent medical condition or to a disturbance in the perception of sleep by the patient without objective evidence of sleep disorder. Disorders of excessive sleepiness may be secondary to sleep-induced respiratory impairment or narcolepsy–cataplexy. Disorders of the sleep/wake cycle are commonly reported as the effect of jet lag or of changing work schedules. Parasomnias are more frequent in children and are usually benign, with the child outgrowing the disorder by adolescence.

22.11 The answer is **A**.

Narcolepsy–cataplexy affects 500,000 individuals in the United States. Narcolepsy–cataplexy has equal prevalence in men and women. The disorder usually occurs by the age of 30 years. The condition tends to be a lifelong affliction and to run in families. Narcolepsy (or precipitously occurring episodes of daytime sleep) becomes associated with cataplexy (temporary loss of muscle tone) in nearly 75 percent of the cases. This disorder can result in significant impairment in the areas of social, vocational, and psychiatric functioning. A characteristic of the condition is that the patient descends rapidly from wakefulness into REM sleep. As patients get older, fragmentation of nighttime sleep occurs.

The treatment of narcolepsy–cataplexy involves the use of stimulant medication or alerting tricyclic antidepressants. The physician should attempt to use the lowest possible effective dose. Frequent drug holidays may also be necessary in order to avoid problems associated with the development of tolerance.

22.12 The answer is **D**.

Sleepwalking, sleep terrors, and functional enuresis are the most commonly reported parasomnias of childhood. These disorders are much more common in boys than in girls and may coexist in the same child. They are also more common in the families of probands than in the general population. Parasomnias are disorders of partial arousal out of the lower levels of NREM sleep. Parasomnia symptoms tend to occur once each night. This fact is helpful in the differential diagnosis with epileptogenic parasomnias, which tend to occur more than once each night. The common parasomnias of childhood also tend to occur during the first two or three hours after initiation of sleep. These disorders are benign, and children tend to outgrow them by the time adolescence is reached.

22.13   The answer is **A**.

Routine clinical interventions for sleep disorders include attention to sleep/wake hygiene, psychoactive drug detoxification, stimulus control, temporal control, and treatment of any associated psychiatric disorders. If routine clinical interventions are not successful in treating the sleep complaints, referral to a sleep laboratory may be necessary. Detailed assessments in the sleep laboratory are necessary in the diagnosis of sleep-disordered breathing and abnormal periodic leg movements. Referral to a sleep laboratory is also necessary for the evaluation of complaints of excessive daytime sleepiness.

22.14   The answer is **C**.

In contrast to the ASDC classification system, the *DSM-III-R* has only two general categories of sleep disorders, namely, dyssomnias and parasomnias. The dyssomnias include the three ASDC categories of disorders of initiating and maintaining sleep, disorders of excessive sleepiness, and disorders of the sleep/wake cycle. The *DSM-III-R* definition of parasomnias specifies that the predominant disturbance is an abnormal event occurring during sleep. The various physical etiologies for hypersomniac conditions are not differentiated in the *DMS-III-R*.

22.15   The answer is **D**.

It is estimated that 10 percent of the individuals complaining of chronic insomnia have myoclonic sleep disorder. The most frequent complaint associated with myoclonic sleep disorder is "restless" legs, where the patient reports painful dysesthetic feelings in the muscles of the thighs or calves. Laboratory assessments of these individuals result in documentation of periodic leg twitches occurring about every 30 seconds. The leg twitches are associated with EEG microarousals, with resultant fragmentation of sleep. The patients complain of nonrestorative sleep, and the bed partners complain of being kicked. Clinical evaluations and interviews can be useful in the beginning stages of diagnosis for this disorder, but a laboratory evaluation is necessary in order for the definitive diagnosis to be made.

There is no agreement regarding the treatment of choice for myoclonic sleep disorder. However, there are data to suggest that propoxyphene may be useful in treating the restless leg syndrome. Other reports indicate that carbamazepine, phenytoin, vitamin E, and both long-acting and short-acting benzodiazepines may also be useful.

22.16   The answer is **B**.
22.17   The answer is **E**.
22.18   The answer is **A**.

22.19   The answer is **D**.
22.20   The answer is **C**.

Narcolepsy–cataplexy is a condition in which the patient complaints are of unintentionally falling sleep during the day, frequently occurring during times when the sleep episode interferes with vocational or social functioning. Narcolepsy–cataplexy is the second most common cause of excessive sleepiness, following only obstructive sleep apnea syndrome in the number of patients it affects. Narcolepsy–cataplexy is best diagnosed in the sleep laboratory where the characteristically rapid descent from wakefulness to REM sleep can be documented. The usual procedure is the multiple sleep latency test (MSLT). In the MSLT, the individual is asked to take four or five daytime naps spread out at two-hour intervals. Narcoleptics can fall asleep in under five minutes and demonstrate two or more sleep onset REM periods. The treatment of narcolepsy–cataplexy involves the use of drugs such as methylphenidate or imipramine. The lowest effective dose should be used and frequent drug holidays should be instituted.

Insomnia associated with central nervous system dependency should always be treated first with detoxification. Detoxification is considered to be a routine intervention for insomnia. The patient may start to use central nervous system depressants in order to self-medicate feelings of anxiety or to relax in order to fall asleep. The danger is that prolonged use of such depressants is associated with lengthening of the sleep onset latency.

Mixed obstructive sleep apnea syndrome occurs in between 50 and 60 percent of patients who complain of excessive daytime sleepiness. Laboratory evaluations of patients with obstructive sleep apnea syndrome show persistent effort in the presence of upper airway occlusion. Obstructive sleep apnea syndrome is more commonly seen in overweight, middle-aged, hypertensive males. In milder forms of the disorder, weight loss may be a sufficient treatment. In moderately severe instances of the disorder, training the patient to sleep on his side instead of his back may be helpful. However, severe cases require aggressive treatment because of the complications of the disorder, including systemic and pulmonary hypertension, cardiac arrhythmias, depression, organic mental syndromes, and impotence. Therefore severe cases may require modified chronic tracheotomy.

Conditioned or learned insomnia is also known as persistent psychophysiological insomnia. It is a condition of difficulty in initiating or maintaining sleep not due to another mental disorder or physical condition. These individuals worry about their sleep problems, sometimes to the extent that they seem obsessed about sleep. Conditioned or learned insomnia may result from another medical condition once the other condition is treated but the insomnia remains. About 15 percent of the individuals in sleep centers with chronic insomnia suffer from psychophysiological insomnia. Interventions include attention to proper sleep hygiene, temporal control, and stimulus control.

Delayed sleep phase syndrome is a condition characterized by an individual falling asleep later than is typical for the context. The body operates on a 26-hour circadian cycle. When that cycle is out of synchronization with the rest of society, a sleep phase syndrome may occur. Delayed sleep phase syndrome is more commonly seen in young adults, and advanced sleep phase syndrome is more commonly seen in older adults. The treatment for delayed sleep phase syndrome involves chronotherapy where a series of 26 or 27 hour cycles is imposed on the individual's sleep patterns until a congruence between the internal clock and the external time sequence is reached.

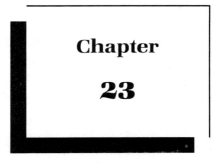

Chapter

23

Eating Disorders

DIRECTIONS: Each of the statements or questions is followed by five suggested responses or completions. Select the one that is the best choice or most complete answer in each case.

23.1 Eating disorders are best conceptualized as:

    A. a collection of behavioral abnormalities secondary to a disease process

    B. a set of abnormal behaviors generated by faulty learning histories

    C. problems in the self-control of eating-related behaviors

    D. syndromes classified on the basis of a cluster of symptoms

    E. psychiatric diseases secondary to disruptions of central nervous system catecholamines

23.2 Which of the following is not part of the current conceptualizations regarding eating behavior?

    A. Eating behavior is an interaction between physiological states and environmental variables.

    B. Normal eating behavior is determined by physiological variables; abnormal eating behavior is learned.

    C. Both normal and abnormal eating behavior are learned.

    D. Ambient temperature has an effect on eating behavior.

    E. The amount of storage tissue affects eating behavior.

23.3 Which of the following statements is not true?

A.   An early animal model of eating behavior involved food deprivation to induce eating.

B.   Microstructural analysis of feeding includes the recording of grooming behavior.

C.   Amphetamines decrease eating rate.

D.   Macroanalysis of eating behavior involves the measurement of long-term eating patterns in free-feeding animals.

E.   The role of stress in eating behaviors has been studied in animals.

23.4 Which of the following statements regarding the study of neurotransmitters in eating behavior is true?

A.   Serotonin facilitates satiety.

B.   High doses of dopamine increase feeding.

C.   Dopamine agonists stimulate eating behavior.

D.   Serotonin injected peripherally facilitates eating.

E.   Dynorphin, an endogenous kappa opioid receptor ligand, inhibits feeding.

23.5 Which of the following statements regarding anorectics is not true?

A.   Anorectics tend to hide food in their pockets and purses.

B.   Anorectics have an intense fear of gaining weight.

C.   Anorectics cut their food into very small pieces.

D.   Anorectics have a disturbance in the way they experience their body weight, shape, or size.

E.   Anorectics avoid all mention or thought of food.

23.6 The epidemiological studies of anorexia nervosa indicate that:

A.   although the reporting has increased, the rate of anorexia nervosa has remained relatively constant in the past 30 years

B.   only between 20 and 30 percent of the anorectic population is male

C.   in the 1970s the annual incidence rate of anorexia nervosa was around 3.7 percent

D.   in the last 30 years, the incidence of anorexia has increased in both the United States and Western Europe

E.   only between 5 and 10 percent of the anorectic population is male

23.7   The immediate treatment goal of therapy for anorexia nervosa is:

    A.   restore the patient to a normal nutritional state
    B.   intervene with the associated depressive affect
    C.   change the long-term eating habits of the patient
    D.   restructure the underlying abnormal personality
    E.   decrease the obsessive thoughts regarding food

23.8   Which of the following statements regarding bulimia is not true?

    A.   The word *bulimia* means binge eating.
    B.   Binge eating signals the presence of a psychiatric disorder.
    C.   The diagnosis of bulimia can be given even if the patient is already diagnosed as anorectic.
    D.   Bulimia can occur in normal-weight individuals.
    E.   Bulimic episodes can be interrupted by abdominal pain or discomfort.

23.9   The prevalence of bulimia nervosa among college and high school students is:

    A.   between .3 and .5 percent
    B.   between .5 and 1 percent
    C.   between .9 and 1.3 percent
    D.   between 2.6 and 5.1 percent
    E.   between 3.8 and 9 percent

23.10   Which of the following was not a result of the use of imipramine in a double-blind study of the treatment of bulimia nervosa?

    A.   reduced frequency of binges
    B.   reduced frequency of use of laxatives
    C.   decreased preoccupation with food
    D.   greater subjective global improvement
    E.   decreased depression

DIRECTIONS: For each of the statements or questions below, one or more of the alternative answers is correct. Choose answer:

    A if only 1, 2, and 3 are correct
    B if only 1 and 3 are correct
    C if only 2 and 4 are correct
    D if only 4 is correct
    E if all are correct

23.11 Which of the following statements regarding the epidemiology of obesity is true?

1. Socioeconomic status (SES) is unrelated to obesity.
2. Low SES men have a lower rate of obesity than higher SES men.
3. There is a higher prevalence of obesity among women as compared with men.
4. Obesity is associated with increased age until age 50.

23.12 What are the components of successful treatment of mild obesity?

1. behavior modification in groups
2. a balanced diet
3. exercise
4. gastric stapling

23.13 The treatment of choice for overweight children is:

1. the use of appetite suppressants
2. psychotherapy to treat poor self-image
3. exercise programs
4. behavior modification

23.14 Poor outcome in the treatment of anorexia nervosa is associated with

1. longer duration of illness
2. younger age of onset
3. poor childhood social adjustment
4. absence of previous psychiatric admissions

23.15 Medical complications in anorexia nervosa:

1. include lowering of serum enzymes
2. are secondary to the starvation state or purging behavior
3. are extremely difficult to reverse
4. may include carotenemia

23.16   Anorexia nervosa may develop following a period of extreme food deprivation that may be due to:

1. dieting in order to enhance physical appearance
2. dieting to increase athletic performance
3. food restriction secondary to severe stress
4. food restriction secondary to severe illness or surgery

23.17   Studies of the role of neurotransmitters in anorexia nervosa have implicated:

1. dysregulation of dopamine
2. dysregulation of serotonin
3. dysregulation of norepinephrine
4. dysregulation of neuropeptides

23.18   Cognitive techniques in the treatment of anorexia nervosa include:

1. decentering
2. modification of the patient's basic assumptions
3. prospective hypothesis testing
4. reinterpretation of body image misperception

23.19   Medical complications of bulimia nervosa:

1. are associated with the abuse of emetics and laxatives
2. may include atrophy of the parotid gland
3. may include electrolyte imbalances
4. may include elevated levels of potassium

23.20   Which of the following are medical complications of obesity?

1. increased rates of prostate cancer in men
2. congestive heart failure
3. increased rates of ovarian cancer in women
4. increased serum creatinine

ANSWERS

23.1 The answer is **D**.

Eating disorders are not diseases with a common cause, standard course, or consistent pathology. Eating disorders are best conceptualized as syndromes. The eating disorders are classified on the basis of whether or not a cluster of symptoms is present. Eating disorders appear to have existed since early in the history of western civilization. For example, there are many contemporary reports of binge eating in Roman times. There are also well-documented cases of anorexia nervosa in descriptions of early Christian saints.

23.2 The answer is **B**.

Current thought regarding eating behavior indicates that a systems conceptualization is perhaps the most useful one. Both normal and abnormal eating behaviors have physiological and environmental determinants. The hypothalamic centers appear to have both facilitatory and inhibitory effects on eating behavior. There appears to be a broad range of neuroregulator interactions that impinge on eating behavior. Satiety appears to be regulated by peripheral mechanisms associated with hormones released by the gastrointestinal and pancreatic systems.

Most investigators accept the idea that eating behavior is under the control of an interaction between an organism's physiological states and enviromental conditions. Included among the physiological variables are various neuropeptides and neurotransmitters. Metabolic rate, metabolic state, condition of the gastrointestinal system, amount of storage tissue, and sensory receptors for taste and smell all affect eating behavior. The pertinent environmental variables include the taste, texture, novelty, accessibility, and nutritional composition of the food; the presence of other people; level of stress; and the ambient temperature of the eating setting.

23.3 The answer is **C**.

There are currently several available models and methodologies for studying eating behavior. Early animal models for studying eating behavior included depriving animals of food in order to induce eating behavior and creating hypothalamic lesions for the same purpose. More recent work has developed techniques for using pharmacological agents to study the structure of feeding behavior. Still other studies have investigated the role of stress on eating in animals by inducing mild levels of stress using methods that include mild tail pinching.

Some studies record related behaviors such as drinking, grooming, locomotor activity, and resting, as well as eating behavior in a form of examination called microstructural analysis. The measurement of long-term free feeding patterns in naive animals that have never experienced food deprivation is called macroanalysis of feeding. Some of these studies have resulted in important information such as that although amphetamines increase eating rate, they inhibit the onset of eating.

23.4   The answer is A.

The adrenergic beta-2 receptors in the perifornical hypothalamus and the alpha-2 adrenergic receptors in the paraventricular nucleus appear to play a role in eating behavior. Serotonin appears to facilitate satiety. On the other hand, dopamine has a less simple relation to eating behavior. Administering low doses of dopamine or dopamine agonists stimulates feeding, but administering high doses of dopamine inhibits feeding. There is also evidence that administration of the endogenous kappa opioid receptor ligand, dynorphin, enhances feeding.

23.5   The answer is E.

Anorectic patients have an exaggerated fear of gaining weight and tend to be preoccupied with thoughts of food and self-denigrating thoughts about how fat they think they are. They express frequent concerns about how fat and flabby they are and spend much time looking at themselves in the mirror. They also tend to demonstrate denial.

Their preoccupation with food is manifested in collecting recipes and preparing elaborate meals for their families. They sometimes spend a great deal of time cutting their food up into very small pieces or rearranging their food on their plates. Anorectics also hoard and hide food. They often carry candy in their pockets or purses. They will attempt to dispose of their food surreptitiously rather than eat it.

Anorectics have a disturbance in the way they perceive their body weight, shape, or size. They feel that they are too fat even when other individuals perceive them as being emaciated. They may try to lose weight by decreasing their food intake. They may also exhibit associated obsessive behavior related to cleanliness.

23.6   The answer is D.

Recent epidemiological studies indicate that there has been an increase in the incidence of anorexia nervosa in the United States and Western Europe in the past 30 years. The average annual incidence rate in Monroe County, New York, increased from 0.35 per 100,000 in the 1960s to 0.64 per 100,000 in the 1970s. In London in the 1970s, the prevalence of anorexia nervosa was one severe case per 200 girls between the ages of 12 and 18. Between 4 and 6 percent of the population of anorectics are male.

Anorexia nervosa can be a very serious disorder. Long-term studies indicate that the morbidity rate is 6.6 percent at 10 years following the termination of treatment. At the 30 year follow-up, the death rate is 18 percent.

23.7   The answer is A.

The immediate treatment goal in anorexia nervosa is to restore the patient to normal nutritional status. Because being severely underweight can result in irritability, depression, and sleep disturbance, this first step can alleviate some of the associated problems. However, treatment cannot stop there. The therapist must obtain the patient's cooperation in a treatment plan.

Treatment of anorexia nervosa is necessarily multifaceted. There needs to be coordination of medical management: behavioral modification; individual, group, and family psychotherapy; and cognitive therapy. Behavior therapy is used to encourage small weight gains. A response prevention technique may be necessary to inhibit purging or vomiting behavior following eating. The cooperation of the family is extremely important in treating this type of problem.

23.8   The answer is C.

The word *bulimia* means overeating. However, the syndrome of bulimia nervosa usually also includes abuse of emetics or laxatives or manual means of eliciting vomiting following the binge episode. This practice has unfortunately become popular among college and high school age girls. Not all binge eating results in a psychiatric diagnosis. Bulimia and anorexia nervosa are distinct enough that it is possible for an individual with the diagnosis of bulimia to also receive a diagnosis of anorexia nervosa. However, many bulimics may have normal weight.

Binge eating is episodic, uncontrolled, rapid ingestion of enormous quantities of food in a short period of time. The bingeing episodes may be interrupted by abdominal pain or discomfort, self-induced vomiting, social interruption, or sleep. The patient often has feelings of guilt, depression, or self-disgust following the bingeing episode.

23.9   The answer is E.

There is a lack of sufficiently well-done studies on the incidence of bulimia. Part of this problem may be due to the fact that bulimia was first described as a distinct clinical entity in the 1980 *Diagnostic and Statistical Manual of Mental Disorders (Third Edition) (DSM-III)*. In addition, the criteria for bulimia in *DSM-III* did not differentiate between occasional episodes of binge eating and the psychiatric disorder of bulimia. The *DSM-III-R* does allow this distinction, and relevant studies may be forthcoming. The prevalence of bulimia nervosa among high school and college students is probably somewhere between 3.8 and 9 percent.

The prevalence of males among bulimics may be between 10 and 15 percent. The average age of onset for bulimia is 18 years. The range is between 12 and 35 years. There is a much higher percentage of social classes 4 and 5 among bulimia nervosa patients as compared with anorexia nervosa patients.

23.10   The answer is B.

Recent studies have demonstrated the utility of antidepressant medication in the treatment of certain bulimia nervosa patients. One double blind study using imipramine resulted in decreases in frequency of bingeing, lowered intensity of bingeing, decreases in preoccupation with food, decreases in levels of depression, and improvement in self-reported subjective global functioning. Another double blind study showed greater effects of desipramine in the frequency and intensity of bingeing episodes. A double-blind study of phenelzine resulted in significantly fewer binges in the treated group.

23.11   The answer is C.

Obesity is the condition of being overweight. Obesity is more common among women than among men. Considering only men, obesity is more common among men of lower socioeconomic status than among those of higher socioeconomic status. Obesity is also more common among children of lower socioeconomic status. The prevalence of obesity increases with age until the age 50.

23.12   The answer is A.

Mild obesity is the condition of being between 20 and 40 percent overweight. Treatment of obesity can be obtained from both nonprofit and commercial programs. The most efficient treatment of mild obesity is group behavioral therapy (behavior modification), institution of a balanced diet, and exercise. Behavioral treatment procedures include self-monitoring, nutrition education, physical activity, and cognitive restructuring. In setting up a behavioral program, it is necessary to conduct a behavior analysis in order to determine the antecedents and consequences of eating behavior. Extreme procedures such as gastric stapling are unnecessary in treating mild obesity.

23.13 The answer is **D**.

The treatment of choice for obesity in children is behavior modification. Both the school and the parents should be enlisted in any behavioral program for children. Although psychotherapy may be helpful for some patients who have related problems, psychotherapy is not generally recommended in the treatment of obesity in children.

23.14 The answer is **B**.

Long-term follow-up studies of the treatment of anorexia nervosa indicate that although there may be improvement in the medical condition of the patient, many still exhibit the characteristic psychological problems associated with anorexia nervosa. Poor outcome in the treatment of anorexia nervosa is related to longer duration of illness and older age of onset. In addition, a history of previous psychiatric admissions, poor childhood adjustment, premorbid personality problems, and disturbed relations between the patient and other family members are also associated with poor outcome.

23.15 The answer is **C**.

Most of the medical complications of anorexia nervosa are consequent to either the starvation state or to purging behavior. Most of the physiological and metabolic changes associated with anorexia nervosa are reversible following resumption of adequate nutrition. Abnormalities such as those in hematopoiesis (e.g. leukopenia and relative lymphocytosis) may be found in patients who are in an emaciated state. Elevation of serum enzymes reflective of fatty degeneration of the liver can be associated with both the emaciated state and the refeeding period.

Carotenemia is also seen in these patients. Amenorrhea is common in anorexia nervosa and may not be directly related to the weight loss. Elevated serum cholesterol levels can occur, especially in younger patients. If vomiting is associated with the anorexia, disturbances in electrolyte levels may result. Patients who abuse laxatives may develop hypokalemic alkalosis.

23.16 The answer is **E**.

It is unknown whether there is a specific etiology and pathogenesis preceding the development of anorexia nervosa. Episodes of anorexia nervosa occur following periods of severe food deprivation. This food deprivation may be due to dieting in order to become more physically attractive; dieting to increase athletic performance or professional competence in ballet dancers, jockeys, and gymnasts; food restriction secondary to severe stress; or food restriction secondary to severe illness or surgery. It is unknown why some individuals can experience these periods of food deprivation and not develop anorexia nervosa and why other individuals do develop anorexia nervosa.

23.17   The answer is A.

Investigations have shown that the neurotransmitters dopamine, serotonin, and norepinephrine have effects on eating behavior, satiety, and appetite. Other studies indicate that a dysregulation of each of these is implicated in the development of anorexia nervosa. However, it should be noted that the studies used indirect probes of neurotransmitter functions and the results may not reflect a central neurotransmitter dysfunction. There may be decreased levels of cerebrospinal fluid norepinephrine in long-term anorectics. There may also be a decreased serotonin turnover in bulimics compared with restricting anorectics.

23.18   The answer is D.

Cognitive therapy techniques for both individual and group therapy are being developed for application to the treatment of anorexia nervosa. First the patient's cognitions are assessed using a self-report format. These cognitions are then examined for distortions in the processing and interpretation of the thoughts. Techniques include operationalizing beliefs, decentering, the use of the "what if" technique, evaluating automatic thoughts, prospective hypothesis testing, reinterpretation of the body image misperception, and examination of the underlying assumptions of the patient followed by modification of the assumptions.

23.19   The answer is B.

There are many medical complications possible in bulimia nervosa, especially if the disorder is accompanied by self-induced vomiting or abuse of laxatives. These patients may develop hypokalemic alkalosis. There may also be electrolyte imbalances including elevated serum bicarbonate, hypochloremia, hypokalemia, and in some cases, lowered serum bicarbonate, which would be a sign of metabolic acidosis.

Dehydration in laxative abusers may result in the generation of aldosterone and further potassium excretion from the kidneys. Patients with electrolyte imbalance will report lethargy, weakness, and sometimes cardiac arrhythmias. Bulimia patients may also show attrition and erosion of the teeth, causing irritating sensitivity, exposed pulp, loss of dental arches, and diminished chewing ability.

Parotid gland enlargement secondary to serum amylase elevations may also be seen in patients who binge and purge. Bingeing may also result in dilatation of the stomach, although this is rare. Self-induced vomiting may result in esophogeal tearing. A very serious condition involves cardiac failure secondary to abuse of ipecac.

23.20 The answer is **A**.

Obesity affects many different functions of the body. Increased body weight may cause problems with blood circulation or, more dangerously, congestive heart failure. Obese individuals are more likely to develop hypertension and diabetes. Pulmonary function can be compromised with resultant hypoventilation, hypercapnia, hypoxia, and somnolence. Obesity may also hasten the development of osteoarthritis. Obesity is also associated with several different forms of cancer, including cancer of the prostate in men and ovarian cancer in women. Obesity is also associated with cardiovascular disease.

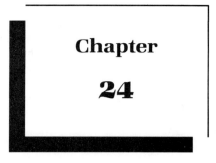

Chapter 24

Psychopharmacology and Electroconvulsive Therapy

DIRECTIONS: Each of the statements or questions is followed by five suggested responses or completions. Select the one that is the best choice or most complete answer in each case.

24.1 According to the prevailing theory regarding the mechanism of action of antipsychotic drugs, the effects of this class of drugs are:

- A. due to the presynaptic inhibition of serotonin
- B. likely to be due to the blocking of the binding of dopamine to the postsynaptic dopamine receptor in the brain
- C. currently unknown regarding neurochemical transmission
- D. due totally to drug side effects
- E. none of the above

24.2 The most significant risk factor for the development of tardive dyskinesia is:

- A. a drug history
- B. the presence of brain damage
- C. increasing age of the patient
- D. time since first exposure to antipsychotic drugs
- E. the presence of an affective disorder

24.3 A "therapeutic window" has been established for which of the following antidepressant medications?

    A. desipramine
    B. amitriptyline
    C. imipramine
    D. nortriptyline
    E. amoxapine

24.4 Which of the following antidepressant medications has been associated with irreversible priapism?

    A. trazodone
    B. amitriptyline
    C. nortriptyline
    D. phenelzine
    E. desipramine

24.5 The most widely studied beta-blocker that has been used for the treatment of aggressive behavior is:

    A. metoprolol
    B. pindolol
    C. nadolol
    D. propranolol
    E. none of the above

24.6 The mortality rate for patients who receive electroconvulsive therapy (ECT) is:

    A. 1 per 1,000
    B. 1 per 100,000
    C. 1 per 10,000
    D. 1 per 5,000
    E. 1 per 500

DIRECTIONS: For each of the statements below, one or more of the alternative answers is correct. Choose answer:

A   if only 1, 2, and 3 are correct
B   if only 1 and 3 are correct
C   if only 2 and 4 are correct
D   if only 4 is correct
E   if all are correct

24.7   Antipsychotic drugs are effective in treating which of the following conditions?

1. steroid psychosis
2. acute manic symptoms
3. organic brain disorders
4. acute exacerbations of borderline personality disorder

24.8   With regard to antipsychotic medications, drug potency refers to:

1. the milligram equivalence of drugs
2. the dosage that has been found to be efficacious in clinical trials and clinical practice
3. the affinities of the drug for the dopamine-2 receptor
4. the relative efficacy of the drug

24.9   Which of the following may be side effects of antipsychotic drugs?

1. dystonic reactions
2. akathisia
3. rabbit syndrome
4. akinesia

24.10   A complete trial of antidepressant medication should include:

1. treatment with therapeutic doses of the drug for a total of six weeks
2. concomitant use of antidepressant and antipsychotic medications
3. treatment with a therapeutic trial dose equivalent of 300 mg imipramine followed by a dose equivalent of 90 mg phenelzine before concluding that the depression is refractory to pharmacotherapy
4. concomitant use of a heterocyclic medication with a benzodiazepine

24.11 The depressed patient who has been refractory to standard antidepressant treatment:

1. may have been given an inadequate therapeutic trial with antidepressants
2. may respond to the addition of lithium carbonate
3. may respond to the addition of another class of antidepressant medication
4. may not be compliant with the medication regimen

24.12 Which of the following statements are true regarding the use of benzodiazepines in the treatment of anxiety?

1. These medications are useful because they do not lead to dependence.
2. These medications may cause sedation and impairment of mental alertness.
3. All benzodiazepines have similar half-lives.
4. All benzodiazepines are equally efficacious.

24.13 Which of the following statements are true regarding lithium therapy?

1. Lithium has been found to be very effective in the prevention of manic and depressive symptoms in patients with bipolar illness.
2. Lithium therapy may be initiated with concomitant neuroleptic therapy.
3. Lithium therapy is effective in the prevention of future depressive episodes in patients with unipolar illness.
4. Rapid-cycling bipolar patients have been found to respond particularly well to lithium therapy.

24.14 Electroconvulsive therapy may be advantageous over other treatment approaches for which patient(s)?

1. patients with delusional depression
2. patients who have suffered recent myocardial infarctions
3. patients whose affective symptoms have not responded to pharmacological treatment
4. patients with space-occupying cerebral lesions

DIRECTIONS: Each of the following questions consists of lettered headings followed by a list of numbered alternatives. Select the single lettered heading that is most closely associated with the appropriate numbered alternative. Each lettered heading may be chosen only once.

Side effects of psychiatric treatment

A. Retrograde amnesia
B. Nephrogenic diabetes insipidus
C. Orthostatic hypotension
D. Acute dystonic reaction

Treatment

24.15 can be caused by tricyclic antidepressants
24.16 can be caused by ECT
24.17 can be caused by antipsychotic medications
24.18 can be caused by lithium carbonate

ANSWERS

24.1 The answer is **B**.

The prevailing theory regarding the mechanism of action of antipsychotic drugs is based on the observation that all of the available medications in this class block the binding of dopamine to the postsynaptic dopamine receptor in the brain. The dopamine-2 (D-2) receptor, which is not linked to adenylate cyclase, is believed to be responsible for the action of antipsychotic drugs. In addition, there are delayed actions of these drugs on presynaptic dopamine activity that closely parallel the time course of the therapeutic action. The above-mentioned findings have been supported by the observation of increased dopamine concentrations and increased number of D-2 receptors in the brains of patients with schizophrenia.

24.2   The answer is **C**.

The most significant and consistently documented risk factor for the development of tardive dyskinesia is increasing age of the patient. Other risk factors may include a history of drug holidays, dose of antipsychotic medication, the time since first exposure to antipsychotic medication, the presence of brain damage, and diagnosis (especially the presence of affective disorders).

24.3   The answer is **D**.

Plasma level studies of antidepressant medications have focused on three principal medications: imipramine, nortriptyline, and desipramine. The American Psychiatric Association Task Force on Laboratory Tests in Psychiatry developed guidelines in 1985 for the use of plasma level monitoring. For an adequate therapeutic trial, plasma levels of imipramine and desipramine should be greater than 200 to 250 ng/ml. A therapeutic window has been observed for nortriptyline, with optimal response between 50 to 150 ng/ml. However, most patients respond to usual levels of antidepressants and do not require level monitoring.

24.4   The answer is **A**.

Trazodone is the only antidepressant that has been associated with priapism, which may be irreversible and require surgical intervention. However, sexual dysfunction is a common occurrence in patients treated with monoamine oxidase inhibitors and most frequently includes anorgasmia and impotence. Because sexual difficulties are not usually voluntarily disclosed by patients, the clinician should inquire about sexual functioning prior to initiating therapy, and also regularly during the course of treatment.

24.5   The answer is **D**.

With regard to the treatment of aggression, propranolol, a lipid-soluble, nonselective beta-adrenergic receptor blocker, has received more study than any of the other beta-blockers. Fourteen papers have reported controlled studies, open trials, or case reports involving its use in aggressive or violent patients. For example, Greendyke et al. reported a randomized, double-blind, placebo-controlled, crossover study of propranolol in 10 patients with organic brain disease secondary to trauma, tumor, alcoholism, encephalitis, or Huntington's disease. Five of these patients showed marked improvement with propranolol, while two showed moderate improvement, and two showed no improvement.

With regard to open trials of propranolol, Williams et al. retrospectively reviewed propranolol treatment of 30 children and adolescents with organic brain dysfunction. The authors reported moderate to marked improvement in greater than 75 percent of the patients.

Eight papers have been published that present case reports of a total of 21 patients whose aggressive outbursts responded to propranolol.

24.6   The answer is C.

The mortality rate of patients with ECT is one per 10,000 patients. The most frequent complaints of patients receiving ECT are memory impairment, headaches, and muscle aches, while the most significant risks associated with ECT are cardiovascular. Ictal and postictal fluctuations in autonomic tone may elicit cardiac arrhythmias of many varieties, including premature ventricular contractions during the immediate postictal period. In addition, patients with preexisting disorders such as space-occupying lesions, or other central nervous system dysfunctions, hypertension, or degenerative bone disease also are at increased risk for serious side effects related to ECT and should receive ECT only after careful evaluation by a nonpsychiatric medical specialist.

24.7   The answer is E.

Antipsychotic drugs are effective in treating psychotic symptoms that result from diverse etiologies such as affective disorders with psychotic features, drug toxicities such as steroid psychoses, and brain disorders such as Huntington's disease or post-head injury. Acute manic symptoms may also be effectively treated with antipsychotic drugs. Patients who suffer from borderline and schizotypal personality disorders may respond to brief treatment with antipsychotics. Patients with psychotic or delusional depression may be successfully treated with a combination of antipsychotic and antidepressant drugs, but not with antipsychotics alone.

24.8   The answer is A.

Drug potency refers to the milligram equivalence of drugs, not to the relative efficacy of the drug. The affinities of the antipsychotic drugs for the human brain D-2 receptors have been studied using radioligand binding techniques. The relative affinities of these agents for D-2 receptors correlate with the dose required to treat psychotic symptoms.

24.9   The answer is E.

Serious side effects of antipsychotic use result from the blockade of the postsynaptic dopamine receptor. The acute dystonic reaction is among the most disturbing adverse drug reactions and may involve the uncontrollable tightening of the face and neck and spasm and distortions of the patient's head and/or back.

Akathisia is an extrapyramidal disorder consisting of unpleasant feelings of restlessness and the inability to sit still. It is a common reaction and most often occurs shortly after the initiation of antipsychotic therapy.

Akinesia is defined by Rifkin as a "behavioral state of diminished spontaneity characterized by few gestures, unspontaneous speech, and, particularly, apathy and difficulty with initiating usual activities." This reaction may be mistaken for depression in patients treated with antipsychotic medications.

The rabbit syndrome consists of fine, rapid movements of the lips that mimic the chewing movements of a rabbit. This side effect occurs late in treatment with neuroleptics and is treated with anticholinergic drugs.

24.10   The answer is **B**.

A complete trial of antidepressant drugs consists of treatment with therapeutic doses of a drug for a total of six weeks. Quitkin has emphasized the necessity of treating depressed patients with a therapeutic trial of a dose equivalent of 300 mg of imipramine followed by a trial of a dose equivalent of 90 mg of phenelzine before concluding that depression is refractory to standard pharmacotherapy.

24.11   The answer is **E**.

A careful review of the clinical history and response to previous treatment often reveals that the depressed patient who has been refractory to treatment with standard antidepressants has had an inadequate therapeutic trial of the drug. Other common sources of treatment "resistance" include patient compliance and physician factors such as failure to educate the patient and his or her family about medication side effects.

24.12   The answer is **C**.

All benzodiazepines used for the treatment of anxiety are equally efficacious. Choice of a specific medication depends on the pharmacokinetics and pharmacodynamics of the drug. Diazepam, chlordiazepoxide, and clorazepate have half-lives that are several days in length. This may allow less frequent dosing than medications such as lorazepam and alprazolam, which have half-lives of 6 to 12 hours. Because of the tendency for benzodiazepines to cause excessive sedation and impairment in mental performance, this class of drugs should be used for as brief a period of time as possible.

24.13   The answer is **A**.

Lithium has been found to be effective in the treatment of many of the affective disorders. Acute manic episodes respond to lithium treatment within 7 to 10 days after initiation. Supplemental antipsychotic drugs are often administered on an acute basis. In addition, lithium has been shown to be effective in the treatment of both manic and depressive episodes in patients with bipolar affective disorders. Rapid-cycling bipolar patients have been reported to not respond well to lithium treatment. Patients with less severe bipolar illness, such as cyclothymia or bipolar II disorder, may also respond favorably to lithium therapy.

24.14   The answer is **B**.

Electroconvulsive therapy may be advantageous over other treatments in a) patients with severe affective disorders who have not responded to appropriate pharmacological treatment, b) patients with delusional depression, c) patients (particularly elderly) who cannot tolerate the side effects of antidepressant or antipsychotic drugs, d) patients whose acute symptoms are so severe that a rapid and dramatic treatment response is required, and e) patients with histories of depressive episodes that have responded to previous ECT treatment.

24.15   The answer is **C**.
24.16   The answer is **A**.
24.17   The answer is **D**.
24.18   The answer is **B**.

Among other side effects (blurred vision and dry mouth), many of the tricyclic antidepressant drugs may lead to significant orthostatic hypotension and cardiac conduction delays that may be critical in patients with a previous history of cardiovascular illness.

When the memory function of patients receiving ECT is studied carefully, it has been found that patients who experience retrograde amnesia have recovered complete memory function six months after treatment. For those patients who do not completely recover memory function, information acquired during the days or weeks prior to initiation of treatment may be permanently lost.

The acute dystonic reaction is one of the most dramatic and frightening side effects of antipsychotic drugs. This reaction most frequently occurs within hours or days of the initiation of therapy and consists of uncontrollable tightening of the patient's head and/or back.

The most noticeable effect of lithium on renal function is vasopressin-resistant impairment of the kidney's ability to concentrate urine. This is called nephrogenic diabetes insipidus and may result in polyuria. Up to 60 percent of patients taking lithium complain of increased frequency of urination.

Chapter

25

Individual Psychotherapies

DIRECTIONS: Each of the statements or questions is followed by five suggested responses or completions. Select the one that is the best choice or most complete answer in each case.

25.1 The goal of psychoanalysis is:

- A. the elucidation of the childhood neurosis as it presents itself in the transference neurosis
- B. regression back to the original precipitating traumatic experience
- C. provision of an effective treatment for severely disturbed patients
- D. acceptance of the patient's "character flaws"
- E. none of the above

25.2 The central principle of the cognitive theory of depression is that symptoms are the result of:

- A. conditioned reactions
- B. underlying neurotic conflict
- C. characteristic distortions in thinking
- D. unresolved oedipal experiences
- E. difficulties in interpersonal relationships

25.3　Which of the following is not characteristic of cognitive therapy, as described by Beck?

　　A.　the use of "collaborative empiricism"
　　B.　the invalidation of cognitive distortions
　　C.　the analysis of "automatic thoughts"
　　D.　the explanation of interpersonal dynamics
　　E.　a focus on irrational beliefs

25.4　The technique by which the therapist acts as an "auxiliary ego" for the patient is generally known as:

　　A.　confrontive psychotherapy
　　B.　rational–emotive psychotherapy
　　C.　supportive psychotherapy
　　D.　short-term psychoanalysis
　　E.　none of the above

25.5　Which of the following is thought to represent a contraindication for psychoanalysis?

　　A.　current preoccupation with resolving a crisis situation
　　B.　resistance to change by the patient
　　C.　the existence of an underlying neurotic style
　　D.　the existence of countertransference feelings in the analyst
　　E.　the existence of transference feelings toward the analyst

25.6　The rule of abstinence as defined in the practice of psychoanalysis refers to:

　　A.　abstinence from sexual activity between the analyst and analysand
　　B.　withholding of the patient's "wished for" gratification by the analyst
　　C.　avoidance of discussion of every-day events between the analyst and analysand
　　D.　condemnation of the analysand's wishes by the analyst
　　E.　none of the above

DIRECTIONS: For each of the statements below, one or more of the alternative answers is correct. Choose answer:

  A if only 1, 2, and 3 are correct
  B if only 1 and 3 are correct
  C if only 2 and 4 are correct
  D if only 4 is correct
  E if all are correct

25.7 The term *psychotherapy* can best be described as:

1. referring to changing behavior through the reorganization of mental structures
2. a term that specifically describes psychoanalytically oriented therapy
3. a generic term for a large number of treatment techniques whose primary means of affecting behavior is through verbal interchange
4. an outmoded form of treatment

25.8 Which of the following are techniques usually associated with psychoanalysis?

1. free association
2. analysis of defenses
3. dream analysis
4. implosion

25.9 Which of the following factors are thought to be important in the selection of patients for short-term anxiety-provoking therapy?

1. above-average intelligence
2. high motivation for change
3. The potential patient must have had at least one meaningful relationship during his or her lifetime.
4. The patient must have a specific chief complaint.

25.10 Which of the following are characteristics of Beck's "thinking disorders of depression"?

1. selective abstraction
2. inexact labeling
3. overgeneralization
4. magnification and minimization

25.11 Which of the following are characteristics of individuals who are likely to be candidates for supportive psychotherapy?

1. good impulse control
2. a history of poor interpersonal relationships
3. good reality testing
4. low capacity for introspection

DIRECTIONS: Each of the following questions consists of lettered headings followed by a list of numbered alternatives. Select the single lettered heading that is most closely associated with the appropriate numbered alternative. Each lettered heading may be chosen only once.

Brief psychotherapy model

A. Focal psychotherapy
B. Short-term anxiety-provoking therapy
C. Time-limited psychotherapy
D. Broad-focus short-term dynamic psychotherapy

Description

25.12 involves a focus on the oedipal conflict and may not be effective in treating patients who suffer from reactive depression following the loss of a loved one
25.13 has been used specifically with patients who suffer from long-standing obsessional and phobic neuroses and is often used with patients who have multiple psychiatric foci
25.14 emphasizes the importance of "finding the appropriate focus from what the patient offers" and "consistently approaching the focal problem with interpretive activity alone"
25.15 emphasizes the variable of time as a specific operative factor in psychotherapy as well as a curative element

ANSWERS

25.1 The answer is **A**.

The goal of psychoanalysis is the elucidation of the childhood neurosis as its manifests itself in the transference neurosis. This process requires a reasonably healthy individual to sustain the treatment. Psychoanalysis has often been criticized because it has most often been used to treat healthy and not seriously psychiatrically ill patients.

25.2 The answer is **C**.

The central principle of the cognitive theory of depression is that symptoms are the result of distortions in thinking. This position contrasts with traditional behaviorism, which views cognitions as irrelevant or unverifiable, and with psychoanalysis, which interprets cognitions in terms of deeper underlying meaning.

According to Aaron Beck, a cognitive theorist, depressed individuals have negative interpretations of the world, themselves, and the future (the negative triad). Depressed individuals typically interpret events as reflecting defeat, deprivation, or disparagement, and see their lives as filled with obstacles and burdens. In cognitive theory, the affective and motivational aspects of depression are not the primary symptoms but rather are secondary to the negative interpretation of events.

25.3 The answer is **D**.

Cognitive therapy, as conceptualized by Beck, is a directive, time-limited psychological treatment based on the following principles: a) that distorted, negatively biased thinking predisposes to and perpetuates depressed mood, b) that relevant thoughts are conscious and can be noticed and reported by the patient, and c) that the depressed mood can be lifted if the patient can be induced to relinquish his or her negative bias and become more logical and reality based in his or her thinking. The therapeutic model for accomplishing this is referred to as "collaborative empiricism," through which the therapist and patient work together to discover the patient's irrational beliefs and thinking patterns associated with his or her depression.

25.4 The answer is **C**.

The principle that underlies the technique of supportive psychotherapy is the principle of "substitutive psychotherapy"—the substitution of capacities by the therapist that the patient lacks. This is sometimes conceptualized as the therapist's acting as an "auxiliary ego" for the patient. The deficient ego capabilities for which substitution is needed may include basic elements of self-perception such as a stable sense of self over time and a clear recognition of boundaries between oneself and others. The auxiliary ego functions of the therapist appear in the form of suggestion, reinforcement, advice, reality testing, cognitive restructuring, and reassurance.

25.5 The answer is A.

Individuals who are in the midst of a personal crisis and are therefore very concerned and focused on the real events in their life should not enter psychoanalysis. Psychoanalysis focuses on the patient's experience of and fantasies of his or her life, rather than on real life events. A crisis situation does not allow the patient the opportunity to explore fantasies in any meaningful fashion.

25.6 The answer is B.

The analyst operates under several rules that facilitate the analysis of the transference. These include the rule of neutrality and the rule of abstinence. The rule of neutrality refers to the rule by which the analyst favors neither the patient's wishes (id) nor the condemnation of these wishes (superego). The rule of abstinence refers to the analyst's withholding gratification from the patient similar to that of the wished for object. Sandler has described transference as the role pressure placed on the analyst to conform to the behaviors of a significant individual in the patient's past. Abstinence is the avoidance of becoming this figure in reality and gratifying the wishes.

25.7 The answer is B.

The term *psychotherapy* is a generic term for a large number of treatment techniques whose primary means of affecting change is through verbal interchange. Psychotherapy is focused on changing behavior through the reorganization of mental structures. Through the process of this reorganization, both perception and behavior change.

25.8 The answer is A.

There are a number of techniques that are usually associated with psychoanalysis. First, free association is a major element in psychoanalysis. Freud has described free association as attempting to report all thoughts that come to mind without censorship and without thinking them too trivial. The analyst also focuses on analyzing the defenses the patient uses to minimize conflict and disturbing affects. Defenses such as intellectualization, denial, repression, and reaction formation are identified and repeatedly interpreted to the patient. Through the analysis of defenses, the transference grows in a manner that can be analyzed. Dream analysis is another important aspect of psychoanalytic treatment. Dreams provide an avenue to the understanding of unconscious phenomena.

25.9   The answer is E.

According to Sifneos, in order to be considered for short-term anxiety-provoking therapy, the patient must be of above-average intelligence and have had at least one meaningful relationship with another person during his or her lifetime. In addition, the patient must be highly motivated for change, not just symptom relief. The patient must have a specific complaint and must be able to identify one conflict area and postpone work on other than the identified area. The ability to do this is taken as an indication of the patient's ability to tolerate anxiety.

25.10   The answer is E.

Among others, Beck has identified the following as components of the "thinking disorders of depression":

Selective abstraction has been defined as the process of drawing conclusions about a given situation or event on the basis of a single detail, to the exclusion of other salient details.

Inexact labeling refers to the tendency to label events in proportion to one's own emotional response to them rather than according to the facts of a situation.

Overgeneralization refers to the tendency to draw a general conclusion about oneself on the basis of a single example.

Magnification and minimization refer to the process of grossly overestimating negative and underestimating positive aspects of situations.

25.11   The answer is C.

The typical candidate for supportive psychotherapy has significant deficits in ego functioning that include poor reality testing and poor impulse control. Poor reality testing refers to difficulty in separating fact from fantasy and a failure to recognize boundaries between oneself and others. Patients with poor reality testing may become psychotic under the stress of psychodynamic therapy and develop psychotic transferences. Poor impulse control refers to a need on the part of the patient to promptly discharge affects through actions that are often destructive to oneself or to others. These patients are not able to contain and examine feelings, as is required in change-oriented psychotherapies, and may bolt from psychotherapy when strong negative affects are aroused.

25.12   The answer is **B**.
25.13   The answer is **D**.
25.14   The answer is **A**.
25.15   The answer is **C**.

Short-term anxiety-provoking Therapy was developed by Peter Sifneos in the 1960s and 1970s. This form of brief therapy focuses on the oedipal conflict and emphasizes the importance of patient selection because of the anxiety-provoking nature of the techniques used. Sifneos further distinguishes anxiety-provoking from anxiety-suppressing therapy (supportive psychotherapy) and emphasizes the ability of the patient to identify one specific chief complaint as being important in selection for treatment. He also emphasizes that the individual must be of above-average intelligence to be efficaciously treated with short-term anxiety-provoking therapy and must have had at least one meaningful interpersonal relationship prior to undergoing this treatment.

Broad-focus short-term dynamic psychotherapy was developed by Habib Davanloo and has been used successfully with patients with an oedipal focus, a loss focus, or multiple foci. Davanloo has been especially interested in treating patients who suffer from longstanding obsessional and phobic disorders. During the therapy session, the emotional experience of the patient in the transference is emphasized. The patient is gently but relentlessly confronted about his or her defenses. The usual techniques of psychoanalytic psychotherapy are employed, including analysis of defenses, transference interpretations, and genetic reconstruction. Davanloo recommends from 5 to 40 sessions.

Focal psychotherapy is an example of applied psychoanalysis that has been developed by David Malan. This form of brief psychotherapy emphasizes the importance of choosing and maintaining a narrow focus in therapy and limiting the therapy to a brief period of time. Malan further emphasizes the importance of "finding the appropriate focus from what the patient offers" and "consistently approaching the focal problem with interpretive activity alone." To Malan, identification of a focal conflict is critical to the successful outcome of the therapy.

Time-limited psychotherapy, as developed by James Mann, focuses on the specific limitation of time in brief psychotherapy. Mann views the variable of time as a specific operative factor in psychotherapy as well as an element in its own curative effect. Usually, psychotherapy is limited to a total of 12 treatment hours. According to Mann, the selection of the central issue of therapy is an extremely important event. Mann looks for an issue that is developmentally and adaptively relevant and has been recurrent over time. The central issue formulated in terms of time, affect, and an image of the self is the "paradigm of the transference" that is expected to emerge in treatment.

Behavior Therapy

DIRECTIONS: Each of the statements or questions is followed by five suggested responses or completions. Select the one that is the best choice or most complete answer in each case.

26.1 Which of the following is not one of the basic principles underlying the conceptual basis for behavior therapy?

    A. Both normal and abnormal behaviors are assumed to be learned.

    B. The social environment is largely responsible for the development and maintenance of behaviors.

    C. Behavior change follows intrapsychic reorganization.

    D. The major focus of treatment is on the behavior problem itself.

    E. Therapy is based on a scientific approach to treatment.

26.2 Which of the following statements is the best synopsis of social cognitive learning theory?

    A. There is a reiterative relationship among environment, behavior, and personal and cognitive processes.

    B. The most effective learning occurs in social situations.

    C. Reinforcement is the automatic effect of reward from others in the social environment.

    D. Affective and adaptive functioning is mediated by the degree of social skills possessed by a person.

    E. Social behavior is largely learned.

26.3 Reciprocal inhibition is:

    A. the antagonistic relation between conflicting behavioral goals
    B. the cancellation of one behavior by its polar opposite
    C. the dampening effect anxiety has on free behaviors
    D. the use of social interactions to inhibit inappropriate behaviors
    E. eliciting a response incompatible with anxiety in the presence of another stimulus that usually elicits anxiety

26.4 Participant modeling occurs when:

    A. a patient is asked to model a behavior for the therapist, thereby increasing the probability that the behavior will occur outside the therapeutic situation
    B. a patient first observes and then attempts a previously difficult behavior, such as an approach to a fearful stimulus
    C. the therapist models appropriate behavior for the patient in a role-play situation
    D. professional confederates (or models) exhibit desired behaviors for the patient under the direction of the therapist
    E. members of a therapy group demonstrate appropriate and desired behaviors for each other

26.5 Long-term studies indicate that the standard psychotherapeutic treatment for phobia should be:

    A. implosion therapy
    B. flooding
    C. uncovering the dynamic meaning of the fear
    D. graded exposure therapy
    E. hypnotherapy

26.6 Which of the following statements regarding exposure therapy is not true?

    A. Couples training in communication skills enhances the effect of exposure therapy.
    B. Exposure therapy is associated with a low dropout rate of 10 percent.
    C. Eighty percent of treated agoraphobics improve with the use of exposure therapy.
    D. Exposure therapy is not useful in the treatment of phobias.
    E. Exposure therapy combined with imipramine appears to have a synergistic effect on panic attacks.

26.7   The behavioral treatment of obsessive-compulsive disorder relies heavily on the technique of:

    A.   positive reinforcement
    B.   in vivo systematic desensitization
    C.   response prevention
    D.   social skills training
    E.   punishment

26.8   Which of the following elements has not been found to be useful in the treatment of mild to moderate obesity?

    A.   self-monitoring
    B.   reinforcement of increased activity level
    C.   slowing of the eating rate
    D.   concentration on short-term goals
    E.   punishment of overeating behavior

DIRECTIONS: For each of the statements or questions below, one or more of the alternative answers is correct. Choose answer:

    A   if only 1, 2, and 3 are correct
    B   if only 1 and 3 are correct
    C   if only 2 and 4 are correct
    D   if only 4 is correct
    E   if all are correct

26.9   Which of the following statements regarding the behavioral treatment of psychotic disorders is not true?

    1. It is adjunctive to pharmacological treatment.
    2. It is directed toward the amelioration of problem behaviors.
    3. It is directed toward the social rehabilitation of the patient.
    4. It has been effective for major depression but not for schizophrenia.

26.10   Behavioral treatment of anorexia nervosa includes which procedure(s)?

    1. reinforcement of weight gain in small increments
    2. feedback of information regarding progress
    3. serving large meals
    4. systematic desensitization to food

26.11   Punishment is:

1. less useful than positive reinforcement because of the side effects of aggressive behavior
2. never used with children
3. used in situations that represent clear danger to the patient without treatment
4. effective only for short periods of time

26.12   The basic components of behavioral treatment for psychosomatic disorders do not include:

1. relaxation training
2. biofeedback
3. control of disturbing cognitions
4. positive reinforcement for symptom-free time periods

26.13   Which of the following behavior therapy approaches has (have) been shown to be useful in the treatment of sleep-onset insomnia?

1. stimulus control
2. positive reinforcement for time spent in bed
3. relaxation training
4. systematic desensitization

26.14   Which of the following statements regarding the token economy is (are) true?

1. It is more effective than traditional treatment in controlling conduct disorders in children.
2. It can be applied in an inpatient but not in a home setting.
3. It has been found to be useful in classrooms.
4. It does not work with psychotic children.

26.15   Studies of the use of behavioral approaches in the treatment of hyperactivity generally indicate that:

1. behavioral approaches are no more effective than medication
2. behavioral approaches result in increases in academic performance
3. the use of stimulant medication increases the effectiveness of behavioral interventions
4. behavioral interventions result in decreases in hyperactive behavior

26.16 Melamed demonstrated that in children about to undergo an aversive medical procedure (surgery), exposure to a film about a child coping with the surgery:

1. increased the children's physiologic arousal immediately following the film
2. was associated with increased requests for pain medication following the surgery
3. was associated with a quicker return to solid food
4. increased the children's apprehension regarding the surgery

26.17 The most effective treatment for agoraphobia with panic includes:

1. relaxation training
2. exposure treatment
3. response prevention
4. drugs

26.18 Self-disclosure to significant others regarding the binge and purge behaviors is a basic component of the behavioral treatment for bulimia because this behavior:

1. helps the patient achieve a feeling of a "clear conscience"
2. induces shame that then acts to punish the bulimic behavior
3. gives the patient a fresh start
4. increases social control over the secretive bulimic behavior

ANSWERS

26.1 The answer is **C**.

Behavior therapy arose out of attempts to provide an empirical basis for psychotherapy. Its theoretical bases are in British associationist theory and in the research conducted in learning by Pavlov. There are four basic principles of behavior therapy. First, behavior therapy assumes that both normal and abnormal behaviors are learned and maintained in the same way. Therefore, methods of changing normal behavior will be useful in changing abnormal behavior. Second, it is assumed that the social environment is the largest influence on the development and maintenance of behavior. As a result, the environment may need to be changed in order for behavior change to be initiated and maintained.

Third, the major focus of treatment is on the problematic behavior itself. An important aspect of pretreatment assessment is specification of the behaviors to be changed. The problematic behaviors are broken down into workable components and the antecedents and consequences of the behaviors are determined. Treatment follows from this assessment. Fourth, behavior therapy is based on a scientific approach to treatment. Treatment procedures must be replicable through description. Treatment is evaluated in a controlled experiment. The active components of the treatment are separated from the inactive nonspecific components of therapy by the additive clinical research design.

26.2   The answer is **A**.

Behavior therapy has a tradition of innovation and change. One of the most influential innovations of recent times is that of social cognitive learning theory as proposed by Bandura. Social cognitive learning theory is based on elements of both Pavlovian and Skinnerian behaviorism. Social cognitive learning theory also posits a reiterative relationship among environment, behavior, and personal and cognitive processes. The environment affects behavior and the person can alter the environment, and in this way the person can alter his or her future behavior.

Under operant behaviorism, reinforcement is the direct effect of reward. Under social cognitive learning theory, reinforcement is a source of information about the potential effects of future behavior, and cognitive processes therefore mediate behavior. The most important cognitive processes that alter behavior are expectations. There are two main types of expectations. Outcome expectations refer to the degree of certainty that a particular behavior will result in a particular outcome. Efficacy expectations refer to the degree of confidence that individuals have in their ability to successfully carry out certain behaviors.

26.3   The answer is **E**.

Joseph Wolpe first proposed the principle of reciprocal inhibition as a way of explaining his theory of the treatment of anxiety. Wolpe had developed an animal model of anxiety by exposing them to fear-inducing situations. He then used food to inhibit the fear response by pairing the food with the fear-inducing situation. Reciprocal inhibition refers to the act of eliciting a response incompatible with anxiety in the presence of a stimulus that usually induces the anxiety response.

In humans, Wolpe used deep muscle relaxation in order to inhibit the anxiety induced by a phobic stimulus. This procedure became an important part of the treatment method known as systematic desensitization. In systematic desensitization, the patient is told to practice deep muscle relaxation while imagining scenes of the situations that usually induce anxiety. The imaginal scenes are presented in a graded hierarchy, beginning with the least fear-arousing situation and ending with the most fear-inducing situation.

26.4   The answer is B.

Bandura employed the technique of observational learning in work with children. He showed that the specific fears of children could be reduced by having them observe nonfearful children interact with the fear-inducing stimulus. Greater effectiveness was obtained when the children watched and then used a gradual approach to the fear-inducing stimulus. This second technique is known as participant modeling. Modeling of the nonfearful behaviors is followed by attempts by the fearful child to imitate the behaviors. Many applications of this technique for the treatment of children have been demonstrated.

26.5   The answer is D.

Although there were many demonstrations of the effectiveness of behavioral treatments for phobic reactions, there were some concerns raised regarding the long-term maintenance of gains. Some of these concerns were raised by behaviorists themselves because of the known effect of removing positive reinforcement. (The behaviors may revert to pretreatment levels.) Therefore long-term studies were conducted in order to determine whether or not the positive effects of a behavioral treatment could be maintained.

Research data indicate that the effects of systematic desensitization on phobias could be maintained for up to seven years following termination of treatment. Long-term studies indicate that the treatment for phobic disorders should include an element of graded exposure and that treatments that do not contain such elements are contraindicated in the treatment of phobias. These studies were extremely important in dispelling the notion that in order to successfully treat phobias the therapist must deal with the intrapsychic conflicts of the patient.

26.6   The answer is D.

Exposure therapy involves the graduated exposure of a phobic individual to the fear-inducing stimulus. Exposure therapy has low drop-out rates estimated at about 10 percent and rates of significant improvement estimated at over 80 percent. Recent empirical studies have shown that involving a spouse or significant other in the treatment process can increase the effectiveness of the treatment. In addition, providing training in couples communication skills lengthens the period over which treatment gains are maintained. It is hypothesized that successful treatment of the phobic individual changes the pattern of interaction with the spouse and communication skills training can minimize the stressful effects of such changes and help the couple adjust to the changes.

26.7   The answer is C.

Obsessive-compulsive disorders involve the reduction of ritualistic, compulsively repetitive behaviors that are irrational because of the lack of observable effect on the situation facing the individual. Theoretical considerations of the anxiety-reducing characteristics of compulsive behaviors, which are construed as avoidance behaviors, have resulted in the application of response prevention methods in the treatment of this disorder. The general idea is that compulsive behaviors do not allow patients a chance to test the reality of their fear. When these patients are prevented from engaging in the compulsive behavior, the lack of relation between the fearful stimulus and the imagined consequence can be observed by them.

Response prevention has been shown to be effective in reducing the frequency of compulsive behaviors, but it does not appear to be effective in treating the fears associated with the stimulus situation. Repeated exposure to the fearful situation is effective in reducing the fears of the patient. In addition, imagined or covert desensitization has been found to be effective in maintaining treatment gains over the long term. Therefore, successful treatment of the obsessive-compulsive disorders includes all three elements: response prevention, exposure, and imaginal systematic desensitization.

26.8   The answer is E.

Mild to moderate obesity is treated with a multifaceted behavioral program, reflecting the complexity of environmental factors that have been implicated in the initiation and maintenance of behaviors related to obesity. Successful behavioral treatment of mild to moderate obesity includes the self-monitoring of eating behavior and of situations that elicit eating behavior; reinforcement of increases in activity level of the patient; reduction of the stimuli associated with eating by decreasing the number of situations in which eating occurs; adherence to a low-fat, high-fiber diet; and use of reinforcement and self-reinforcement to achieve short-term goals.

Treatments that include the above elements have been found to be more effective than traditional diets, psychotherapy, or pharmacological approaches. The weight losses in these programs are usually modest, with the average patient losing .5 kg per week and a treatment course of 16 weeks resulting in a loss of between 8 and 10 kg. Group behavioral therapy appears to be more effective than individual therapy in the treatment of mild to moderate obesity. Maintenance of treatment gains (in this case, of weight loss) depends on the continued practice of behaviors learned during the course of therapy.

26.9   The answer is A.

Behavioral approaches to the treatment of psychotic disorders are adjunctive to pharmacological approaches. Behavioral treatments of psychotic disorders are directed at the remediation of specific problem behaviors and toward the social rehabilitation of the psychotic patient. They have been found to be effective in the treatment of both schizophrenic and depressive disorders. The methods used to behaviorally treat psychotic disorders are derived from the methodology of operant conditioning.

Because psychotic disorders can present with such a wide array of problematic behaviors, an important aspect of behavioral treatment is the specification of the target problem behaviors. Behavioral techniques can be directed at problem behaviors that do not improve with medication or at the limitations in social and vocational skills resulting from the psychotic disorders.

The use of a token economy, whereby tokens are given contingent on the production of behavioral change, has been shown to be effective in the treatment of chronic patients. A social learning treatment program has been shown to be more effective than the traditional milieu treatment of chronic patients. Patients in a social learning treatment required less medication, showed greater improvement in a wide range of prosocial behaviors, and maintained their treatment over a longer period of time.

26.10   The answer is A.

The goal of behavioral treatment of anorexia nervosa is the restoration of normal body weight. This treatment typically occurs in an inpatient setting. After normal weight is attained, the focus of treatment turns toward treating the factors that are found to have been maintaining the eating disorder. Three factors appear to be useful in the behavioral treatment of anorexia nervosa: 1) reinforcement of weight gain in small increments, 2) feedback of information regarding the progress of the individual by communicating the daily weight and caloric intake, and 3) serving large meals even though that patient may at first not eat most of the food served. These behavioral programs are conducted in the context of a carefully negotiated therapeutic contract and a well-designed treatment milieu.

26.11   The answer is **B**.

There are three general procedures in operant conditioning. The first is positive reinforcement, in which a positive reward is given to the patient contingent on demonstration of a specified behavior. The second is negative reinforcement (sometimes confused with punishment), in which the patient's emitting a desired target behavior is followed by removal of an unpleasant stimulus from the patient's environment. The third is punishment, in which the patient's emitting an undesired behavior is followed by application of an unpleasant stimulus or situation.

The use of punishment is problematic for practical and ethical reasons. The practical reasons include the empirical observation that punishment is often followed by aggressive behavior on the part of the patient. The ethical reasons include the fact that punishment carries the risk of a side effect of harm to the patient. Therefore, punishment is used only when positive reinforcement has not been effective or when the problem behaviors emitted by the patient represent danger to the patient, such as self-mutilation behaviors. The use of punishment requires the supervision of an oversight committee at the institution where the procedures are used.

26.12   The answer is **D**.

Psychosomatic disorders have been found to be amenable to the application of behavioral treatments. Many psychosomatic disorders, including asthma, essential hypertension, sleep disturbance, and peptic ulcer, are thought to be exacerbated by high levels of anxiety and arousal. Relaxation training including deep muscle relaxation, meditation, hypnosis, and biofeedback have all been found to be effective in treating a wide range of psychosomatic disorders. The relative effectiveness of the different techniques seems to vary by patient, rather than by disorder. The effect of stressful situations on psychosomatic symptoms appears to be mediated by disturbing cognitions, and control of these cognitions has also been used in treating psychosomatic disorders.

26.13   The answer is **B**.

Sleep disturbance is often associated with different psychiatric disorders. However, sleep-onset insomnia without other associated psychiatric disorders is also a common problem. Although sleep-onset insomnia will frequently respond to sedative hypnotic agents in the short term, the long-term use of these pharmacologic agents has undesirable effects. Two behavioral treatments have been found to be effective in the treatment of sleep-onset insomnia. The first is relaxation training, which is assumed to reduce the level of anxiety and other cognitive and arousal problems that interfere with the initiation of sleep. The second is stimulus control.

Stimulus control treatments are based on the premise that sleep onset is usually signalled by a narrow range of stimuli. When these stimuli also become associated with outcomes other than sleep, there is said to be loss of stimulus control over the initiation of sleep. The treatment involves removing distracting stimuli such as television, books, and food from the bed and bedroom. Then the patient is told to get out of bed if he or she does not become drowsy within 10 minutes. The patient is instructed not to return to bed until he or she feels drowsy. If the patient does not fall asleep within 10 minutes, the process is repeated. Recent studies indicate that although both treatments are effective in reducing sleep-onset latency, stimulus control is more effective than relaxation training.

26.14   The answer is B.

The token economy is a system whereby small tokens are given as reinforcement for the production of desired behaviors. Although these tokens have no intrinsic value, they can be saved and "cashed in" for objects or activities that have more overtly recognizable reinforcing characteristics. The token economy has been implemented in the treatment of inpatient chronic psychotic patients as well as in the home treatment of child problem behaviors and in the classroom treatment of disruptive behaviors. It has been found to be effective in both the reduction of problem behaviors and in the increase of prosocial behaviors.

The use of the token economy has been found to be more effective than traditional therapy in treating conduct-disordered children. In one study, the use of a home token economy was associated with a 67 percent reduction in deviant behavior, compared with a 34 percent reduction when traditional therapy was used with conduct-disordered children.

26.15   The answer is C.

Attention deficit disorder (ADD) with and without hyperactivity is often associated with learning disorders and presents a significant problem in this country. It is estimated that five percent of the children in the United States have ADD. There is a history of nearly three decades of studies demonstrating the effectiveness of behavioral treatment of ADD. Usually the behavioral treatment is aimed at the problematic academic behavior. Behavioral treatment results in increased academic performance, decreased deviant behavior, and relatively long-term maintenance of therapeutic gains.

The use of medication, in particular methylphenidate, is associated with decreases in hyperactivity. However, medication does not appear to increase academic performance. One study comparing medication with behavioral treatment of ADD showed some interesting results. Methylphenidate resulted in reduction of hyperactive behavior, but not improvement in academic performance. The hyperactive behaviors increased once the medication was withdrawn. Subsequently, a behavioral treatment was implemented with the result that not only was academic performance improved, but hyperactive behavior decreased. Other studies have indicated that the addition of stimulant medication to a behavioral program has little effect on the treatment gains effected by the behavioral program.

26.16   The answer is B.

Behavioral pediatrics is the application of behavioral techniques in the treatment of pediatric medical problems. Many of these applications have occurred in the treatment of chronic diseases that require behavior changes in the child for the adequate medical management of the disease. Successful applications have occurred in the areas of insulin-dependent diabetes and hemodialysis.

Melamed has conducted a series of studies addressing the effectiveness of modeling in treating children who are about to undergo aversive medical procedures such as surgery. In one study, children facing surgery were exposed to a film about a child who successfully copes with hospitalization and medical treatment. The effect of the modeling procedure film was to increase the children's physiological arousal immediately following the viewing. However, the children exposed to the modeling film had lower levels of arousal prior to surgery than did children exposed to a placebo film about an unrelated topic. Fewer of the children who received modeling required postsurgical pain medication or complained of side effects. More of the children exposed to the modeling film returned more quickly to eating solid food.

26.17   The answer is C.

Agoraphobia with panic requires a more complex set of treatment considerations than does agoraphobia without panic and other specific phobias. Agoraphobia without panic and simple phobias can be successfully treated with a variant of exposure treatment. However, studies indicate that agoraphobia with panic is more effectively treated when exposure treatment is combined with the use of imipramine.

26.18   The answer is D.

Bulimia nervosa is a disorder that is being seen with increasing frequency since the late 1970s. In this disorder the patient demonstrates a cyclic pattern of overeating or bingeing followed by the health-threatening use of laxatives or emetics. The behavioral treatment of bulimia involves reinforcement of the consumption of three adequate meals each day, slow introduction of the feared binge food to the diet, challenge to the patient's distorted cognitions regarding food, self-disclosure of the bulimic behaviors to significant others, and a relapse prevention program. The self-disclosure is intended to increase social control over the bulimic behaviors. It does not have any relation to clearing the conscience, inducing shame, or generating the false image of a fresh start without adequate behavioral control.

Chapter

27

Hypnosis

DIRECTIONS: Each of the statements or questions is followed by five suggested responses or completions. Select the one that is the best choice or most complete answer in each case.

27.1 Which of the following refers to the process through which routine experiences that would ordinarily be conscious occur out of conscious awareness?

    A. suggestibility
    B. desensitization
    C. dissociation
    D. implosion
    E. systematic sensitization

27.2 Which of the following is not true regarding hypnosis?

    A. Hypnotized individuals tend to accept uncritically instructions given to them while in a trance.
    B. Hypnotized individuals are actually in a sleeplike state while in a trance.
    C. Power spectral electroencephalograms of hypnotized individuals show a pattern consistent with resting alertness.
    D. Approximately one out of four individuals is not hypnotizable.
    E. None of the above.

27.3 In general, individuals in what age group are more likely to be hypnotizable?

    A. individuals in late childhood
    B. elderly individuals
    C. middle-aged individuals
    D. young children
    E. individuals in their 30s

27.4 Which of the following statements is true regarding the relationship between hypnotizability and psychiatric disorders?

    A. Hypnotizability is unrelated to psychopathology.
    B. High hypnotizability is associated with serious psychiatric disorders.
    C. Low hypnotizability is associated with serious psychiatric disorders.
    D. Physically abused children often lose the ability to dissociate themselves from stressful situations.
    E. None of the above.

27.5 Which of the following statements is true regarding the hypnotizability of patients with schizophrenia and affective disorders?

    A. Schizophrenic patients have generally demonstrated somewhat lower hypnotizability and the absence of very high hypnotizability.
    B. Schizophrenic patients have demonstrated very high hypnotizability.
    C. Patients with major affective disorders have been found to score lower than schizophrenics on measures of hypnotizability.
    D. Individuals with generalized anxiety disorder have been associated with inhibition of hypnotic responsiveness.
    E. At this point in time, no meaningful statements can be made concerning the relationship between these disorders and hypnotizability.

27.6   Which of the following represents a major application of hypnosis in legal settings?

    A.   the use of confabulation in court
    B.   the application of testimony of witnesses hypnotized while testifying in court
    C.   the use of hypnosis for the purpose of "refreshing" recollections of witnesses and victims of crimes
    D.   the use of testimony of witnesses who have been hypnotized prior to testifying in court
    E.   the use of hypnosis as a "lie detection" procedure in court

27.7   Clinical experience suggests that which of the following patient groups is likely to obtain some benefit from the application of hypnosis to weight control?

    A.   individuals who are markedly obese
    B.   individuals within 30 percent of their ideal body weight
    C.   individuals within 10 to 20 percent of their ideal body weight
    D.   individuals with whom dietary and exercise programs have not been successful
    E.   Hypnosis has not been found to be useful in weight control.

DIRECTIONS: For each of the statements below, one or more of the alternative answers is correct. Choose answer:
    A   if only 1, 2, and 3 are correct
    B   if only 1 and 3 are correct
    C   if only 2 and 4 are correct
    D   if only 4 is correct
    E   if all are correct

27.8   Hypnosis is a form of:

    1. sleep
    2. broadened attention
    3. helplessness
    4. concentration

27.9   Hypnosis involves:

    1. absorption
    2. dissociation
    3. suggestibility
    4. inattention

27.10 Hypnosis has been successfully used in the treatment of:

1. aviophobia
2. alcoholism
3. smoking
4. schizophrenia

27.11 The use(s) of hypnosis in the treatment of psychosomatic symptoms includes:

1. helping the patient to ignore the symptom
2. helping the patient control the symptom
3. proving to the patient that the symptom is psychological in origin
4. facilitation of a differential diagnosis

27.12 Factors associated with the diagnosis of multiple personality disorder include:

1. a history of physical abuse in childhood
2. a concurrent diagnosis of schizophrenia
3. high hypnotizability
4. drug abuse

DIRECTIONS: Each of the following questions consists of lettered headings followed by a list of numbered alternatives. Select the single lettered heading that is most closely associated with the appropriate numbered alternative. Each lettered heading may be chosen only once.

Principles of psychotherapy in the use of hypnosis

A. Condensation
B. Congruence
C. Control
D. Confession

Description

27.13 can make the overwhelming aspects of a traumatic event more manageable by giving them concrete, symbolic form and by facilitating restructuring of the experience by joining previously disparate images

27.14 structures the patient's experience so that the patient has the opportunity to terminate the session when he or she feels overwhelmed

27.15   attempts to integrate traumatic material into consciousness in such a way that patients can tolerate experiencing the memories as part of themselves

27.16   helps patients distinguish between misplaced guilt and real guilt for acts performed

ANSWERS

27.1   The answer is **C**.

The intense absorption experience associated with hypnosis means that even routine experiences that would ordinarily be conscious may occur out of conscious awareness. Even complex emotional states or sensory experiences may be dissociated during hypnosis. These experiences may range from the simple, such as a hand feeling that it is not as much a part of the body as usual, to the complex, such as a fugue episode lasting for a period of hours or even months. Such experiences can be both induced and reversed with the structured use of hypnosis.

27.2   The answer is **B**.

The hypnotized individual is not asleep, but rather is awake and alert. Like the individual who is asleep, the hypnotized person has suspended peripheral awareness, but unlike the individual who is asleep, focal attention is intense and is carefully controlled. In fact, the power spectral electroencephalograms of hypnotized individuals show a pattern consistent with resting alertness rather than sleep.

While hypnotized individuals do not lose the ability to evaluate instructions given to them, they do tend to accept uncritically instructions given to them while in a hypnotic trance, suspending the usual conscious editing function that raises the question "Why?" when an instruction is given to them. Thus, the hypnotized individual is likely to be more accepting of instructions, no matter how irrational.

27.3   The answer is **A**.

Hypnotizability varies from individual to individual. Hypnotizability is highest in late childhood and declines gradually throughout adulthood. About one in four adults is not hypnotizable.

27.4   The answer is **B**.

There is accumulating evidence that high hypnotizability is associated with some serious psychiatric disorders. Clinicians have long observed that it is unusual to find a patient with a severe dissociative disorder such as a fugue state, psychogenic amnesia, or multiple personality disorder who is not highly hypnotizable. The recent literature on multiple personality disorder indicates that these patients have two things in common: high hypnotizability and a history of severe physical abuse during their childhood years. This has led to the recognition that the capacity to dissociate psychological from physical experience is mobilized during and after periods of extreme physical distress such as assault.

27.5   The answer is **A**.

As far back as 1937, Copeland and Kitching observed that presumably psychotic patients who were hypnotizable were not genuinely psychotic. Since that time, more than 20 studies have been conducted to investigate the relationship between hypnotizability and major psychiatric disorders. These studies have generally shown somewhat lower, and the absence of very high, hypnotizability among schizophrenics. In addition, patients with major affective disorders have been found to score higher than schizophrenic patients but lower than normals on indices of hypnotizability.

27.6   The answer is **C**.

A major application of hypnosis in the legal setting has been for the purpose of refreshing the memories of witnesses and victims of crimes.

However, there has been serious criticism of the use of hypnosis in forensic applications. One is "confabulation," or the possibility that the hypnotized individual will make up material out of a desire to please the hypnotist or as a result of being in the nonrational hypnotic state itself. The other is referred to as "concreting," or the process of emerging from the hypnotic trance with an enhanced conviction that one's memories are correct.

Courts have been uniformly unwilling to admit the testimony of individuals hypnotized while testifying. Recently, courts have also begun to exclude testimony of witnesses who have been hypnotized previously.

27.7   The answer is **C**.

Although long-term outcome studies are currently lacking, clinical experience suggests that patients who are within 10 to 20 percent of their ideal body weight are likely to obtain some benefit from restructuring techniques such as self-hypnosis in addition to careful attention to diet and exercise.

27.8   The answer is **D**.

The word *hypnosis* is derived from the Greek root "hypnos," which means sleep. However, the hypnotized individual is not asleep but rather is awake and alert. Hypnosis is not a form of broadened attention but rather a state of focused attention, with intense absorption in the trance state and suspension of peripheral awareness. Although the hypnotized individual is more likely to uncritically accept information provided to him or her during the trance, the individual is not at all helpless during the hypnotic trance.

27.9   The answer is **A**.

Hypnosis involves the processes of absorption, dissociation, and suggestibility. Absorption refers to a tendency for the hypnotized individual to undergo spontaneous absorbing experiences such as the experience of being "caught up" in a movie to the extent that awareness of being in a theatre (peripheral awareness) is temporarily lost. Dissociation refers to the process by which routine experiences that would ordinarily be conscious occur out of conscious awareness. Suggestibility refers to the tendency of the hypnotized individual to uncritically accept instructions in trance.

27.10   The answer is **B**.

Hypnosis has been employed as an adjunctive tool with a variety of habit control strategies, primarily for smoking cessation. Specifically with regard to smoking cessation, it has been used to 1) provide a substitute relaxation for the momentary respite that accompanies the inhalation of a cigarette, 2) enhance self-observation and self-monitoring, 3) provide positive reinforcement for behavior change, 4) diminish the positive reinforcement provided by smoking itself, and 5) facilitate cognitive restructuring of the smoking habit. Recent emphasis has been on teaching the patient to use self-hypnotic strategies rather than having multiple sessions with a therapist.

Hypnosis has also been successfully used as a treatment for phobic disorders. For example, patients with aviophobia (fear of airplane flight) can be taught to combine the physical sense of floating with the concept of floating with the airplane. They can then focus on the idea of the plane as an extension of their body instead of feeling trapped by the airplane, and concentrate on the difference between the possibility and the probability of a crash.

Hypnosis has not been found to be an effective treatment of alcoholism or of major psychiatric disorders such as schizophrenia.

27.11 The answer is **C**.

In general, hypnosis for patients who suffer from psychosomatic disorders is useful in two senses, one diagnostic and one therapeutic. First, patients who are highly hypnotizable are more likely to have conversion symptoms than are individuals who are not highly hypnotizable, especially if hypnotic induction tends to bring on the symptom, worsen it, or ameliorate it. Hence, hypnosis may provide important information concerning differential diagnosis between conversion disorder and other conditions.

With regard to the control of psychosomatic symptoms, hypnosis can be useful as a relaxation strategy since it can help the individual master anxiety associated with physical dysfunction. In particular, hypnosis has been found to be quite effective in helping asthmatics and can be used as a "first resort" rather than medication when an attack is coming on. Patients who suffer from stress-induced bowel disease may also obtain relief from symptoms by imagining (in trance) something soothing in their gut.

27.12 The answer is **A**.

The recent literature on multiple personality disorder indicates that these patients have two things in common: high hypnotizability and a history of severe physical abuse as a child.

27.13 The answer is **A**.
27.14 The answer is **C**.
27.15 The answer is **B**.
27.16 The answer is **D**.

Condensation refers to the process of finding an image that condenses a crucial aspect of the traumatic experience. This representation can make the overwhelming aspects of the trauma more manageable by giving them concrete, symbolic form. Furthermore, it can facilitate a restructuring of the experience by joining previously disparate images, for example, linking the pain associated with the death of a friend in combat with the happiness experienced during some earlier shared time.

The principle of control involves structuring the hypnotic experience so that patients are given the opportunity to terminate the working through when they feel they have had enough, can remember as much from the hypnosis as they care to, and feel they are in charge of the self-hypnosis experience.

The principle of congruence refers to the process of facilitation of the integration of dissociated or repressed traumatic material into conscious awareness in such a way that the patient can tolerate experiencing the memories as part of himself or herself, so that the traumatic past is not disjunctive and incompatible with the present.

The principle of concentration is useful in reinforcing the boundaries of the traumatic experience and the painful affect associated with it. By focusing sharply defined attention on the loss, the inference is made that when the hypnotic state is ended, attention can be shifted away from the traumatic experience.

L Chapter

28

Family Therapy

DIRECTIONS: Each of the statements or questions is followed by five suggested responses or completions. Select the one that is the best choice or most complete answer in each case.

28.1 What is the relation between concurrent family therapy and individual therapy

A. There is no need for individual therapy if family therapy is taking place.
B. It is difficult to go to family work once individual therapy has begun.
C. It is difficult to go to individual work once family therapy has begun.
D. Family and individual therapy are orthogonal; it doesn't matter which one comes first.
E. Family therapy should always be accompanied by individual therapy.

28.2 Which of the following were not among the prewar American originators of family therapy?

A. George Herbert Mead
B. Harry Stack Sullivan
C. Franz Boas
D. Ruth Benedict
E. Arthur MacMillan Stetson

28.3 What is the relation between family therapy and couples therapy?

- **A.** Family therapy grew out of and replaced couples therapy.
- **B.** Family therapy and couples therapy differ in their conception of the etiology of psychopathology.
- **C.** Family therapy and couples therapy share many techniques.
- **D.** Family therapy takes up where couples therapy leaves off.
- **E.** Family therapy is qualitatively different from couples therapy.

28.4 A basic tenet of behavioral marital therapy is:

- **A.** Couples therapy begins with the clarification of communication.
- **B.** The therapist needs to be able to control the contingencies of the marital relationship.
- **C.** The role of the therapist is to help the couple identify behaviors that annoy each partner.
- **D.** All marital behavior should be explicitly contracted.
- **E.** Shared behaviors have a higher value than nonshared behaviors.

28.5 The treatment of choice for sexual problems such as impotence, vaginismus, anorgasmia, and premature ejaculation is:

- **A.** strategic family therapy
- **B.** emotionally focused couples therapy
- **C.** paradoxical instructions
- **D.** educational–behavioral couples therapy
- **E.** the use of sex surrogates

28.6 Resistance in family therapy is related to:

- **A.** shifting alliances among the family members
- **B.** the natural homeostasis of the family unit
- **C.** the unconscious desire of one or more family members to fail
- **D.** inability of the family to communicate the nature of the problem to the therapist
- **E.** none of the above—resistance is not a useful concept in family therapy

28.7   Structural family therapy places emphasis on:

    A.   observing the family interactions in order to identify the pathological "culprit"

    B.   resolving unresolved intergenerational issues

    C.   inducing enactments of altered behavior sequences between family members

    D.   uncovering the symbolic meanings of family communications

    E.   expression of emotion

DIRECTIONS: For each of the statements or questions below, one or more of the alternative answers is correct. Choose answer:

    A   if only 1, 2, and 3 are correct

    B   if only 1 and 3 are correct

    C   if only 2 and 4 are correct

    D   if only 4 is correct

    E   if all are correct

28.8   Emotionally focused marital therapy views marital dysfunction as:

    1. related to deficits in bargaining and problem-solving skills

    2. due to unexpressed unconscious needs

    3. related to unresolved intergenerational conflicts

    4. a problem in the way in which the couple expect to meet each other's needs for intimacy

28.9   Psychoanalytic marital therapy focuses on:

    1. the long-term goal of personal development

    2. change in partner interactional behaviors

    3. achievement of intimacy

    4. changing the pattern of relationships via straightforward and paradoxical instructions

28.10   Studies of divorce counseling show that it results in:

    1. a higher level of satisfaction with the agreement

    2. reduction in the amount of later litigation

    3. an increase in joint custody agreements

    4. a decrease in expense

28.11 Studies indicate that behavioral family therapy with adolescent "soft" delinquents and conduct disorders:

    1. was superior to individual therapy
    2. was superior to other forms of family therapy
    3. resulted in less pathology among siblings and mothers of the target adolescents
    4. resulted in symptom substitution

28.12 Compared with other family therapies, systemic family therapy makes relatively heavy use of:

    1. interpretation of underlying meaning in communication
    2. understanding the relations of the family members by analyzing seating arrangements
    3. resolving intergenerational conflicts
    4. the concept of a team of consultants

DIRECTIONS: Each of the following questions consists of lettered headings followed by a list of numbered alternatives. Select the single lettered heading that is most closely associated with the appropriate numbered alternative. Each lettered heading may be chosen only once.

Family therapist

    A. Murray Bowen
    B. Nathan Ackerman
    C. Ivan Boszormenyi-Nagy
    D. Virginia Satir

Description

28.13 placed emphasis on the liberating influence of the experience of emotion
28.14 focused on the validation of differences among family members as a starting point of personal growth
28.15 focused on differentiating oneself from multigenerational entanglements
28.16 placed emphasis on resolving obligations among family members

ANSWERS

28.1 The answer is **B**.

Family therapy and individual therapy can be seen as complementary rather than as being in competition. Some clinicians may find that it is easier to make a complete evaluation of a presenting problem by meeting with more than just the identified patient. An evaluation conducted in such a group meeting has the additional benefit of helping to provide information regarding whether individual, couple, or family therapy is needed. However, it should be noted that it is easier to move to individual therapy once family therapy has been initiated than it is to move to family therapy once individual therapy is begun.

28.2 The answer is **E**.

Conjoint psychotherapy began in earnest following World War II. Even before that time, the trends in the child guidance movement, marriage counseling, and orthopsychiatry were laying the groundwork for the family therapy approach. Family therapy had its theoretical beginnings in various academic movements. Included among these was the social psychology of George Herbert Mead and the interpersonal psychiatry of Harry Stack Sullivan. Two other important prewar influences on family therapy were the anthropologist Franz Boas and his student Ruth Benedict. In particular, Ruth Benedict and her colleague Margaret Mead showed the influence of child-rearing behavior and cultural variables on later adult behavior. It was Margaret Mead's husband, Gregory Bateson, who gave family therapy the first theory of relationship patterns by describing relationships as either symmetrical (competitive and disruptive) or complementary (stabilizing), at least in small groups.

28.3 The answer is **C**.

Family therapy and couples therapy are highly interrelated conceptually and in terms of practical technology. Although distinctions are often made between them, they are more similar to each other than either is to individual therapy. For example, both couples therapy and family therapy involve similar permutations of individual therapy issues such as privacy, confidentiality, and neutrality. They also share similar conceptions of the causes of psychopathology, although there may be differences among various schools of thought as to the emphasis placed on different etiological variables.

28.4   The answer is **A**.

The basic idea of behavioral marital therapy is that couples therapy begins with the clarification of communications. Behavioral marital therapy views marital discord as being due to deficits in skills of communication, compromise, and problem solving, as well as being due to problems in reinforcing the partner's desirable behaviors. The therapist's task is to clarify the contingencies governing each partner's behaviors and to help the couple to learn more appropriate ways of influencing each other's behavior. Although one role of the therapist may be to help the couple to identify behaviors that annoy each other, this is not a primary function.

Under behavioral marital therapy, conflicts or disagreements are worked out via a process of clear communication and compromise under the general principle that the relationship should remain symmetrical and fair. Other important aspects of conflict resolution include the techniques of listing options, negotiating, and problem solving. Behavioral marital therapy seeks to help the couple systematically improve the quality of their shared behaviors, but places no relative value on shared versus private behavior, except as either interferes with the relationship.

28.5   The answer is **D**.

Empirical research has shown that the treatment of choice for the sexual dysfunctions listed in the *Diagnostic and Statistical Manual of Mental Disorders (Third Edition-Revised)* is an educational–behavioral approach. The earliest evidence was provided by a gynecologist and a psychologist (Masters and Johnson). Their reports of success were greeted by skepticism by the family and couples therapists who felt that only approaches that concentrated on the underlying psychopathology could succeed in treating problems such as vaginismus, impotence, anorgasmia, and premature ejaculation.

Despite the initial skepticism, attempts at replicating the methods of Masters and Johnson were much more successful than the traditional approaches, although not quite as successful as the initially reported 90 percent success rate. Treatments derived from the work of Masters and Johnson begin with joint and individual interviews, proceed to didactic instruction about practical techniques, and move to practice sessions. In the meantime, group sessions may offer social support. One technique is to instruct the clients not to engage in sex until the new methods have been mastered, relieving the pressure to perform.

28.6   The answer is **B**.

Even if the family agrees to attempt changes in interactional behavior or communication, the members may not follow through on actually exhibiting the behavior agreed upon. The most commonly invoked reason for this inability to change is related to one of the oldest concepts in family therapy, group homeostasis. In any family, including a dysfunctional family, there is a system of feedback mechanisms that contributes to the stability of the family as a unit. Usually this homeostatic stability is healthy and protective to the family. However, in some instances this stability can be pathological when it makes change to a more healthy system difficult. In those circumstances, this tendency to remain stable is known as resistance.

One of the techniques suggested to counter resistance involves finding a set of forces in the family that can be mobilized for the purpose of change rather than for resistance. When resistance occurs, strategic therapists redefine the problem in such a way as to make it soluble. Another technique is for the therapist to suggest the opposite of what is actually desired so that resistance is organized against the paradoxical instructions and toward the desired response.

28.7   The answer is **C**.

Structural family therapists carefully observe the particulars of family interactions in order to uncover the social structure of the family in which the behavioral sequences occur. (The idea of identifying a "culprit" is not a useful one.) Some of the factors that structural therapists observe include the seating arrangement of the therapy session, the order of speech and topics, who interrupts whom, and the symmetry and synchrony of movement. In this way the therapist can infer the composition of subgroupings in the family.

Once the structure is understood, the therapist can suggest alternate ways for the behavioral sequences to proceed. Salvador Minuchin and his group at the Philadelphia Child Guidance Clinic have developed this idea most thoroughly. This research group has demonstrated the effectiveness of structural methods in the treatment of many psychosomatic disorders in children and adolescents, including unstable diabetes, asthma, anorexia nervosa, and bulimia.

28.8   The answer is **D**.

Emotionally focused marital therapy views marital discord as being due to problems in the way the couple expect to meet each other's needs for intimacy. It is the behavioral marital therapists who view dysfunction as being related to deficits in problem-solving skills, the psychoanalytic family therapists who view family dysfunction as related to unexpressed unconscious needs, and the followers of Murray Bowen who conceptualize family discord as being the result of intergenerational entanglements.

A main assumption of emotionally focused marital therapy is that all people have a need to be part of a bond of attachment. However, a couple may not clearly understand how to help each other to meet these needs. Also involved here are the ambiguous feelings associated with intimacy such as those due to vulnerability and fear of rejection.

28.9   The answer is **B**.

Psychoanalytic marital therapy has goals that are similar to the goals of individual psychoanalytic therapy. The main goals are the achievement of intimacy and the more long-term goal of personal growth. Also similar to individual psychoanalytic therapy is the extremely long course of treatment in psychoanalytic marital therapy. Another emphasis is on the role of unconscious motivation as a determinant of interactions between the couple. Our culture has a general expectation that personal fulfillment will be partly found in marriage, and the goals of psychoanalytic marital therapy seem consonant with that cultural expectation. However, there are no outcome studies to suggest that psychoanalytic marital therapy is actually effective.

28.10   The answer is **E**.

Divorce is a fact of life in our modern society. Because of the high rate of divorce, the process of separating and finding new ways of relating to all of the constituent members of a marriage (for example, children, in-laws) has importance. Divorce can be a financially expensive and emotionally draining experience. Some family therapists (or lawyers with training in family therapy) have devised methods for coping with the divorce process in a way that avoids the adversarial roles usually taken in the legal arena.

Although divorce counseling may not be effective when a couple is extremely belligerent or oppositional, empirical studies of the effectiveness of divorce counseling are very encouraging. Divorce counseling and mediation tend to result in a higher level of satisfaction with the agreement, a reduction in the amount of later litigation, an increase in joint custody agreements, and a reduction in the overall cost of the process.

28.11   The answer is **A**.

Behavioral family therapy is problem oriented and seems to work best when there is some form of general agreement about the identified problem. This problem may be a child with a conduct disorder, a high rate of aversive and argumentative behavior among the family members, or truancy in a child. Empirical studies indicate that behavioral family therapy was superior to other forms of family therapy as well as to individual therapy in the treatment of "soft" adolescent delinquents and conduct disorders. This superiority held up at 18-month and 3-year follow-ups. In addition, there was less pathology exhibited by mothers and less trouble with sibling behavior due to behavioral family therapy. There was no evidence of substitution reported in these studies.

28.12   The answer is **D**.

Systemic family therapists focus on the family as a system even more so than other types of family therapists. This approach characterizes those therapists who were influenced by Gregory Bateson and by the Milan group. Assessment consists of a circular questioning technique in which the presenting problem becomes part of the larger picture of interconnected issues and concerns.

Systemic family therapists also make relatively heavy use of the method of a team of consultants. The consultants view the proceedings through a one-way mirror and provide new insights and valuable observations to the therapists. The therapists can accept or reject the suggestions from the consultants, and the family can view the suggestions as coming from sources alternate to the therapists.

28.13   The answer is **B**.
28.14   The answer is **D**.
28.15   The answer is **A**.
28.16   The answer is **C**.

Nathan Ackerman taught the importance of experiencing frank emotions such as sexual feelings, aggressive feelings, or feelings associated with relationships such as dependency in the therapy sessions. He felt that this was a liberating experience. He used affect as a guide to the development of the family and challenged the family's defenses against emotional expression. His personal style of warmth and giving was probably a factor in the success of his methods.

Virginia Satir's work focused on the role of family interactions in the growth and development of the individual members. This therapy requires the clear communication of feelings and the recognition of individual differences among the family members. She used a series of experiential exercises in order to help family member recognize and act on the experience of others. Her exercises have influenced both the family therapy field and the Encounter movement.

Murray Bowen posits the process of maturation as being the differentiation of the self from the entanglements with others. This is a task that requires active work. Bowen suggests that responses sometimes be delayed so that a plan rather than impulsive responding takes place. He also proposed that emotions have their source in the family and recognizing this source can help subdue their force. Bowen was the founder of the Family Institute of Georgetown in Washington, D.C.

Ivan Boszormenyi-Nagy founded the Contextual school of family therapy and developed its theory and methods in collaboration with his partner Geraldine Spark. His therapy was based on a theory of interpersonal and intergenerational dynamics at the base of which is the concept of exchange. Over time indebtedness or obligation builds up between family members. The goal of his therapy was to discharge these obligations even if they had not been recognized when the family entered therapy.

Chapter 29

Group Therapy

DIRECTIONS: Each of the statements or questions is followed by five suggested responses or completions. Select the one that is the best choice or most complete answer in each case.

29.1 Which of the following statements regarding group therapy is not true?

    A. Group therapy has been shown through multiple outcome studies to be a highly effective form of treatment.

    B. It is a form of therapy that reaches significant numbers of psychiatric patients.

    C. It is being increasingly used in the lay setting through specialized and self-help groups.

    D. It is appropriate for only a narrow range of patients and clinical settings.

    E. It focuses on interpersonal relations and their effect on psychopathology.

29.2 Perhaps the most important advantage of group over individual therapy is:

- **A.** It provides expediency in dealing with several patients simultaneously.
- **B.** It makes use of unique therapeutic properties not shared by other therapies.
- **C.** It is a cost-effective method of treating patients.
- **D.** It is an efficient mode of patient contact.
- **E.** Because the other group members contribute to the therapy of the patient, it is less demanding of the therapist.

29.3 Which of the following is a correct list of the three interrelated characteristics used to categorize groups?

- **A.** the setting of the group, its duration, and its goals
- **B.** the gender of the group leader, the goals of the group, and the "psychological mindedness" of the members
- **C.** the setting of the group, its duration, and the gender of the group leader
- **D.** the goals of the group, the "psychological mindedness" of the members and the size of the group
- **E.** the goals of the group, its setting, and the "psychological mindedness" of the members

29.4 Which of the following statements regarding membership criteria of a group is not true?

- **A.** Membership criteria vary widely from group to group.
- **B.** Membership criteria are intimately related to the goals of the group.
- **C.** An important criteria is the ability of a member to perform the group task.
- **D.** One criteria might be the ability of the patient to handle a group experience.
- **E.** Motivation for change plays no role in membership criteria.

29.5 Long-term interactional groups place a lesser emphasis on which therapeutic factor?

- **A.** instillation of hope
- **B.** catharsis
- **C.** imparting information
- **D.** development of socializing techniques
- **E.** group cohesiveness

29.6   Corrective recapitulation of the primary family group can be of capital importance in which type of group?

- **A.**   self-help groups
- **B.**   interactional groups
- **C.**   inpatient groups
- **D.**   outpatient groups
- **E.**   recovery groups such as Alcoholics Anonymous

29.7   Group cohesiveness is:

- **A.**   an important mechanism of change
- **B.**   important only in interactional groups
- **C.**   important only in the early stages of a group's history
- **D.**   a necessary precondition for change, but not a mechanism of change
- **E.**   a peripheral feature of group success

29.8   The ideal size for a prototypic interactional group is:

- **A.**   between 15 and 20 members
- **B.**   less than five members
- **C.**   undetermined—there is no ideal size
- **D.**   9 to 12 members
- **E.**   seven to eight members

DIRECTIONS: For each of the statements or questions below, one or more of the alternative answers is correct. Choose answer:

- **A**   if only 1, 2, and 3 are correct
- **B**   if only 1 and 3 are correct
- **C**   if only 2 and 4 are correct
- **D**   if only 4 is correct
- **E**   if all are correct

29.9   Modifying forces that can influence the therapeutic mechanisms in any group include:

1. the type of group
2. the stage of therapy
3. individual differences among patients
4. the gender of the group leader

29.10   Interpersonal learning:

1. is a cardinal feature of self-help groups
2. occurs when behavior patterns arising in the social microcosm of the therapy group are examined
3. occurs mainly in lower functioning groups
4. requires explication of members' reactions to behavior in the group

29.11   Disagreement or conflict between co-therapists:

1. should be avoided in lower functioning groups
2. should be addressed only out of session
3. can be helpful in the later stages of higher functioning groups
4. is never appropriate

29.12   In choosing members for a longer term outpatient group, helpful rules of thumb include:

1. choosing at least one member who is likely to be deviant from the group norms
2. choosing members for homogeneity in ego strength
3. choosing one member who will be dominant and serve as an unofficial co-therapist
4. choosing members for heterogeneity in problem areas

29.13   A cognitive approach to group therapy preparation has among its goals:

1. to provide a rational explanation about group process to the patient
2. to describe what sorts of behavior are expected in group
3. to establish a contract about attendance
4. to raise expectations about the effects of the group

29.14   The leader can influence the process of norm setting by:

1. giving explicit instructions about appropriate group behavior
2. giving social reinforcement for norm-congruent behavior
3. modeling desired behavior
4. punishing inappropriate behavior

29.15   Common problems in group therapy include:

1. membership problems
2. subgroupings
3. conflict
4. absenteeism

29.16 Therapist transparency:

1. refers to the process whereby the therapist becomes a passive observer or "transparent" to the group members
2. involves the therapist's providing feedback about his or her reaction to patient group behavior
3. is inappropriate in higher functioning groups
4. is related to therapist self-disclosure

DIRECTIONS: Each of the following questions consists of lettered headings followed by a list of numbered alternatives. Select the single lettered heading that is most closely associated with the appropriate numbered alternative. Each lettered heading may be chosen only once.

Group therapy techniques

A. Providing structure
B. Direct support
C. Working in the here-and-now
D. Structured exercises

Description

29.17 entails acknowledging openly the efforts, intentions, strengths, positive contributions, and risks of an individual
29.18 can be used as an accelerating technique
29.19 uses a lucid and confident personal style
20.20 is a precondition for interpersonal learning

ANSWERS

29.1   The answer is **D**.

Group therapy has unfortunately been neglected in the training of most psychiatrists. This is especially undesirable because large numbers of psychiatric patients receive some form of group therapy treatment. Multiple outcome studies have shown that group therapy can be an extremely effective component in the treatment of psychopathology.

There has been increasing interest in the use of groups in lay settings as well as in clinical settings. Self-help and peer support groups have become common methods of treating everyone from substance abusers to post-cardiac-surgery patients. Group therapy has many different forms and is appropriate for a wide variety of patients.

29.2   The answer is **B**.

There are several practical aspects of group therapy that make it an attractive form of treatment. Because a number of patients can be seen in a single session, group therapy has the advantage of expediency. Seeing a number of patients in a single session is a more economic use of staff time and therefore has greater cost-effectiveness than does individual therapy. A recent analysis of nine studies indicated that group therapy is an efficient means of treating patients.

In addition to the expediency, efficiency, and cost-effectiveness, group therapy has the advantage of being able to use unique therapeutic properties, such as social support and immediate feedback on behavior, that are not available in individual forms of treatment. Group therapy does not relieve the therapist of having to work during therapy because the therapist takes an active role in monitoring and directing the process.

29.3   The answer is **A**.

There are a large number of different forms of group therapy, from self-help groups to long-term interaction outpatient groups and acute crisis drop-in groups. However, most groups can be categorized using the three interrelated characteristics of group setting, duration of the group, and the goals of the group.

The setting of the group can be inpatient or outpatient. Groups can also be conducted in a retreat setting, in a counseling center, or in a medical setting. The setting of the group has an influence on the types of behavior and interactions appropriate to the group and on the membership of the group.

The duration of the group is usually defined prior to starting the group. Some inpatient psychiatric groups are continuous, with new replacements for members who have been discharged from the hospital or who improve beyond the norm of the group and are transferred. Most outpatient groups have a time-limited format.

The goals of a group vary along a continuum that is related to the type of group. Long-term interactional groups may have personality change as their goal. Short-term inpatient groups may have restoration of function as their goal. Other goals include support in "kicking" a habit, general social support, education, or behaviorally focused changes.

29.4   The answer is **E**.

Membership criteria of a group are directly related to the goal of the group. The general principle is that potential group members must be able to work with the group toward reaching the goals of the group. Exclusion criteria include variables that would interfere with reaching the group goals. For example, a person who tends to dominate a group may not be a viable candidate unless the therapist can control this person's tendency. Someone who is unable to partake in the group interaction, for example, a paranoid person, would also be inappropriate. Finally, potential group members should possess the motivation for change.

29.5   The answer is **C**.

Self-help groups place a relative emphasis on the therapeutic factor of imparting information. Long-term interactional groups place a relative deemphasis on imparting information. Giving advice or objective information is not as important here as other factors such as the instillation of hope, which is actually important in a wide variety of groups. Long-term interactional groups rely on group cohesiveness, or the attraction that members feel for each other and for the group, in order to help make the group interactions meaningful. Long-term interactional groups can also use the development of socializing techniques to help members learn about their maladaptive social behavior. Catharsis, or the ventilation of emotions, can be effective when a group has sufficient cohesiveness to allow real sharing of emotional material.

29.6   The answer is **B**.

Corrective recapitulation of the primary family group can occur in interactional groups where members relate to each other in a manner similar to their previous interactions with parents and siblings. Here the maladaptive social behaviors become apparent in the group setting. What is important is that, in interactional groups, not only is this behavior recapitulated, but there is also an opportunity to correct the maladaptive patterns by examining and challenging the roles of the members and by the therapist encouraging members to try new behaviors.

29.7   The answer is D.

Group cohesiveness refers to the attraction that members feel for each other and for the group. Characteristics of a cohesive group include acceptance of each other, support for each other, and an inclination of the members to form meaningful relationships with each other. Group cohesiveness is a necessary precondition for change rather than a mechanism of change. It is an essential feature of successful groups regardless of the type of group. Although group cohesiveness tends to develop over the course of the group, its presence plays an important role throughout the entire course.

29.8   The answer is E.

The ideal size for a prototypic interactional group is around seven or eight members. The lower limit is probably about 4 or 5 members, the maximum probably 12. The important factor here is to have a size that allows maximal interaction among group members but still provides diversity of the interactions with a large enough number of members.

Other groups may have different ideal sizes. Alcoholics Anonymous often has groups of up to 80 members. A large therapeutic community such as a residential halfway house may have up to 15 members in order to use group pressure and interdependence to instill a sense of responsibility to the community.

29.9   The answer is A.

There are three basic modifying forces that affect the therapeutic factors in group therapy. These factors are the type of group, the stage of therapy, and individual differences among the group members. The type of group affects the choice of factors because some types of groups may be better suited to use catharsis. For example, long-term interactional groups tend to use catharsis, interpersonal learning, and self-understanding—factors that would be inappropriate to a lower functioning inpatient group.

Some therapy factors are more appropriate at some stages of treatment than at other stages. The instillation of hope, guidance, and universality are very important in the early stages of interactional groups. Later, catharsis may be applicable.

The individual differences among patients also play a role in therapeutic factors. Higher functioning patients can derive more benefit from interpersonal learning than can lower functioning patients. Catharsis may not be helpful to the patient who has problems with impulse control and affective modulation.

29.10   The answer is C.

Interpersonal learning does not usually occur in self-help groups or groups composed of lower functioning patients. Interpersonal learning is often overlooked by leaders and requires substantial therapist skill in order to be used effectively. Interpersonal learning can occur because members of a group tend to reproduce in the group the maladaptive social behaviors that are problematic in the outside environment. A person who is arrogant and domineering in outside life will replicate those behaviors in the group setting. However, in the group setting there is an opportunity for group members to provide corrective feedback by sharing their reactions to the problematic behavior. In this way the patient can begin to realize the effect of one's behavior on others and, it is hoped, learn to change. Interpersonal learning is a cardinal feature of longer term higher functioning, interactional groups.

29.11   The answer is B.

There is not complete agreement among clinicians regarding whether co-therapists should openly reveal their differences during group sessions. However, some general guidelines are available. Lower functioning groups are not composed of members who are stable enough to be exposed to conflict between the therapists. Also, early in the course of any group, the members may rely on the authority of the therapists and may need to feel that the therapists represent a unitary sense of accuracy in decision making. Later, in higher functioning groups, the fact that the therapists are being honest and open about their disagreements can provide some powerful modeling for the honesty of the group members. If the members witness the therapists respectfully disagreeing and coming to a successful resolution, they can have more of a sense of the realistic possibilities in conflict resolution.

29.12   The answer is C.

When choosing members of a group, the therapist first needs to decide which patients are likely to benefit from group therapy. Then the therapist needs to decide which patients will work well together. The patients should be motivated to change and should have the persistence to remain in group until the group is terminated. Members should have a commitment to the therapy process. A rule of thumb is to choose members who are homogeneous in ego strength and heterogeneous in problem area. Some specialty groups that are symptom oriented such as bulimia groups may have some homogeneity of problem area, but in general it is desirable to choose patients who are sufficiently different to allow meaningful sharing.

29.13   The answer is **E**.

After group members are chosen, but before the group begins, the therapist must prepare the potential members for the group experience. Misconceptions about the group experience, such as that it is diluted therapy or that frightening confrontation occurs, need to be dispelled. Potential members may also be apprehensive about the prospect of self-disclosing shameful material or concerned about being "infected" with the problems of the other group members. A cognitive approach to group therapy preparation seeks to 1) provide a rational explanation about group process, 2) describe the normative behavior in a group, 3) establish a contract about attendance, 4) raise expectations about the effects of the group, and 5) predict some of the problems, discouragements, and frustrations that may occur early in the course of group therapy.

29.14   The answer is **A**.

Every group, whether therapeutic or not, has a characteristic culture that includes rules for normative behavior. In order to provide and maintain the therapeutic environment, the group therapist must take an active role in building the group culture. One way to accomplish this goal is to explicitly communicate the group behavior norms. The therapist states, and if necessary repeats, the expectations regarding group behavior. Explicit communication occurs more frequently in the early stages of the group therapy. Later the therapist may use social reinforcement to encourage and reward examples of appropriate group behavior. Social reinforcement can occur as the result of smiling, giving a subtle nod, or through the use of body language to signal approval. The therapist can also influence the group culture by modeling appropriate behavior. By being honest and open, the therapist provides an example for the members to follow.

29.15   The answer is **D**.

Group therapy, like any other human endeavor, has potential problems that must be faced in order for the therapy to be successful. Membership problems are a group of issues that require the attention of the therapist. Membership turnover, tardiness, and absenteeism threaten the stability and integrity of the group. A large degree of turnover affects the cohesiveness of the group. Having to deal with tardiness and absenteeism directs the attention and energy of the group away from the therapy task at hand.

Subgrouping can occur when some of the members of the group form implicit or explicit subgroups. This can occur when members meet outside of the group setting, which is why extracurricular socialization should be discouraged. When members form a subgroup, they are less likely to give honest feedback to each other and may "gang up" on group members who do not belong to the subgroup. Group members who do not belong to the subgroup may develop feelings of envy or inferiority.

Conflict will almost always occur during group therapy. The task of the therapist is to direct the conflict resolution in the service of the group goals. Each group can handle different levels of conflict, and the therapist needs to titrate the level appropriate to the goals of the group and the ability of the members to handle conflict.

29.16   The answer is C.

Therapist transparency involves the personal self-disclosure of the therapist. The therapist can react to the patient in an honest (nonjudgmentally frank) manner, thereby revealing something of his or her own personal nature. The therapist needs to monitor the stage of the group members to be sure that they can handle therapist transparency. Lower functioning groups may not be able to deal effectively with much therapist transparency; nor may groups that are still in the early stages of therapy. It is important to note that the therapist does not need to be completely self-disclosing. In fact, the degree of self-disclosure should also be judged against the degree to which it will help or hinder the group process.

29.17   The answer is C.
29.18   The answer is A.
29.19   The answer is D.
29.20   The answer is B.

Providing structure is a technique that is especially applicable to group work in inpatient settings. The therapist can provide structure by making explicit the spatial and temporal boundaries of the group. Use of a clear, lucid, and confident personal style can also provide structure for the confused or anxious patient. Another method of providing structure is to give each session a clearly communicated, explicit sequence.

Direct support can be provided as a modification of the basic group techniques that are appropriate for inpatient and lower functioning groups. In an inpatient setting, the therapist must learn to be able to provide support quickly and directly. One way of giving direct support is to openly acknowledge a member's efforts, intentions, strengths, positive contributions, and risks. It is important to give positive support to each member of the group. It is also important for the therapist to help the patient obtain support from the group.

Working in the here-and-now is of paramount importance for interactional groups, but it also possesses importance for all groups. As part of working in the here-and-now, the members must interact with each other in both a cognitive and an affective manner. They must interact in a way that involves direct emotional experience and expression, but they must also be able to cognitively evaluate that emotional interchange in order to come to some understanding so as to be able to change their behavior. One effective way of initiating work in the here-and-now is to provide an in-group analogue for an out-group problem and then to work on the analogue.

Structured exercises are group activities where the members follow a set of defined rules that are usually prescribed by the therapist. For example, the therapist may suggest that two group members interact in a way that circumvents their usual methods of interaction. These exercises may take a few minutes or they may take up most of the group session's time. They may involve the whole group or some subset of the group members with the other members witnessing and commenting on the action. Structured exercises can be viewed as accelerating devices.

Chapter 30

Treatment of Children and Adolescents

DIRECTIONS: Each of the statements or questions is followed by five suggested responses or completions. Select the one that is the best choice or most complete answer in each case.

30.1 Which of the following statements regarding the evaluation of the child patient is not true?

    A. If a physical examination has not been conducted in the past six months, one would be necessary.

    B. If pharmacological treatment is anticipated, laboratory tests may be necessary.

    C. Information from the school is always useful and sometimes necessary.

    D. A psychological evaluation including intelligence and achievement tests is often useful.

    E. A neurological evaluation is always necessary to rule out a central nervous system etiology.

30.2 Which of the following statements regarding treatment planning is not true?

    A. Treatment planning is almost always based on the diagnosis.
    B. It is important to incorporate a variety of treatment modalities.
    C. The efficiency and the benefit/risk ratio should be considered in choosing a treatment.
    D. Parents should be consulted in the choice of treatment strategies.
    E. An important component of treatment planning is a consideration of the target symptoms.

30.3 Which of the following statements regarding the prediction of stimulant responsivity is true?

    A. Research has helped determine the differential responsivity of hyperactive children to stimulants.
    B. Neither neurological soft signs nor electroencephalogram activity predicts stimulant responsivity.
    C. Electroencephalogram activity but not neurological soft signs helps predict stimulant responsivity.
    D. Neurological soft signs can help predict which stimulant would be most effective in a given child.
    E. Because most hyperactive children will respond to stimulants, pharmacotherapy is the treatment of choice.

30.4 Which of the following statements regarding the effectiveness of antidepressant medication in children is true?

    A. The study of antidepressants to treat depressed adolescents indicates a higher success rate than for adults.
    B. Antidepressants tend to exacerbate obsessive-compulsive disorders in children.
    C. Antidepressants are only as effective as placebo in the treatment of school avoidance.
    D. Imipramine may be effective in treating some children with attention deficit disorder.
    E. Antidepressants are the first choice of treatment for enuresis.

30.5 Appropriate treatment for a 10-year-old with attention deficit disorder may include all of the following except:

    A. stimulant medication
    B. special class in school
    C. low-sugar diet
    D. training for parents in behavior management techniques
    E. social skills training

30.6 In the psychopharmacological treatment of prepubertal children:

    A. doses of medications for some drugs should be determined by milligram per kilogram guidelines

    B. children metabolize psychotropic drugs at the same rate as adults

    C. tricyclic antidepressants should be given once a day

    D. side effects are usually easy to detect

    E. information regarding the correct use of drugs can be found via reference to the *Physicians' Desk Reference*

30.7 The initial treatment of choice for primary nocturnal enuresis is:

    A. behavioral training using a chart with rewards or the bell and pad system

    B. waking the child up several times during the night to urinate

    C. punishing the child when he or she wets the bed

    D. imipramine

    E. psychoanalysis

30.8 Which of the following statements regarding the use of lithium in children is true?

    A. Lithium is ineffective in treating children with aggressive behavior.

    B. Following treatment of an acute episode of mania in a child, doses can be lowered but maintenance treatment is necessary.

    C. Children generally experience side effects at higher serum levels than do adults.

    D. A welcome side effect of lithium is its controlling effect on acne.

    E. Therapeutic levels of lithium are the same for children as for adults.

30.9 Which of the following statements regarding treatment approaches for children is true?

    A. Insight-oriented approaches tend to be the most effective treatment for a wide range of noncompliant behaviors.

    B. Child psychoanalysis is the most thoroughly evaluated psychiatric treatment for children.

    C. The choice of a treatment modality is most highly determined by the training and expertise of the clinician.

    D. Because of their focus on symptoms, behavioral treatments tend to be ineffective short-term answers.

    E. Behavior therapy is the most thoroughly evaluated psychiatric treatment for children.

30.10 Which of the following characteristics has not been found to be associated with less positive outcome in parent training?

    A. low socioeconomic status
    B. the signs of incipient characterological deficits in the child
    C. parental depression
    D. marital conflict
    E. lack of a social support network

DIRECTIONS: For each of the statements or questions below, one or more of the alternative answers is correct. Choose answer:

    A if only 1, 2, and 3 are correct
    B if only 1 and 3 are correct
    C if only 2 and 4 are correct
    D if only 4 is correct
    E if all are correct

30.11 In what ways does the psychiatric treatment of the child differ from that of the adult?

    1. Children are more often brought to therapy by someone else.
    2. Electroconvulsive therapy is virtually never used in children.
    3. Play therapy techniques are commonly used for children, but rarely for adults.
    4. There is no difference, except for adjusting the level of abstract verbal communication to one comprehensible to the child.

30.12 Which of the following statements regarding the use of magnesium pemoline in treating attention deficit disorder is true?

    1. Pemoline is longer acting than most other commonly used stimulants.
    2. Pemoline requires multiple daily doses.
    3. The half-life of pemoline increases with chronic administration.
    4. Pemoline is structurally similar to methylphenidate but dissimilar to dextroamphetamine.

30.13 Which of the following are side effects of the therapeutic use of stimulants?

    1. lowering of the seizure threshold
    2. mild dysphoria with social withdrawal
    3. precipitation of a movement disorder such as tics
    4. risk of addiction

30.14 Tricyclic antidepressant doses should be decreased if which of the following are found?

1. pulse is over 130
2. systolic blood pressure is over 140 mm Hg
3. diastolic blood pressure is over 85 mm Hg
4. the electrocardiogram P-R interval is longer than .22 seconds

30.15 Which of the following statements regarding organic therapies is (are) true?

1. Megavitamin therapies are generally more effective than nutritional therapies.
2. Nutritional therapies are effective only when a diagnosis of attention deficit disorder is accompanied by signs of hyperactivity.
3. Megavitamins are more effective for treating schizophrenia and autism than for treating conduct disorders.
4. Neither megavitamin nor nutritional therapies have been found to be effective.

30.16 Which of the following statements regarding individual psychotherapy for children is (are) true?

1. Studies indicate that individual therapy is more effective than no therapy.
2. Direct but gentle questioning of the child provides much needed information regarding the therapy process.
3. Dynamically oriented therapy is not effective for the treatment of disruptive behavior disorders.
4. Children with conduct disorders are more effectively treated with individual therapy than with group therapy.

30.17 Which of the following statements regarding behavior therapy is (are) true?

1. The goal of the behavior therapies is to change current responses that interfere with adaptive functioning.
2. In behavioral therapy, symptoms are seen as results of bad habits, faulty learning, or inappropriate environmental responses to behavior.
3. Behavior therapy is the most effective treatment for simple phobias, enuresis, encopresis, and a wide range of noncompliant behaviors.
4. Generalization of changes is a central problem in behavior therapy.

30.18 Residential psychiatric treatment may be indicated for:

1. acutely depressed children
2. chronic behavior problems such as aggression, running away, substance abuse, or school phobia
3. treatment of attention deficit disorder
4. treatment of self-destructive acts that the home and community cannot manage

30.19 Issues associated with pharmacological treatment that have differential salience for treating children versus treating adults include:

1. metabolism and kinetics
2. compliance
3. developmental toxicology
4. determination of the risk/benefit ratio

30.20 Side effects of therapeutic stimulant use unique to pemoline include:

1. night terrors
2. lip licking
3. increased lip biting
4. potential precipitation of Tourette's syndrome

ANSWERS

30.1 The answer is **E.**

The pretreatment evaluation of the child or adolescent with psychiatric problems is a necessary precondition for treatment. This evaluation should include a complete history from the parents or guardian. This includes a social, developmental, school, medical, and family history. The child should also be interviewed in order to obtain information related to subjective states and attitudes toward the symptoms. If a complete medical evaluation has not been conducted in the last six months, it should be done at that time. If pharmacological treatment is expected, other laboratory tests may be necessary. Information from the school is always useful and is necessary when there is question regarding learning, school behavior, or peer relations. Another important aspect is a psychological evaluation including intelligence and achievement testing for questions related to learning and other tests as indicated. However, projective tests should not be used diagnostically. The neurological evaluation is conducted only if indicated.

30.2   The answer is A.

Psychiatric treatment of children and adolescents is not diagnosis specific. Therefore the diagnosis should not be the primary determinant in treatment planning. In planning a treatment, it is important to obtain information regarding the strengths and weaknesses of both the family and the child. Treatment planning is also affected by aspects of the social environment including the school, neighborhood, and social support network. The best treatment is a combination of treatment modalities. If the primary clinician is not sufficiently competent in a needed treatment approach, referral should be made to another professional for that aspect of treatment. Treatment planning is also based on the predicted efficiency and calculated risk/benefit ratio of different treatment forms.

The choice of a treatment strategy is largely influenced by the determination of target symptoms. Social skills training may be effective in treating withdrawn children while carefully managed contingencies may be more effective in treating noncompliant behaviors. The parents should be consulted in any decisions regarding treatment, both because they are responsible for the health of the child and because their compliance is often essential to success of any treatment attempt.

30.3   The answer is B.

When the symptoms of inattention, impulsivity, and hyperactivity cannot be attributed to another cause, the use of stimulants may be indicated. The first course of action is to try alternate methods of treatment.

Unfortunately, there are no reliable methods of predicting response to stimulants. Neither neurological soft signs nor electroencephalogram activity predicts responsivity. Nor are there any data to suggest the differential effectiveness of different types of stimulants in treating these children. Important considerations in decisions regarding the use of stimulants include the willingness of parents to monitor medication and to attend appointments.

A substantial number of children will not respond to the initially tried stimulant. As many as 20 percent of these nonresponders will respond to some other stimulant. Given the large proportion of stimulant nonresponders and the possibility of side effects, behavioral management strategies and other psychologically based treatments should be considered.

30.4   The answer is **D**.

The differences between children and adults in response to pharmacotherapy are highlighted in a consideration of the effects of antidepressants. It appears that the use of imipramine for adolescents with carefully diagnosed major depression is effective but at a much lower rate than for adults. Some reports indicate that amitriptyline or imipramine may be effective in treating depression in children, but well-controlled studies indicate that these drugs may be no more effective than placebo. Imipramine appears to be more effective than placebo in treating school avoidance or phobia. Antidepressants may also be an effective short-term treatment for enuresis, but they are not the treatment of choice. Tricyclic antidepressants are occasionally used to treat night terrors and somnabulism. Although it is not the drug of first choice in the treatment of attention deficit disorder, imipramine may be effective in some children. Finally, clomipramine may be effective in treating obsessive-compulsive disorders in children; however, it is not currently available.

30.5   The answer is **C**.

Optimally, treatment of the hyperactive child is multidimensional. Although medication may be helpful in controlling some of the symptoms, it is insufficient in treating the whole constellation of associated problems. Special school classes may be necessary to help overcome the disruptions in acquisition of knowledge and academic skills. Training parents in the application of behavioral management strategies is extremely helpful in helping to control the undesirable behavioral symptoms associated with attention deficit disorder. A family therapy approach may be necessary if dysfunctions in familial relations are present. Social skills training can help remediate deficits in social interactional behaviors. Dietary approaches have not been found to be helpful in controlled studies.

30.6 The answer is **C**.

There are special considerations in the pharmacological treatment of children with psychiatric problems. Although children's absorption, distribution, protein binding, and metabolism of stimulants resembles that for adults by the time the child is three years old, other psychotropic drugs are metabolized by children at different rates than they are for adults. For example, because children have a larger liver size relative to body size than do adults, they tend to metabolize antidepressants more quickly. As a result, children may need a higher weight-corrected dose of imipramine, and doses divided into three times a day may be necessary. Adolescents may be given a single daily dose of tricyclic antidepressants.

Partly because of the problems in getting children to accurately self-report physiological, cognitive, and emotional changes, the detection of medication side effects is more problematic for children. Parents should be carefully trained in monitoring medications effects. The physician is better advised to consult current literature for possible side effects than to consult the *Physicians' Desk Reference*, which may either be insufficiently critical or contain information that is out of date.

30.7 The answer is **A**.

When enuresis occurs only at night, it may be due to delayed maturity. In these cases, waiting for the child to outgrow the problem would be effective. In the meantime, the psychiatrist can discourage the parents from using ridicule or punishment. Also in these cases, restriction of liquids or awakening the child to urinate in the middle of the night have not been found to be effective.

When the older child has a problem with enuresis, the use of behavioral training using a chart with rewards for successfully dry nights may be effective. Another successful method involves the use of conditioning via the bell and pad system.

30.8 The answer is **E**.

Lithium is effective in the treatment of acute manic episodes in children. However, once the acute episode is successfully treated, medication should be terminated after three to six months, and the patient should be monitored for signs of relapse. Lithium is excreted via the kidneys. Because children have more efficient kidney function than do adults, higher doses for body weight may be necessary. Unfortunately, there is evidence to suggest that children experience side effects at lower serum levels than do adults. In addition to the side effects present in adults, the side effect of hypothyroidism is more serious for growing children than for adults. In treating adolescents, it is important to remember that lithium tends to aggravate acne. There is some evidence to suggest that lithium may be useful in the treatment of aggressive behavior in children.

30.9   The answer is D.

The choice of treatment modalities should be based on the target symptoms, the ability of the child's social environment to implement and monitor treatment, and the benefit/risk ratio associated with different treatment modalities. The choice of treatment should not be based on the training or bias of the clinician. If the clinician is not sufficiently trained in a needed approach, referral to an appropriate professional should be made for that aspect of treatment.

Behavior therapy (and not psychoanalysis) is the most thoroughly evaluated treatment modality for children. Behavior therapy (and not insight-oriented therapy) is the most effective treatment for simple phobias, enuresis, encopresis, and a wide range of noncompliant behaviors. Although behavioral treatment may require consistent programs for extended periods of time, the effects of successful behavior treatments are not necessarily time limited or "short term."

30.10   The answer is B.

A benefit of behavior modification techniques is that they can be taught to parents who can then implement them outside of the therapy sessions. The degree to which instructions are clearly communicated and understood plays a large role in their eventual effectiveness. Behavior modification techniques are not a panacea, and there are some limitations to their implementation. Lower socioeconomic status of the parents, parental psychopathology such as depression, the presence of marital discord, and the lack of a social support network are all associated with a less positive outcome for behavior modification techniques. If these characteristics are present, special considerations should be made to help ensure success.

30.11   The answer is A.

Psychiatric treatment of children is very different from psychiatric treatment of adults. One major difference is that the child is brought into therapy by someone else. Therefore, there are at least two clients: the parent and the child. The parent's desires may be in conflict with the child's needs. Children are more dependent on other people to meet their basic needs than are adults. Children have fewer choices regarding residence or activities.

The communication with children should take into account the cognitive and emotional developmental level of the child. Play therapy that allows nonthreatening and sometimes nonverbal communication of concerns is almost never used with adults, but may be common in some child treatment settings. Electroconvulsive therapy is almost never used with children.

30.12   The answer is B.

Magnesium pemoline is structurally similar to both methylphenidate and dextroamphetamine. It is a mild central nervous system stimulant that is longer acting than other stimulants. Therefore, it can usually be given in a single daily dose. Pemoline also has less abuse potential. The half-life pemoline increases with chronic use.

30.13   The answer is C.

Most of the stimulants have similar side effects. Dose-related side effects such as anorexia, weight loss, irritability, and abdominal pain usually disappear after a few weeks. One of the reported side effects of therapeutic stimulant use is mild dysphoria with subtle social withdrawal. A few children may develop a mild to moderate clinical depression. Use of stimulants is associated with small decreases in expected weight gain and a variable effect on height. There have also been reports of small and not clinicially significant effects on pulse and blood pressure. Black adolescent males may be at higher risk for increases in blood pressure. One of the more serious side effects is the possible precipitation of a movement disorder such as tics or Tourette's syndrome.

Less common side effects include dry mouth, dizziness, nausea, euphoria, nightmares, constipation, lethargy, anxiety, hyperacusis, and fearfulness. Talkativeness has been reported as an effect of withdrawal from high doses. It does not appear that stimulants lower the seizure threshold.

30.14   The answer is E.

When using tricyclic antidepressants, it is important to remember that pharmacokinetics are different for children than they are for adolescents. Children have a smaller fat/muscle ratio and therefore have a decreased volume of distribution. Lesser volumes of fat mean that children do not store as much tricyclic antidepressant in body fat in response to excessive dosages.

Because of the danger of dose-related side effects, it is important to monitor the cardiovascular system in children at pretreatment, at initiation of treatment, and at dose changes, as well as at periodic evaluations. The doses should be decreased if pulse goes over 130, if systolic pressure is over 140 mm Hg, if diastolic pressure is over 85 mm Hg, if the electrocardiogram PR interval is longer than .22 seconds, or if the QRS interval is more than 130 percent of baseline.

30.15 The answer is **D**.

In the recent past, there has been much focus on nontraditional treatments for childhood psychiatric problems. Many of these nontraditional treatments center on restricting sugar in the diet of hyperactive children or on the use of megavitamins to treat hyperactivity, schizophrenia, autism, and learning disabilities. In addition, an ethiologic role of certain additives in producing hyperactivity or other childhood behavioral problems has been suggested. Controlled studies indicate a lack of support for these approaches. One study indicated that five percent of hyperactive children were helped by the Kaiser-Permanente diet, but the changes were not as dramatic as those seen in children who were treated with stimulants. Although restricting the amount of sugar in a child's diet may be a good idea in the United States where sugar may be overrepresented in most people's diets, it should not be used as a treatment for hyperactivity. The use of megavitamins is much more problematic because of the possibly toxic effects of large doses of many vitamins.

30.16 The answer is **B**.

In general, studies indicate that individual therapy is more effective than no treatment in alleviating childhood and adolescent psychiatric problems. However, with a few exceptions there are not many data available to suggest the relative effectiveness of different types of treatment approaches. There are strong suggestions that dynamically oriented therapy is not effective in the treatment of the disruptive behavior disorders. Children with conduct disorders may be more effectively treated in group or family settings than in individual settings.

Some of the special problems in treating the child involve the ability of the child to provide relevant information via an interview. The clinician needs to obtain collateral information from parents and teachers. Another set of methods for obtaining relevant subjective information is contained in the repertoire of play therapy techniques. There the child can express threatening material via the use of proxy dolls without having to admit certain feelings and experiences directly to the therapist.

30.17   The answer is E.

In general the goal of behavior therapy is to change the presenting behavioral responses that interfere with adaptive functioning. This goal is achieved by using approaches based on empirically derived psychological principles. Behavior therapists view symptoms as being the result of bad habits, faulty learning, or inappropriate environmental responses to behavior, that is, inadvertant reinforcement of maladaptive behavior patterns.

Behavior therapy is the most effective treatment for simple phobias, enuresis, encopresis, and many different forms of noncompliant behavior. A central concern in behavior therapy is the generalization of treatment gains to settings other than the treatment setting. An entire theory of generalization has been proposed, with the most important point being that generalization procedures need to be planned and incorporated into the treatment early in the course of therapy.

30.18   The answer is C.

Treatment of children should occur in the least restrictive environment. Therefore, inpatient treatment should be viewed as a last resort. Indications for residential treatment include behavior problems such as aggression, truancy, substance abuse, school phobias, running away, and self-destructive acts that have not been well managed or tolerated by the family or community. Sometimes the child's deviant behavior exists in a vicious cycle, engendering maladaptive behavior in the caregiver and further problems exhibited by the child.

Short-term hospitalization may be required when there is evidence to suggest an immediate physical danger to self or others. Alternatively, a crisis in the adult environment may make it temporarily impossible for the usual caregiver to provide a safe and therapeutic environment.

30.19   The answer is E.

Psychopharmacological treatment of children presents special problems and concerns that may not be present in the treatment of adults. One important concern is that of developmental toxicology. Certain drugs may have marked interactions with growth and developmental processes. It is extremely important that drugs not interfere with the processes of normal development, either in a physiological sense or in a social or cognitive sense.

Metabolism and pharmacokinetics may be very different in children. Actively growing tissue may affect drug uptake. The proportional size of organs and tissue masses varies with age, an important consideration especially for those drugs that are concentrated in certain organs.

Determining outcome, both beneficial and side effects, is more problematic for children than for adults. For example, the placebo effect appears to be greater in children than in adults. Children may not possess the cognitive requirements to accurately report physical and emotional feelings. The condition of a child is more variable across time than that of an adult.

Compliance is more complicated in children, partly because the cooperation of two people, the child and the adult caretaker, is required. Refusal of treatment is more common in children than in adults who can more readily understand the need for treatment.

30.20 The answer is **A**.

Magnesium pemoline is a long-acting mild central nervous system stimulant. It shares several of the potential side effects found in stimulant use, including decreases in expected weight gain and effects on pulse and blood pressure. Side effects seen only with the use of magnesium pemoline include night terrors and lip licking and biting. There have also been reports of elevated liver function studies, epigastric pain, or jaundice.

Chapter 31

Suicide

DIRECTIONS: Each of the statements or questions is followed by five suggested responses or completions. Select the one that is the best choice or most complete answer in each case.

31.1 The process of examination of the patient's medical and psychiatric history that often involves evaluation of the suicide victim's volitional intent is referred to as:

- **A.** psychiatric postmortem
- **B.** psychological reconstruction
- **C.** psychological autopsy
- **D.** volitional postmortem
- **E.** volitional determination hearing

31.2 The ratio of attempted to completed suicides as estimated by the *Harvard Medical School Mental Health Letter* (1986) is:

- **A.** 8 to 15 attempts to 1 completed suicide
- **B.** approximately 25 attempts to 1 completed suicide
- **C.** five attempts to one completed suicide
- **D.** three attempts to one completed suicide
- **E.** none of the above

31.3 Statistically, what percentage of the total number of people who attempt suicide complete the act at a later time?

- **A.** 50 percent
- **B.** 10 percent
- **C.** two percent
- **D.** 25 percent
- **E.** 70 percent

31.4 Of the affective disorders, the category most frequently associated with suicide is:

- **A.** unipolar type I
- **B.** bipolar type I
- **C.** unipolar type II
- **D.** bipolar type II
- **E.** bipolar type III

31.5 The lifetime suicide rate for alcoholics has been estimated to be:

- **A.** approximately 15 percent
- **B.** approximately 40 percent
- **C.** approximately five percent
- **D.** approximately two percent
- **E.** approximately 50 percent

31.6 Which of the following central nervous system metabolites has been found to be associated with violent suicide?

- **A.** dopamine
- **B.** norephinephrine
- **C.** 5-hydroxyindoleacetic acid
- **D.** catecholamines in general
- **E.** imipramine

DIRECTIONS: For each of the statements below, one or more of the alternative answers is correct. Choose answer:
  A   if only 1, 2, and 3 are correct
  B   if only 1 and 3 are correct
  C   if only 2 and 4 are correct
  D   if only 4 is correct
  E   if all are correct

31.7   Which of the following statements are true regarding suicide?
  1. Men are more likely to commit suicide than women.
  2. Suicide among women is more common on the east coast than it is on the west coast.
  3. Suicide is more common in American Indians than in other ethnic groups.
  4. Women are more likely to complete the suicide act than are men.

31.8   Which of the following is true regarding the relationship between suicidal behavior and psychiatric illness?
  1. The lifetime risk of suicide in the schizophrenic patient is similar to the risk for patients who suffer from depression or alcoholism.
  2. The overwhelming majority of suicide victims have a concomitant psychiatric illness at the time of the suicide.
  3. Dissolution of marriage through divorce is a common event preceding suicide in alcoholics.
  4. Seriousness of suicide intent has been found to correlate with hopelessness about the future.

31.9   Which of the following are true regarding possible genetic factors and suicide?
  1. The association between suicide and a family history of suicide has been recognized for a long time.
  2. Suicide is virtually nonexistent in the Amish population.
  3. Recent studies of Amish and Danish populations suggest a direct link between genetic factors and suicide.
  4. There is no evidence of a direct genetic link between suicide and inherited characteristics.

31.10 Which of the following animal models has (have) been used to explain the possible basis of suicidal behavior?

1. cognitive dissonance
2. learned helplessness
3. behavioral contrast
4. social separation

31.11 Freud described suicide as:

1. an attack on an internalized object that has become a source of ambivalence
2. a manifestation of previously unrecognized libidinal impulses
3. being directed to the self physically but toward a loved object in the psychological sense
4. almost always being related to fixation at the genital stage of development

31.12 Statistically, individuals who complete suicides are:

1. male
2. affected with depression or alcoholism
3. likely to use a rapid, effective means of suicide
4. likely to make the attempt in isolation

31.13 In assessing suicidality, the following considerations are of importance:

1. a thorough mental status exam that includes a careful examination of thought processes, depressive symptoms, and suicidal ideation
2. the creation of a supportive relationship between the patient and the physician
3. a thorough evaluation of whether or not the patient has a plan for committing suicide
4. an interview conducted in a slow deliberate manner without rapid-fire questioning

DIRECTIONS: Each of the following questions consists of lettered headings followed by a list of numbered alternatives. Select the single lettered heading that is most closely associated with the appropriate numbered alternative. Each lettered heading may be chosen only once.

Durkheim's proposed societal influences on suicidal behavior

A. Egoistic
B. Altruistic
C. Anomic

Description

31.14 was said to occur during times of economic prosperity, when individual freedoms were unencumbered by demands for basic sustenance.
31.15 was thought to stem from excessive individualism and from the decreasing influence of prevailing sociologic norms.
31.16 was thought to occur in response to societal expectations.

ANSWERS

31.1 The answer is **C.**

There is no single, acceptable definition of suicide. Without a suicide note it may be quite difficult to determine whether the cause of death is accidental or is a result of suicide. Generally, coroners and medical examiners are conservative in reporting a death as a suicide. For example, most deaths by drug overdose are reported as accidental. This no doubt reflects an attempt to spare family members unnecessary emotional trauma. In addition, a death by suicide may impact on legal issues such as insurance benefits. There also remains a significant stigma attached to committing suicide, and consequently, coroners rarely investigate suspicious accidents. Overall, the above-mentioned factors often result in an underreporting of suicidal death. Psychological autopsies can help to correct this problem.

A psychological autopsy involves an extensive examination of the patient's medical and psychiatric history as well as interviews with survivors concerning the victim's volitional intent prior to the act. Unfortunately, this is a time-consuming process and is rarely undertaken in a comprehensive or systematic manner.

31.2　The answer is **A.**

Conservative estimates suggest suicide attempts occur 8 to 15 times more frequently than completed suicides (*Harvard Medical School Mental Health Letter*, 1986). Also, attempted suicides often include a wider variety of self-destructive behaviors, ranging from life-threatening acts to less dangerous gestures aimed at gaining attention.

31.3　The answer is **B.**

Statistically, 10 percent of the total number of people who attempt suicide complete the act at a later time. Any suicide attempt should be approached as if it represents a subacute form of suicide as an illness and requires referral to an appropriate mental health treatment center. An important predictor of completed suicide is whether or not there has been a previous attempt. Even suicide "gestures" should not be dismissed lightly, especially if adequate historical information or information concerning the patient's level of emotional support is unavailable.

31.4　The answer is **D.**

Of the illnesses subsumed under the classification of affective disorders, the category most frequently associated with suicide is the bipolar type II group. Suicide figures in this diagnostic category have ranged to 51 percent in several well-defined studies. While the impact of lithium therapy on the control of bipolar type I patients is well documented, the type II patient may be denied a therapeutic trial of lithium because of a lack of typical manic symptoms. Hence, hypomanic episodes alternating with periods of depression may go unrecognized and therefore untreated with lithium since the bipolar nature of the disorder is never recognized.

31.5　The answer is **A.**

Substance abuse in general, and alcoholism in particular, is the second most often encountered psychiatric diagnosis found among patients who commit suicide. In fact, the risk for male alcoholics who have had psychiatric hospitalizations has been placed at 75 times that of the general population within the five-year period following the last psychiatric admission. Generally, most studies predict a lifelong suicide rate of 15 percent for all alcoholics, a figure strikingly similar to the lifetime risk of suicide in depressives.

31.6   The answer is C.

Recent biological studies of psychiatric phenomena have focused on the possible role of central nervous system metabolites, particularly the catecholamines and the indolamines. However, conclusive evidence for their etiologic significance has been lacking.

The question concerning the relationship between central nervous system metabolites and suicidal behavior is a separate issue from that of the involvement of these substances in other psychiatric disorders and separate measurements distinct for suicidality have been suggested. For example, Asberg reported a bimodal distribution of serotonin metabolites, particularly 5-hydroxyindoleacetic acid (5-HIAA) in the cerebrospinal (CSF) fluid of depressed patients. Those patients displaying the lower levels of 5-HIAA were found to be suicide prone by especially violent means such as firearms, hanging, or jumping off high places. In addition, Von Praag compared several different groups featuring violent and suicidal behavior, and his results supported the hypothesis that low CSF 5-HIAA may be correlated with dysregulation of aggression in suicidal behavior.

31.7   The answer is B.

The publication "Suicide: An Update" (1986) provides a wide range of statistical information on suicide. For example, suicide rates remain the highest for individuals over the age of 65. This age group comprises 11 percent of the total population but accounts for 17 percent of all suicides. For the age-adjusted group ages 15 to 44, there is an important and wide variation of male suicide rates by geographic distribution, with the western mountain states having a higher rate of suicide than that of the middle Atlantic states. Overall, the western states, including both the mountain and Pacific regions, have the highest rate of suicide among females. In addition, men are three times more prone to suicide than are women, and elderly men as a group are 10 times more prone to commit suicide than are women. With regard to suicide rates for various ethnic groups, the American Indian has a higher suicide rate than whites at any age. Although as a group blacks commit suicide less frequently than whites, young black males commit suicide twice as frequently as their white counterparts.

31.8   The answer is **E**.

The overwhelming majority of suicide victims suffer a concomitant psychiatric illness at the time of the act, with well-controlled, diagnostically oriented retrospective studies confirming figures as high as 93 to 94 percent. Affective illness, usually major depression, has been identified in 40 to 80 percent of the victims in a consecutive series of studies. More specifically, seriousness of suicidal intent has been found to correlate with one aspect of depression—hopelessness about the future—than with the degree of depression per se.

The lifetime risk of suicide in the schizophrenic patient is 15 percent, similar to the risk for the patient with depression or alcoholism.

With regard to the relationship between suicidality and alcoholism, dissolution of marriage through divorce or an angry separation is the most common event preceding suicide in an alcoholic.

31.9   The answer is **A**.

The relationship between suicide and a family history of suicide has been recognized for some time. Whether the act is produced from a genetic aberration passed from generation to generation or by modeling of suicidal behavior as a coping style is controversial. The psychiatric illnesses most often associated with suicide (depression, alcoholism, schizophrenia) display evidence for their own genetic transmission. Beyond this, it is also possible that suicide is not simply a symptom of another disorder but a genetic defect itself. This has been supported by studies of both Amish and Danish populations.

31.10   The answer is **C**.

Of the laboratory-based animal models of psychiatric illnesses, two of the best known are the learned helplessness model for rats and the social separation model of primates. In the learned helplessness model, rats exposed to uncontrollable electric shock exhibit deficits in learning tasks, spontaneity, and appetitively motivated tasks—symptoms that would respond to treatment with tricyclic antidepressant medications. Although these behaviors would not necessarily be suicidal in the laboratory, they would impair survival in the wild.

With regard to the social separation model, primates separated from their mothers at birth show deficits in locomotor, exploratory, and social behaviors. Under stress, these animals are observed to self-mutilate to a far greater degree than normally raised primates.

31.11   The answer is **B**.

In general, aggression toward the self following the internalization of frustration or disappointment related to a loved one is a prominent psychoanalytic theory of suicidal behavior. Freud described suicide as a murderous attack on an internalized object that has become a source of ambivalence. Since the loved object has become introjected by the individual, the act of suicide is directed to the self physically but toward the loved one in a psychological sense.

31.12   The answer is **E**.

Statistically, the individual who completes suicide is 1) a male in any age category who is 2) afflicted with depression and/or alcoholism, 3) uses a rapidly effective means of suicide, and 4) makes the attempt in isolation. The typical person who attempts but does not complete the suicide is 1) a female who is 2) generally under 35 years of age, 3) frequently has no previously diagnosed psychiatric illness, 4) conducts the suicidal act in a more public setting, and 5) uses means that are generally less lethal.

31.13   The answer is **E**.

The assessment of suicidal potential requires an intensive physical and psychiatric evaluation with a special focus on risk factors. Accurate assessment should include a complete mental status examination in crisis to include an especially careful examination of thought processes, vegetative signs of depression, and suicidal ideation. In addition, approaching the issue of suicide in a slow deliberate manner may assist in establishing a trusting relationship with the patient and therefore allow a more truthful interchange. It is also extremely important to assess whether or not the individual has an actual plan for committing suicide.

31.14   The answer is **C**.
31.15   The answer is **A**.
31.16   The answer is **B**.

Anomic suicide was said to occur during times of economic prosperity, when individual freedoms and personal choices were unencumbered by demands for basic sustenance such as food; a diminution of the influence of society's traditional organizational pattern such as family life was also judged to contribute to anomic suicide.

Egoistic suicide was thought to stem from excessive individualism and from decreasing influence of prevailing sociologic norms, such as the waning influence of the church. In contrast, events that were enacted "for the good of all" such as participation in a nationalistic war were found to lead to a decrease in suicide.

Altruistic suicide was described as resulting from a response to a cultural expectation, such as the act of the widow in India throwing herself on her dead husband's funeral pyre.

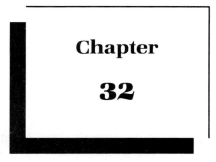

Chapter

32

Violence

DIRECTIONS: Each of the statements or questions is followed by five suggested responses or completions. Select the one that is the best choice or most complete answer in each case.

32.1 There is much concern regarding violent acts perpetrated by psychiatric patients. What percentage of patients presenting to psychiatric hospitals have shown violent behavior just before admission?

    A. less than one percent
    B. about four percent
    C. between five and seven percent
    D. between 14 and 16 percent
    E. about 10 percent

32.2 Which of these statements regarding the relation of sex chromosome abnormalities to violent behavior is true?

    A. XXY chromosome abnormalities are associated with an increase in violent behavior.
    B. XYY chromosome abnormalities are associated with an increase in violent behavior.
    C. There is no association between XXY or XYY chromosome abnormalities and violent behavior.
    D. XXY abnormalities are associated with increases in violent behavior; XYY abnormalities are associated with decreases.
    E. XYY abnormalities are associated with increases in violent behavior; XXY abnormalities are associated with decreases.

32.3 Which of the following statements regarding the relation between violence and drugs is not true?

  A.   There is a strong relation between alcohol use and certain types of homicide involving disputes.
  B.   Opiate drug abuse is directly related to violent behavior.
  C.   Amphetamines are associated with violent behavior.
  D.   Cocaine is associated with violent behavior.
  E.   Hallucinogen abuse is associated with violence.

32.4 Which of the following statements regarding the relation of environmental variables to violent behavior is not true?

  A.   Physical crowding may be related to violence.
  B.   The number of bystanders may be inversely correlated with the level of violence.
  C.   Extremely uncomfortable warm temperatures decrease violence.
  D.   The warmer it is, the more likely violence may occur.
  E.   An increased number of persons without crowding may lead to more social control and decreased levels of violence.

32.5 Which of the following should not be offered during an interview conducted to predict dangerousness with a previously violent patient?

  A.   statements designed to encourage insight into the patient's current level of hostility
  B.   comments that describe the patient's current presentation in a neutral manner
  C.   soft-spoken statements
  D.   calming, nonjudgmental comments on the current situation
  E.   a chair for the patient to sit in

32.6 A number of organic mental disorders are associated with violent behavior. Which of the following is not among the central nervous disorders that have been associated with violent behavior?

  A.   Alzheimer's disease
  B.   paretic hemiparesis
  C.   Wilson's disease
  D.   normal pressure hydrocephalus
  E.   postconcussional syndrome

32.7 A number of personality disorders are associated with violent behavior. Which of the following has the best prognosis?

    A. borderline personality disorder
    B. paranoid personality disorder
    C. intermittent explosive disorder
    D. histrionic personality disorder
    E. schizoid personality disorder

32.8 Borderline personality disorder and intermittent explosive disorder have some traits in common. Which of the following are not associated with borderline personality disorder?

    A. instability of interpersonal relationships
    B. episodic violence
    C. profound mood problems
    D. depressed affect for long periods of time
    E. identity problems

DIRECTIONS: For each of the statements or questions below, one or more of the alternative answers is correct. Choose answer:

    A   if only 1, 2, and 3 are correct
    B   if only 1 and 3 are correct
    C   if only 2 and 4 are correct
    D   if only 4 is correct
    E   if all are correct

32.9 Which of the following are indications for the emergency use of seclusion or restraint?

    1. to prevent imminent harm to others
    2. as part of an ongoing behavior treatment program
    3. to prevent serious disruption of the treatment program
    4. at the patient's request

32.10 The American Psychiatric Association task force on the use of seclusion and restraint recommended

    1. specific techniques of approaching patients
    2. written guidelines and a manual for the use of procedures in a given setting
    3. the use of certain restraint devices
    4. education of the staff and rehearsal of the procedures

32.11 Which of the following statements regarding a patient in seclusion or restraints is true?

    1. A physician should visit a patient every 12 hours.
    2. The patient should be observed by the nursing staff every 15 minutes.
    3. After 72 hours, review of the case by persons outside the treatment unit should occur.
    4. No patient should be left in restraints longer than 15 minutes.

32.12 The neuroleptics are the most common form of sedative used in an emergency situation. However, use of these drugs may be contraindicated in which cases?

    1. toxic metabolic confusional states
    2. violent schizophrenics already on neuroleptic prescriptions
    3. patients intoxicated with alcohol
    4. agitated, depressed patients

32.13 The use of lithium carbonate has not been recommended for the treatment of violent behavior in which patients?

    1. violent patients with bipolar affective disorder, mania
    2. violent patients with personality disorders
    3. violent patients with premenstrual syndrome
    4. violent patients with paranoid schizophrenia

32.14 Propranolol has been recommended for the treatment of violent behavior in patients with:

    1. head trauma
    2. seizure disorders
    3. Wilson's disease
    4. Korsakoff's psychosis

32.15 The phrase "differential reinforcement of other behavior" when applied to the behavioral treatment of violent behavior refers to:

    1. positive reinforcement to reward nonassaultive behavior
    2. social skills training
    3. giving rewards for the emission of violence-incompatible behaviors over increasing time periods

ANSWERS

32.1 The answer is **E.**

There has been much publicity surrounding the violent acts per-petrated by psychiatric patients. Both television and newspaper reports detail stories regarding patients who may have been discharged from a psychiatric facility and subsequently committed a violent act. However, these reports provide publicity for events for which the actual frequency may be low. Many more violent acts are associated with robbery than with psychiatric disorders. Studies of the incidence of violent acts by psychiatric patients indicate that approximately 10 percent of the patients admitted to a psychiatric service may have committed some form of a violent act just prior to admission.

32.2 The answer is **C.**

Perhaps because of the observed greater frequency of violent acts committed by males, there has been a past focus on the relation between violent behavior and abnormalities involving the sex chromosomes X and Y. A double-blind controlled study found no relation between either XXY or XYY chromosomal abnormalities and violent behavior. Other studies have investigated other aspects of the relation between violent behavior and genetics. However, a recent study failed to show any relation between violence committed by adopted men and violent be-havior in either the adopted or the biological parents.

32.3 The answer is **B.**

Opiate drug use is not directly related to violent behavior. Instead, the relation appears to be indirect, since narcotic drug abusers tend to engage in violent criminal behavior in order to obtain money to support their drug habits. There are several studies that link other forms of drug abuse and violent behavior. For example, there is a relation between alcohol use and violent behavior to settle disputes. Many other forms of drug abuse appear to be related to violent behavior. Included in this category are the amphetamines, cocaine, hallucinogens, and minor tran-quilizers.

32.4 The answer is **D.**

There have been a number of studies investigating the relation be-tween environmental variables and violent behavior. Physical crowding tends to increase the frequency with which violent behavior occurs.

Increases in the number of people without an increase in crowding may actually decrease the level of violence by increasing social control. Increasing the number of bystanders available for surveillance and intervention may decrease the frequency of violent behavior.

The relation between temperature of the environment and level of violent behavior is more complex. Moderately uncomfortable temperatures result in increases in violence. However, extremely hot, uncomfortable temperatures actually decrease the level of violent behavior.

32.5   The answer is **A**.

The previously violent patient or potentially violent patient requires special considerations in an interview situation. The interviewer should appear to be calm and in control. The interviewer should speak in a manner that is neither provocative nor judgmental. One can begin by making concrete comments about obvious facts, for example stating that the patient looks angry. Interpretations regarding insight or dynamic considerations do not have a place in these situations. Both the interviewer and the patient should be seated. There should be adequate space between the two individuals so that the patient does not feel crowded. Direct eye contact should be avoided because it might be seen as a challenge to the patient.

32.6   The answer is **B**.

Violent, aggressive behavior is associated with multiple disorders of the central nervous system. These disorders include traumatic injuries, infections, and congenital disorders. The traumatic injuries associated with violent behavior include birth trauma, adult injuries, and postconcussional syndrome. Infections include encephalitis and postencephalitic syndrome, brain tumors, Alzheimer's disease, Wilson's disease, multiple sclerosis, and normal pressure hydrocephalus have all been associated with violent behavior. Other central nervous system disorders secondary to body system dysfunction that have been implicated in violent behavior include hypoglycemia, electrolyte imbalance, hypoxia, uremia, vitamin insufficiencies, systemic infections, systemic lupus erythematosus, porphyria, and industrial neurotoxins.

32.7   The answer is **C**.

Personality disorder patients have a wide range of possible dysfunctional behavior, including violent behavior. In general, patients with personality disorders tend to act out their problems rather than talk about them. The patients with the best prognosis are those patients with intermittent explosive disorder. These patients have multiple discrete episodes of loss of control involving violence directed at another person or involving destruction of property. Although it is sometimes possible to identify precipitants to the violent act in these patients, the violence is out of proportion to the events precipitating it. The violence can last from minutes to an hour and may be associated with the use of alcohol. Frequently, the patient expresses remorse following the incident.

32.8   The answer is D.

Borderline personality disorder has some characteristics in common with the intermittent explosive disorder. Both disorders will exhibit episodic violence. However, for borderline personality disorder, the episodic violence is associated with broad instability in interpersonal relations. As well as violent acting out, the borderline personality patient will act out in sexual terms and will also show other impulsive behaviors such as overeating, spending sprees, suicide attempts, stealing, and alcohol and drug abuse. The borderline personality disorder will also exhibit disturbances of identity and mood.

32.9   The answer is E.

The use of seclusion and restraints is controversial because of the potential for abuse. Court rulings have indicated that the principle of least restrictive treatment should regulate interventions aimed at all patients including the violent patient. A task force of the American Psychiatric Association has suggested several indications for the use of seclusion and restraints. Violence need not actually have occurred, but may be imminent. Seclusion and restraints may be used to prevent imminent harm to the patient or others when other means of intervention are not available. They may also be used to prevent serious disruption of the treatment program or significant damage to the environment, as part of an ongoing behavioral program, to decrease the stimulation that the patient receives, or at the patient's request.

32.10   The answer is C.

The American Psychiatric Association task force on the use of seclusion and restraints did not recommend specific procedures, techniques, or equipment. However, they did recommend that an institution should have written guidelines for the use of seclusion and restraints and a manual for the use of these two procedures. The task force also recommended that the guidelines be approved by the institution's lawyer, administration, and state. Staff should receive education in the use of the procedures and actual rehearsal of the procedures. There should also be a mechanism for providing feedback from the staff regarding problems with the guidelines so that revisions could be made.

32.11 The answer is **A**.

When the patient is first put in seclusion or restraints, he or she should be visited by a physician. A physician should see a patient in seclusion or restraints at least once every 12 hours. The patient should be observed by the nursing staff every 15 minutes with written documentation of the patient's behavior and status. After 72 hours of continuous restraint or seclusion, the case should be reviewed by a person not involved in the case. Nursing staff should visit the patient in the room at least once every two hours. The patient should be allowed to use the toilet every four hours.

Meals for the patient should be served at the same time as the rest of the patients receive their meals. No forks or knives, even plastic ones, should be allowed in the room. When the patient is in four-point restraints, each extremity should be released or loosened every 15 minutes. Patients restrained on their back should be observed constantly in order to check for aspiration.

32.12 The answer is **B**.

Medication in the treatment of violent behavior can be divided into medication in the emergency situation and medication in the long-term treatment and prevention of violent behavior. Neuroleptics are the most commonly used type of medication in the emergency treatment of violent behavior. However, depending on the diagnosis of the patient, there are special considerations that must be made in the use of these medications. When treating patients with organic mental disorders, the sedative or anticholinergic effects of the neuroleptics may worsen delirious or toxic metabolic confusional states. Similarly, the use of neuroleptics is contraindicated in cases of intoxication with alcohol or sedatives.

32.13 The answer is **D**.

The use of lithium carbonate for the treatment of mania is well known. However, lithium has also been recommended for the treatment of violent behavior in retarded individuals, for the treatment of violence in patients with personality and conduct disorders, and for violent patients with premenstrual syndrome. These recommendations are in need of controlled studies in order to back up the suggestions with empirical data regarding their effectiveness.

32.14   The answer is **E.**

Propranolol, a beta-adrenergic blocking agent, has been recommended in the treatment of violent behavior in patients with traumatic head injury, seizures, Wilson's disease, Korsakoff's psychosis, mental retardation, minimal brain dysfunction, and other organic mental disorders. The response time to propranolol varies between two days and more than two weeks. Side effects include lowered blood pressure, pulse rate, and, less frequently, respiratory problems including wheezing or bronchospasms. Other reported side effects include nightmares, ataxia, and lethargy.

32.15   The answer is **A.**

Differential reinforcement of other behavior is a behavioral method by which the frequency of undesirable behavior is decreased by increasing the frequency of desired behavior. The general idea is that there is a finite amount of behavior that can be emitted by the patient. When punishment is inappropriate or when the undesired behavior is a low-rate phenomenon, the patient can be rewarded for emitting behavior that is desired. Examples of differential reinforcement of other behavior in the application to decreasing violent behavior include positive reinforcement to reward nonassaultive behavior and social skills training to increase the likelihood that the patient will express negative emotions in a more acceptable fashion. The differential reinforcement of other behavior also includes giving rewards for demonstrations of violence-incompatible behavior over gradually increasing periods of time. Seclusionary time-out is an example of punishment.

Chapter 33

Psychiatry and the Law

DIRECTIONS: Each of the statements or questions is followed by five suggested responses or completions. Select the one that is the best choice or most complete answer in each case.

33.1 Which of the following subareas is not considered part of the area of law and psychiatry?

    A. peer review
    B. informed consent
    C. advertising
    D. relationships with nonphysician health care providers
    E. worker's compensation

33.2 Psychiatry in the practice of law is not concerned with:

    A. consultation directed toward the ends of the legal system
    B. the patient's welfare
    C. competency to stand trial
    D. child custody
    E. personal injury

33.3 The difference between psychiatry and law hinges on several points. However, these differences are not related to:

    A. the extent to which a person's mental status is impaired
    B. the type of logic used
    C. a focus on rights versus a focus on needs and welfare
    D. concepts of causation
    E. empirical evidence versus precedent

33.4 Different forms of competency issues can be raised prior to trial and are collectively known as criminal competencies. Which of the following is not included among them?

    A. competency to waive Miranda rights
    B. competency to testify
    C. testamentary competency
    D. competency to be executed
    E. competency to be sentenced

33.5 A psychiatrist asked to evaluate a defendant's competency to stand trial primarily directs attention to the defendant's mental condition at the time of:

    A. the alleged crime
    B. release from custody of the criminal court
    C. sentencing on the criminal charge
    D. the present examination
    E. the criminal arrest

33.6 In 1983 legislation related to the special verdict of insanity, the U. S. Congress enacted an insanity defense based on:

    A. the volitional capacity of a defendant
    B. the cognitive capacity of a defendant
    C. both the volitional and the cognitive capacities of a defendant
    D. the diminished mental capacity of a defendant
    E. the diminished mental capacity and volitional capacity of a defendant

33.7 A psychiatric disorder that impairs a defendant's criminal competency is:

  A. schizophrenia
  B. irreversible dementia
  C. any psychiatric disorder that presents with sufficient cognitive impairment or communicative capability
  D. organic affective disorder
  E. organic amnesia

33.8 The past psychiatric practice of a retired psychiatrist without a current malpractice insurance policy is covered for liability as long as his or her former policy was of the:

  A. occurrence type
  B. claims type
  C. exclusive type
  D. pure loss type
  E. ultimate net loss type

33.9 Which of the following is not one of the criteria proposed by Delgado-Escueta regarding the determination of whether a seizure resulted in a specific crime?

  A. The diagnosis of epilepsy is established by an experienced neurologist.
  B. The presence of epileptigenic automatism is documented by electroencephalogram telemetry and closed circuit TV.
  C. The criminal act should be consistent with documented ictal behavior.
  D. The occurrence of aggressive behavior should diminish under appropriate medication.
  E. A neurologist should provide the clinical judgment that the criminal act was the result of a seizure disorder.

33.10 A successful tort action must maintain which of the following elements?

  A. A legal duty was owed the plaintiff by the defendant.
  B. The defendant breached a legal duty.
  C. The plaintiff was damaged.
  D. The injury occurred as a result of an action by the defendant.
  E. The defendant is able to provide recompense.

DIRECTIONS: For each of the statements or questions below, one or more of the alternative answers is correct. Choose answer:

A if only 1, 2, and 3 are correct
B if only 1 and 3 are correct
C if only 2 and 4 are correct
D if only 4 is correct
E if all are correct

33.11 Which of the following statements regarding the right to refuse psychotropic medication is (are) true?

1. Courts agree that a voluntary inpatient has an absolute right to refuse medication in a nonemergency.
2. Courts agree that a committed individual has an absolute right to refuse medication in a nonemergency.
3. Courts agree that an inpatient does not have the right to refuse medication in an emergency.
4. In most states, an inpatient's right to refuse medication is determined at a civil commitment hearing.

33.12 The 1976 *Tarasoff* decision:

1. specified a legal duty to warn a potential victim
2. is invoked after a serious threat to property or person
3. pertains to serious threats of suicide
4. pertains only to therapists within California

33.13 Which of the following statements regarding the standard of care in malpractice suits is (are) true?

1. Standards of care are derived from local considerations.
2. A physician with some other specialty will be judged by psychiatric standards in the treatment of a mental disorder.
3. Specialists and generalists are held to the same standards of care.
4. Standards of care are derived from national considerations.

33.14 Exceptions to the disclosure requirements of informed consent include:

1. an emergency situation
2. when the patient waives his or her right
3. when the physician believes disclosure would be detrimental to the patient
4. when the patient is incompetent to give consent

33.15   Criteria for civil commitment typically include the presence of:

1. refusal of voluntary admission
2. serious mental illness
3. danger to property
4. danger to others

33.16   Testamentary competence involves the ability of an individual to write a will. Requirements of testamentary competence include:

1. an awareness that a will is being signed
2. understanding of the identity of the heirs
3. familiarity with the extent of property to be willed
4. absence of undue influence of others

33.17   According to the zone of physical danger rule, a bystander to a personal injury is:

1. entitled to recover for his or her own emotional distress
2. must have suffered physical injury in order to recover damages
3. must be placed in danger of physical injury in order to recover damages
4. must bring his or her legal claim within one year of injury

33.18   Successful defenses against a claim of abandonment include:

1. proof that the patient was responsible for the termination of treatment
2. proof that the patient failed to inform the physician of concurrent treatments obtained elsewhere
3. proof that the patient failed to seek treatment from a referred care provider
4. proof that during treatment the standard of care was met

33.19   Professional liability may be risked in the case of psychopharmacology when injury results from the use of psychotropic medication and when:

1. there was failure to disclose relevant information to the patient and/or guardian
2. there was a failure to obtain an adequate history
3. there was a failure to monitor and treat side effects
4. there was a failure to consult with the relevant experts

33.20   Sexual activity between therapist and client may not be defended on the basis that:

1. it was necessary to the treatment of a sexual dysfunction
2. it was necessary to the treatment of a gender disorder
3. it occurred outside the office and therefore outside the therapeutic relationship
4. it was a necessary corrective emotional experience

ANSWERS

33.1   The answer is **E**.

The area of law and psychiatry refers to the legal regulation of psychiatry. The various types of law that regulate psychiatry include constitutional, statutory, and regulatory law. Historically, psychiatry had been self-regulated. However, there has been a shift to external and governmental control over psychiatric practice. Most states now have mental health codes or laws.

There are several subareas that can be considered to be part of law and psychiatry. For example, issues related to informed consent to examination and treatment, voluntary and involuntary treatment, malpractice, liability for acts to third parties, and confidentiality are all part of law and psychiatry. Other subareas include evidentiary privilege, record keeping, billing practices, employment contracts, staff privileges, peer review, advertising practices, relationships with nonphysician health care providers, and insurance for health care.

33.2   The answer is **B**.

Psychiatry in the practice of law is also known as forensic psychiatry. This area is concerned with the application of psychiatry to legal issues for legal purposes. Any psychiatric interventions here are related to legal issues in which the patient is involved, whether voluntarily or involuntarily. The psychiatric activity is undertaken toward the ends of the legal system, not toward the ends of the patient.

A forensic psychiatrist may be called on to provide psychiatric services in areas of competency, such as competency to stand trial, competency to be sentenced for a crime, or competency to be executed. The forensic psychiatrist may also be asked to provide information related to criminal responsibility for an alleged offense. Similarly, the forensic psychiatrist may be asked to provide information related to testamentary competency, competency to manage one's financial affairs, child custody, termination of parental rights, personal injury, or workman's compensation. Generally, the forensic psychiatrist serves some party other than the patient, such as the court or an attorney. While the general psychiatrist is concerned with the welfare of the patient, the forensic psychiatrist is concerned with the legal rights of the patient.

33.3   The answer is A.

Professional activity involving both psychiatry and the law is not lightly undertaken. The psychiatrist who seeks to undertake this activity should be familiar with the differences between the two fields. Psychiatry and law are derived from different ideological and conceptual fields. Although psychiatry relies on deductive reasoning, the law relies on inductive reasoning. Psychiatrists operate in an atmosphere of cooperation among professionals, but lawyers operate in an adversarial system. Psychiatrists are generally concerned with the welfare and needs of the client, and lawyers are concerned with the rights of a client. The scientific basis of psychiatry derives from empiricism. The basis of the law is legal precedent. The activity of law may be directed at correcting past wrongs, and psychiatry is directed at the control of present and future events.

The legal system holds that an individual has free will in his or her behavior. Although psychiatry may basically agree with this concept, psychiatry is also cognizant of the determinism brought about by biological and psychological factors. The law admits of differing levels of certainty, but psychiatry does not articulate among levels of certainty. Psychiatrists may depend heavily on information derived from an individual in the environment of the client, but the law does not allow hearsay evidence.

33.4   The answer is C.

When an individual is charged with a crime, several issues of competency may be raised prior to trial. These issues are referred to as criminal competencies. They include competency to waive Miranda rights, competency to testify at trial, competency to stand trial, competency to be sentenced, and competency to be executed. These issues of competency arise when a lawyer (either defense or prosecuting) or a judge suspects that the mental condition of the defendent will interfere with the ability of the defendant to participate in the trial process.

33.5   The answer is D.

The determination of a defendent's competency to stand trial has at issue the mental status of the defendant at the time of the present examination. The issue of competency to stand trial has its origins in the common law concept of a prohibition against trying an individual in absentia. The defendant needs to be competent in order to provide his or her lawyer with information necessary to the defense, especially where that information is known only to the defendant. The defendant cannot be said to have been fairly tried unless the defendant is able to understand the defenses, their consequences, and the nature of the proceedings against him or her. Retribution and individual deterrence cannot be said to have been well served if the defendant did not understand why the trial occurred. Finally, the judicial process may be demeaned if the defendent is disruptive.

33.6   The answer is B.

One of two standards for determining criminal competency is used in state courts. The first standard, used in about half of the states is the traditional M'Naughten standard. Using the M'Naughten standard, a defendant can use a defense of insanity if he or she can prove that at the time of the alleged crime, the defendant did not know the nature and quality of the act because of a defect of reason from a disease of the mind. The second standard is that recommended by the American Law Institute and adopted by most of the remaining states. This standard adds a clause to the M'Naughten standard and states that the defendant must not have the capacity to appreciate the criminality of the act or the capacity to conform his or her behavior to the requirements of the law.

In 1983 the U.S. Congress enacted a law that determined the criminal insanity test for federal courts. This test requires that a defendant appreciate the wrongfulness of his act at the time of the alleged crime. Therefore, it is a test of the cognitive capacity of the defendant to understand the nature of his or her act.

33.7   The answer is C.

There is no psychiatric disorder that will a priori allow a defendant to be judged incompetent to stand trial. However, any psychiatric disorder that presents significant impairment in cognitive or communicative capabilities may be determined to affect the defendant's criminal competency. Although functional psychiatric disorders predominate in the distributions of disorders evaluated for criminal competency, it is not unusual for a psychiatrist to be called on to evaluate an accused criminal with irreversible dementia, cerebral vascular disease, head trauma, organic affective disorder, or substance-induced organic mental disorder.

There are three general methods by which a psychiatric disorder may be used in a successful defense against charges of criminal activity. The first method involves evidence that the psychiatric disorder present at the time of the alleged crime negated the mens rea (criminal intent) required for the crime. The second method involves evidence that the defendant's mental condition at the time of the crime can relieve the defendant of responsibility through the verdict of insanity. The third method involves the use of evidence regarding a psychiatric disorder in order to find the defendant guilty but mentally ill.

33.8   The answer is A.

There are a large variety of malpractice insurance policies available, and they all have varying levels of coverage. Probably the most all-inclusive type of coverage is known as the occurrence variety. With this type of policy, the past psychiatric practice of a retired physician without a current malpractice policy is covered for liability. Therefore, as long as the policy was in place at the time of the alleged event, the insurance company must cover the losses, regardless of when the claim is filed. As might be expected, this type of coverage is extremely expensive for the insurance company.

Another type of coverage is known as claims-made coverage. Here, the insurance policy covers only those claims reported during the policy year. Unfortunately, the insured individual is then responsible for any claims filed after the policy is no longer in effect. Claims-made insurance policies are cheaper than occurrence policies for the first five years of coverage. After that period of time, the costs tend to even out.

33.9   The answer is D.

Some cases involving the determination of criminal responsibility have involved attempts to use the defense of epilepsy. However, ictal violence is probably a very rare event. It is much more likely that stereotypical behavior may occur ictally, although it is possible that stereotypical behavior of a defensive nature may involve criminal activity.

Delgado-Escueta and his colleagues have attempted to standardize practice in this area by proposing five criteria that must be met in order for a determination to be made that a violent crime was the result of an epileptic seizure. First, the diagnosis of epilepsy must be made by an experienced neurologist who is competent in seizure disorders. Second, the presence of an epileptogenic automatism must be documented by electroencephalogram telemetry and closed-circuit TV. Third, ictal aggression must be verified in a videotaped seizure with concomitant seizure activity in the electroencephalogram record. Fourth, the patient's aggressive or violent acts must be consistent with the history of ictal behavior. Fifth, a neurologist should provide the clinical judgment that the criminal activity was the result of a seizure episode. It is not necessary to prove that the occurrence of the behavior diminishes under medication.

33.10   The answer is E.

Tort law refers to the law of civil wrongs. The defendant sues to recover damages from the plaintiff for the occurrence of physical or emotional harm. A psychiatrist may be involved in one of two types of tort actions: personal injury or professional negligence. A successful tort action requires four separate components. First, a legal duty must be owed the plaintiff by the defendant. Second, the defendant must have breached that duty. Third, the plaintiff should have suffered damage. Fourth, the injury must have occurred as the result of the defendant's breach of duty.

Usually monetary compensation is allowed for negligently inflicted injuries as well as for their emotional consequences. The damages due for emotional or psychological consequences are known as parasitic torts and are less frequently the cause of monetary compensation than are physical injuries.

33.11   The answer is B.

Involuntary psychiatric hospitalization requires the determination that an individual has a mental illness and is in need of treatment. However, even after an individual is civilly committed, he or she can refuse treatment, including treatment in the form of psychotropic medication in certain instances. Both voluntary and civilly committed patients have the right to refuse medication in a nonemergency if they are competent.

There are three general models used to determine the treatment of civilly committed patients who refuse medication. In the first model, the medical model, the decision to override the patient's refusal is made by the treating physician or another physician, either one on the staff of the same medical facility or a physician from the community. In the second, or administrative, model, a committee composed of physicians, nurses, patient advocates, and administrators determines the disposition. In the third model, the judicial model, the patient has to be declared incompetent before the refusal can be overridden.

The usual criterion for determining the disposition of refusal of medication in nonemergencies is incompetence. However, other considerations include the prognosis with and without medication, the presence of chronic danger to self and others, and the risk of significant medication side effects. Inability to participate in the treatment plan without medication, the likelihood that medication will shorten hospitalization, the religious beliefs of the patient, and the consideration of least restrictive treatment are also variables entering into the determination decision.

33.12   The answer is D.

Professional negligence in psychiatry refers to the duty of the physician to the patient. A related issue is the duty of the physician to other individuals, for example, the duty to protect. The most famous case involving this issue was the Tarasoff case. In this case, the therapist was sued by the parents of a woman who was killed by an outpatient. The ultimate decision of the California Supreme Court was that the therapist has a duty to protect an intended victim if that victim can be readily identified and in those cases in which the ultimate victim is in close proximity to the intended victim. Although strictly speaking, the Tarasoff case applies only to therapists in California, the ruling is likely to influence cases in other states.

33.13   The answer is C.

Malpractice is professional liability or negligence in conduct of professional duties. Court decisions regarding malpractice are measured against the concept of standard of care. Standards of care are determined on a national, rather than a local, basis. When a specialist practices outside the area of expertise, he or she is held to the same standards as apply to the area of care. For example, a cardiologist treating depression is held to the same standard of care as a psychiatrist treating depression. However, specialists are usually held to a higher standard of care than are general practitioners.

No medical professional is expected to guarantee results. However, the physician is expected to exercise the same degree of skill, care, diligence, and judgment as would another physician in a similar situation. Malpractice cases are governed by the law of civil torts.

33.14   The answer is E.

Informed consent can only be given by a legally competent patient or by a surrogate. In obtaining informed consent, the physician is required to inform the decision-maker of the nature and purpose of the intended treatment as well as of the anticipated benefits and risks associated with the intended treatment. In addition, the physician is required to provide information regarding alternative treatments and, in some cases, the prognosis without treatment.

There are four conditions under which a physician may forego obtaining informed consent. The first such instance is when obtaining consent may delay, jeopardize, or prevent treatment, resulting in substantially adverse consequences to the patient. The second instance is when the patient waives the right to consent or to the information. The third instance is when the physician believes that disclosure of the information may be significantly detrimental to the condition of the patient. The fourth instance is when the patient is legally or functionally incompetent to make the decision. In the fourth instance, the physician must obtain informed consent from a surrogate decision-maker.

33.15   The answer is C.

Earlier, civil commitment was dependent on determination of the presence of a mental illness in need of treatment. The criteria for civil commitment are still in evolution. However, most current conceptions require the presence of a serious mental illness and the presence of danger to self or others. The criteria of dangerousness can be vague in definition and application. Some legal jurisdictions have also requested the presence of an overt act of violence or attempted violence. Other jurisdictions may include damage to property (but not danger to property) or psychological harm to the patient. Other criteria have included the availability of treatment at the facility in question, the treatability of the patient, and the unwillingness or inability of the patient to consent to hospitalization.

33.16   The answer is E.

In a general sense, the competence of an individual pertains to the understanding of the nature and consequences of his or her behavior in a given situation. In particular, the requirements of testamentary competence include an awareness that a will is being signed. In addition, the individual must be able to assess the quality and the quantity of the estate and must be able to identify the heirs. Finally, the individual must be free from undue influence from others.

33.17   The answer is **B**.

Personal injury cases refer to attempts to obtain redress of harm visited on an individual by the actions of another. In some cases, the plaintiff can recover monetary damages for emotional distress if he or she was placed in physical danger while witnessing physical harm to another individual. This is known as the zone of physical danger rule.

33.18   The answer is **A**.

Abandonment refers to the termination of treatment when the decision is made by a physician in disagreement with the patient. A patient proves abandonment when it can be shown that the decision to terminate treatment was unilateral and without referral to another treatment possibility. Successful defenses against claims of abandonment can be accomplished if the physician can prove that the patient was responsible for the termination of treatment, if the patient failed to inform the physician of medication side effects or of treatment obtained from another source, if the patient failed to pay the bill or comply with the terms of treatment, or if the patient failed to obtain treatment from the referred second care provider.

33.19   The answer is **E**.

The risk of professional liability in the prescription of psychotropic medication can occur if the patient suffers injury secondary to the physician's negligence. The other requirements for professional liability in these cases include a failure by the physician to obtain an adequate history, a failure of the physician to provide relevant information to the patient or surrogate decision-maker, and a failure by the physician to obtain adequate laboratory testing or physical examination prior to treatment. Other considerations include use of a drug with unknown efficacy in the treatment of the disorder in question; prescription of a drug or drug combination when not indicated, in the wrong dosage, or for the wrong treatment interval; or failure to recognize, monitor, and treat side effects. Finally, professional liability is risked when there is a failure to consult the appropriate experts.

33.20 The answer is **E**.

Sexual feelings between physician and patient may be unavoidable, and in some cases may work to the benefit of the patient. However, sexual behavior between psychiatrist and patient is unethical. Sexual activity between psychiatrist and patient may not be defended on the basis that it was necessary to the treatment of sexual dysfunction or gender disorder or that it was a necessary corrective emotional experience. Nor can sexual interaction be defended on the basis that the interaction occurred outside the office and was therefore outside the therapeutic relationship.

Chapter 34

Ethics and Psychiatry

DIRECTIONS: Each of the statements or questions is followed by five suggested responses or completions. Select the one that is the best choice or most complete answer in each case.

34.1 Ethics are described by the American Medical Association Council on Ethical and Judicial Affairs as follows:

- A. a system of moral philosophy
- B. a method of settling ethical dilemmas
- C. a code of etiquette for physicians
- D. a code of moral principles, customs, and policies for physicians
- E. a system of values relating to right or wrong conduct

34.2 Observing ethical rules of conduct is important for a psychiatrist because:

- A. they provide an assurance of predictability to the patient
- B. they will protect the psychiatrist from malpractice suits
- C. they lead to the good life
- D. they will keep the psychiatrist out of legal difficulties
- E. none of the above

34.3 The key value in the Hippocratic Oath is:

    A. look after your patients
    B. do not harm
    C. take care of society
    D. do not overcharge
    E. cure the patient

34.4 Sexual contact between a psychiatrist and patient:

    A. is sometimes therapeutically beneficial
    B. should not always be considered to be unethical
    C. helps the patient better define reality
    D. usually occurs between a male therapist and female patient
    E. none of the above

34.5 The most common source of breach of confidentiality usually occurs from:

    A. the third-party carrier
    B. the psychiatrist
    C. employee assistance departments
    D. the patient
    E. the medical records clerk

DIRECTIONS: For each of the statements below, one or more of the alternative answers is correct. Choose answer:

    A if only 1, 2, and 3 are correct
    B if only 1 and 3 are correct
    C if only 2 and 4 are correct
    D if only 4 is correct
    E if all are correct

34.6 The Hippocratic Oath has been criticized for the following reasons:

    1. It is too paternalistic.
    2. It is too "patient centered."
    3. It ignores responsibilities to society.
    4. It ignores patient rights.

34.7 Psychiatrists practicing in a pluralistic society face:

    1. a variety of different value systems among values
    2. the task of converting patients to their values
    3. therapeutically the need to be nonjudgmental
    4. diffusion of values

34.8 Psychiatric diagnosis can:

1. stigmatize the patient
2. constrain the patient's freedom
3. undermine the patient's family relationships
4. create unemployment problems for the patient

34.9 Electroconvulsive therapy:

1. is an unethical form of treatment
2. produces less memory impairment with unilateral administration
3. should be legally outlawed
4. has a very low mortality rate

34.10 The Current Opinions of the American Medical Association Council on Ethical and Judicial Affairs (1986) has offered the following guidelines on advertising medical services:

1. Advertising in an aggressive manner is permissible so long as advertisement of services does not involve the use of the mediums of television or radio.
2. Advertising should be designated to communicate information in a straightforward, dignified, and readily comprehensible manner.
3. "Yellow pages" advertisement is strictly forbidden.
4. Any advertisement or publicity, regardless of format or content, should be true and not misleading.

DIRECTIONS: Each of the following questions consists of lettered headings followed by a list of numbered alternatives. Select the single lettered heading that is most closely associated with the appropriate numbered alternative. Each lettered heading may be chosen only once.

Ethical principle

A. Primum non nocere
B. Do not abandon
C. Accountability and informed consent
D. Exploitation of the doctor–patient relationship
E. Breach of confidentiality

Description

34.11 may be threatened by increasing efforts at cost containment by insurance carriers

34.12　requires the discussion with the patient of relevant aspects of treatment (charge for services, who else will have access to the records, and conditions of disclosure of the details of therapy)

34.13　is the principle that if breached may be because of undue involvement of the psychiatrist in the patient's financial affairs as well as sexual contact between the physician and patient

34.14　is the backbone of the Hippocratic tradition

34.15　requires that patients be forewarned in advance of the psychiatrist's plans to leave town

ANSWERS

34.1　The answer is **D**.

The American Medical Association defines ethics as "matters involving moral principles or practices; customs and usages of the medical profession; and matters of policy not necessarily involving issues of morality in the practice of medicine."

34.2　The answer is **A**.

Rules of conduct are essential parts of the practice of psychiatry because they are evolved from the basic moral principle of "do your duty." This involves expectations of what the patient can count on from the physician and what he or she has a right to believe will be forthcoming. Nowhere in medicine is this moral expectation more important than in psychiatry.

34.3　The answer is **B**.

The Hippocratic tradition, which exerts a major influence on present-day medical ethics, originated in the fifth century B.C. This oath provides written expression of the resolve of the physician to avoid actions which could be damaging or destructive to the patient. This principle is embodied in the dictate "Primum non nocere" (first do not harm).

34.4   The answer is **D**.

Clearly, the most sensationalized form of patient exploitation is un-due intimacy or sexual contact between the psychiatrist and patient. A recent survey of psychiatrists revealed a small segment (six percent) who have reported sexual or inappropriately intimate contact with patients. This study reports approximately the same prevalence as surveys con-ducted 10 years earlier. The overwhelming majority of such relationships occur between male psychiatrists and female patients.

34.5   The answer is **B**.

Psychiatric practice in the United States offers many opportunities for breach of confidentiality. The primary source is the psychiatrists themselves, most often carelessly with colleagues and others. Many psychiatrists practice in multiple roles, including consultation, therapy, and forensic evaluation, offering increased access to private information about patients and families that can be easily shared without consent.

34.6   The answer is **E**.

In recent years, the Hippocratic oath has been criticized as encour-aging a paternalistic attitude in the doctor–patient relationship, ignoring patient rights, and ignoring the physician's responsibility to society.

34.7   The answer is **B**.

Medical ethics can be complicated because the psychiatrist lives in a pluralistic society with diverse and conflicting values. Psychiatry is governed by a humanistic code well summarized by Barton and Barton: "Preserve life, relieve suffering, seek to restore wholeness of those who seek help, be beneficent and just, be honest and keep promises, obey the law, do your duty."

34.8   The answer is **E**.

The social attitudes concerning psychiatric illness and the stigma often associated with psychiatric treatment place the patient in a position of vulnerability in seeking treatment. In fact, the very act of diagnosis can spell a loss of personal freedom, the use of potentially dangerous medications, and a stigmatizing label. Legal and social disadvantages such as loss of credibility as a employee or parent are also a threat. Furthermore, the very nature of emotional disorders damages the au-tonomy of the patient and creates an extra risk of undue dependency on or sensitivity to the doctor–patient relationship.

34.9   The answer is **C**.

Electroconvulsive therapy (ECT) is no longer employed in many state hospitals for fear of litigation. At one point this form of treatment was banned by law in Berkeley, California. However, current data on electroconvulsive therapy document that with the use of modern techniques such as unilateral treatment, it is a very safe treatment with practically no mortality and practically no morbidity.

34.10   The answer is **C**.

The Current Opinions of the American Medical Association Council on Ethical and Judicial Affairs (1986) has offered the following guidelines on the use of advertisement for psychiatrists: "The form of the communication should be designed to communicate the information contained therein to the public in a direct, dignified and readily comprehensible manner. Aggressive, high pressure advertising and publicity may create unjustified medical expectations. Any advertisement or publicity, regardless of format or content, should be true and not misleading."

34.11   The answer is **E**.
34.12   The answer is **C**.
34.13   The answer is **D**.
34.14   The answer is **A**.
34.15   The answer is **B**.

A serious and insidious infringement on privacy comes from insurance carriers, peer review activities, and case management reviews related to payment for psychiatric services. More and more information is required to justify payment for the kind of treatment, days in the hospital, and duration of treatment. Although the ethical psychiatrist strives to protect confidentiality of the patient and shares with the patient when confidentiality is violated, efforts toward cost containment pose a real threat to the doctor–patient relationship.

The issue of informed consent is as important in establishing the treatment contract between doctor and patient as is the protection afforded research subjects under the law. Patients increasingly expect to know the details of the treatment contract. Information concerning the doctor's billing practices, policy regarding missed appointments, side effects of psychoactive medications, charges for telephone consultation, and who will have access to the patient's records are but a few of the details of importance. The ethicality of the psychiatrist depends on whether or not he or she has discussed these points with the patient. The key component in this relationship is the word *knowing*. Mills has outlined three elements in the patient's knowing. These include the patient's competency, the ability to understand rationally; the patient's knowledge of the circumstances of treatment or research; and his or her voluntarily entering the treatment/research contract without coercion or improper inducement.

Although somewhat less spectacular than sexual misconduct between the psychiatrist and patient, ethical questions of undue influence in financial matters are also very important. Examples of this include offering a relative of the therapist a job, outright bequest of money, or offering to include the therapist in the will. Not only do these place obstacles in the therapeutic process, but they also represent an exploitation of the relationship.

The principle of Primum non nocere (first do not harm) is the backbone of the Hippocratic tradition. Therapeutic interventions in medicine are fraught with potential harm. Psychiatry is no exception. Three kinds of potential harm are particularly important with regard to psychiatric treatment: hospitalization against the patient's will, pharmacotherapy, and the use of somatic treatments. Hospitalization is potentially harmful because it constrains the patient's fundamental right to freedom. Medications may produce permanent side effects, habituation and addiction, or may be employed in a suicide attempt. The somatic therapies, especially electroconvulsive therapy and psychosurgery have been subject to legal criticism and constraint.

The principle of "do not abandon" clearly states that the physician shall be free to choose whom to serve but that it is unethical to abandon the patient. Patient should be forewarned, either before the consultation begins or well in advance, of the therapist's leaving the therapy situation. If the therapist must terminate the therapeutic relationship, adequate effort should be made to refer the patient elsewhere.

Chapter 35

Psychiatry and Culture

DIRECTIONS: Each of the statements or questions is followed by five suggested responses or completions. Select the one that is the best choice or most complete answer in each case.

35.1 Society is defined as a group of human beings who live together in a system of:

- A. hermits
- B. social relationships
- C. families
- D. political affiliations
- E. none of the above

35.2 Environment refers to physical circumstances of climate, natural resources, and:

- A. social relationshps
- B. activities
- C. altitude
- D. health
- E. geography

35.3 The imposed etic view refers to a collection of observations about a culture that may be characterized as:

    A. objective
    B. distortions
    C. reasonable
    D. thorough
    E. nomothetic

35.4 The longer and more intimate the mother–son symbiosis is, the more likely it is that the boy will become:

    A. androgynous
    B. feminine
    C. masculine
    D. a transvestite in adult life
    E. psychotic in adult life

35.5 Recent research has challenged the old assumptions that American blacks possess:

    A. significant self-hatred
    B. high IQs
    C. dependency traits
    D. musical talent
    E. a higher rate of schizophrenia than non-blacks

35.6 As Puerto Ricans acculturate to New York City, their willingness to express their subjective distress:

    A. remains the same
    B. has increased
    C. has rapidly increased
    D. has decreased
    E. none of the above

35.7 An example of a culture-specific syndrome would be:

    A. meningitis
    B. epilepsy
    C. falling-out
    D. schizophrenia
    E. affective disorder

35.8 Migration causes stress primarily because of the encounter with:

   A.   different family values
   B.   a similar language
   C.   religion
   D.   educational systems
   E.   different social customs

35.9 In the acculturation process, marginality represents:

   A.   a negative view of life
   B.   emphasis on seeking friendship with the dominant group
   C.   emphasis on self-respect
   D.   a good approach to political detente
   E.   none of the above

DIRECTIONS: For each of the statements below, one or more of the alternative answers is correct. Choose answer:

   A   if only 1, 2, and 3 are correct
   B   if only 1 and 3 are correct
   C   if only 2 and 4 are correct
   D   if only 4 is correct
   E   if all are correct

35.10   Problems with attempts to establish the frequency of psychiatric disorders across cultures include:

   1. lack of agreement about diagnostic categories
   2. a lack of well-prepared interviewers who may not use the language of their respondents
   3. difficulty coordinating accurate health care surveys in the United States
   4. the narrow interpretation of schizophrenia in the United States compared with other countries

35.11   The following represent explanations for the finding that blacks in the United States are overdiagnosed in some diagnostic categories and underdiagnosed in other categories:

   1. erroneous diagnoses that may be caused by social differences between patient and clinician
   2. stereotypes of black patients
   3. controversy relating to the use of traditional intelligence tests in black populations
   4. stereotypes of psychopathology expected of blacks

DIRECTIONS: Each of the following questions consists of lettered headings followed by a list of numbered alternatives. Select the single lettered heading that is most closely associated with the appropriate numbered alternative. Each lettered heading may be chosen only once.

Culture-specific syndrome

A. Ataque
B. Amok
C. Koro
D. Bulimia

Description

35.12 is often characterized by anxiety, hyperventilation, confusion, and pseudoepileptic movements; there may also be screaming or violence
35.13 was traditionally associated with Malaya but has also been described as occurring in Africa, and in New Guinea. It is characterized by sudden, unprovoked rage.
35.14 is most common among middle-class white females although it has also been observed among black females from similar socio-economic circumstances
35.15 is quite rare and has been described among the Cantonese and Malayans and manifests itself as an oppressive fear that one's penis is shrinking

ANSWERS

35.1 The answer is **B**.

Leighton and Murphy have defined "society" as a group of human beings who live together in a system of social relationships.

35.2   The answer is C.

The term "environment" refers to physical circumstances of climate, altitude, natural resources, and the presence or absence of noxious agents. In the context of cultural psychiatry, the effect of the environment on behavior is thought to be especially important. For example, a tropical climate has considerable influence on the games played by adolescents and favors the use of the outdoors over indoor play. Similarly, a colder climate may influence the behavior of young lovers in that activities out of doors would be limited by the outside temperature.

35.3   The answer is B.

An important problem inherent to cultural or transcultural psychiatry arises from distortions regarding the population under study. For example, someone from culture A who makes observations about culture B is likely to do so from the perspective of culture A. The concept of "etic" refers to culture-general or universal approaches to the viewing of psychiatric problems. Consequently, observers from culture A may impose their cultural perspectives on the observations about culture B. The result is a "pseudoetic" or imposed etic view that may represent a collection of distortions about culture B.

35.4   The answer is B.

A significant example of the study of developmental issues in cultural psychiatry has been the elaboration of theories of masculinity. Stoller and Herdt posited the hypothesis that the longer and more intimately and pleasurably established was a mother–son symbiosis, the more likely it would be that the boy would become feminine. These investigators used New Guinea observations to test their hypothesis, examining an isolated tribe called the Sambia. This tribe was studied because they hold maleness and warriorhood in high esteem and because each male is viewed as being essential to communal productivity and military defense. The Sambia were found to establish a strong and prolonged bond between mother and son. However, the males of the tribe undergo a unique and elaborate ritual to break the bond, and ultimately develop into strong heterosexual males.

35.5   The answer is A.

The impact of culture on intrapsychic development has been an important theme in cultural psychiatry, and this has been particularly evident in research focused on the development of self-concept among minority groups in the United States. It is an old hypothesis that blacks possess significant self-hatred. This lack of a self-concept has been thought to be reinforced by the white dominant American culture that has defined blackness as being inferior. However, this assumption has recently been challenged on methodological grounds.

35.6   The answer is D.

In regard to the basic notion of how culture may affect the expression of distress, studies of Puerto Ricans have been particularly interesting. Rates of reported symptoms among Puerto Ricans seem to have remained high at all socioeconomic classes and were noted to be higher when compared to respondents from other cultural groups. More specifically, it has been found that the severity of the psychiatric symptom scores of the Puerto Ricans surveyed in New York City varied inversely with the length of time the individual had lived in the city. From this finding, it was concluded that culture seemed to account for the Puerto Ricans' willingness to express their subjective distress; and, as they acculturated to New York, their traditional response style has tempered.

35.7   The answer is C.

Considerable work has been done on the description of syndromes psychiatrists consider either to be unique to certain cultures or to occur with increased frequency among a defined group of people. One example of this is the syndrome referred to as "falling out" seen in black Americans. This syndrome is characterized by collapse without loss of bowel control or biting of the tongue.

35.8   The answer is A.

It is no secret that migration has long been regarded as a cause of psychopathology. The movement of individuals from a culture where they may be surrounded by family, friends, and familiar institutions to a different geographical area that distances them from their usual supportive environment has generally been seen as stressful. Such dislocation of people from their own cultural group has frequently been a contributory element to the emergence of psychopathology in the individual. For example, Canino and Canino have described the process of acculturation for Puerto Ricans who migrate to the United States. They described the traditional, normal enmeshment pattern of the Puerto Rican family as characterized by the presence of an authoritarian father and submissive, self-effacing mother. However, the Puerto Rican family that has migrated to the United States has to confront poverty, discrimination, minimal political influence, as well as a host of cultural values that are different. The mother may be encouraged to abandon her submissive role and consequently foster a more autonomous role in the adolescent daughter, thus challenging traditional family values.

35.9   The answer is **A**.

Berry and Kim have constructed a theoretical model that has been useful in understanding how stress influences the type of acculturation outcome. In this model, marginality is an adaptational response to stress and represents a hopeless and negative view of life. Individuals who subscribe to this view of life are likely to be functioning on the periphery of life.

35.10   The answer is **A**.

Attempts to establish the frequency of psychiatric disorders across cultures have been fraught with difficulties. Significant issues arise from the fact that researchers and clinicians have been unable to agree on diagnostic categories. For example, it has been well established that schizophrenia tends to be a broader category in the United States than it is in other countries. Also, in the United States, significant problems have been associated with health care surveys of the minority populations, specifically for Spanish-heritage Americans, Afro-Americans, Native Americans, and Asians. Difficulties have also been associated with technical problems associated with the preparation of interviewers who may not speak the language of their respondents.

35.11   The answer is **E**.

Several reasons have been given for alleged errors in diagnosis of blacks in the United States. First, social and cultural differences between the patient and clinician might account for erroneous clinical work. These differences are manifested in the areas of vocabulary and style of communication. Stereotypes of black psychopathology have also been evoked as being partially responsible. Another explanation for diagnostic differences between blacks and other populations has been the use of psychological tests in general and intelligence tests in particular. Currently, controversy exists with regard to the use of these tests with black patients. Some researchers have made the point that there is nothing wrong with using these tests despite the fact that most psychological tests were developed for use with nonminority populations. Others have taken the opposing view that intelligence testing with blacks should not be undertaken and that more "culture fair" test instruments should be developed and used.

35.12   The answer is **A**.
35.13   The answer is **B**.
35.14   The answer is **D**.
35.15   The answer is **C**.

Puerto Rican syndrome, or ataque, is characterized by anxiety, hyperventilation, confusion, and pseudoepileptic movements. There may also be hallucinations, screaming, violence to others or to the self, and mutism. Usually, the episode is self-limited and may last only minutes. At other times it is more severe and may last as long as several days, thereby causing diagnostic confusion with an acute schizophreniform reaction or atypical psychosis.

The syndrome of amok has traditionally been associated with Malaya, but has also been described as occurring in Africa, and in Papua New Guinea. It is characterized by a sudden, unprovoked rage that leads to the individual aimlessly running around with a weapon that is used to kill animals or people. Sometimes, the perpetrator kills himself. Those who have been captured have claimed no memory for the episode.

Bulimia has been argued to be most common among middle-class American white females, although it seems to be appearing also among black females from a similar socioeconomic background. This syndrome is characterized by excessive food intake with subsequent self-induced vomiting. It has also been associated with depression and with anorexia. This syndrome is considered by many to be an American culture-bound disorder because it is rare in other parts of the world.

Koro is a rare syndrome described among the Cantonese and Malayans. It manifests as a severely oppressive fear an individual has that his penis is shrinking and will disappear into his abdomen. It has been argued that this syndrome has been seen in different cultures and is nothing more than a culture-influenced delusion that is part of schizophrenia.

Chapter 36

Geriatric Psychiatry

DIRECTIONS: Each of the statements or questions is followed by five suggested responses or completions. Select the one that is the best choice or most complete answer in each case.

36.1 The first priority in assessing patients with cognitive dysfunction is:

    A. an inquiry for symptoms of depression or delirium
    B. the physical examination
    C. review of medications
    D. a computed tomographic scan
    E. a full-scale neuropsychological examination

36.2 Individuals with chronic, progressive dementias who reside in the community constitute approximately what percentage of the elderly population?

    A. 25 percent
    B. five percent
    C. 50 percent
    D. one percent
    E. 15 percent

36.3   The fundamental cause of Alzheimer's disease is:

A.   previous head trauma
B.   brain tissue autoimmune disease
C.   currently not known
D.   a slow virus
E.   a breakdown of the blood–brain barrier

36.4   The classical form of late-onset primary paranoid disorder is referred to as:

A.   catatonia
B.   hebephrenia
C.   nuclear schizophrenia
D.   paraphrenia
E.   late-onset schizophreniform disorder

36.5   Pseudodementia refers to:

A.   a reversible dementia that is secondary to depression
B.   a short-lasting delirium, usually caused by medication toxicity
C.   a chronic condition in which cognitive impairment is less global than in the full dementia syndrome
D.   a state usually attributable to schizophrenia
E.   none of the above

DIRECTIONS: For each of the statements below, one or more of the alternative answers is correct. Choose answer:

A   if only 1, 2, and 3 are correct
B   if only 1 and 3 are correct
C   if only 2 and 4 are correct
D   if only 4 is correct
E   if all are correct

36.6   Which of the following are true regarding dementias?

1. They occur after normal intellectual maturity has been reached.
2. There is usually a deterioration in social functioning.
3. There is usually deterioration of memory, orientation, general intellectual, and specific cognitive abilities.
4. Dementias are always progressive.

36.7 Alzheimer's disease is characterized by the following changes in the brain:

1. neurofibrillary tangles
2. degeneration of postsynaptic muscarinic receptor sites
3. degeneration of cholinergic pathways from the nucleus basalis to the temporal lobe
4. a decrease in amyloid levels in the nerve fibers

36.8 Which of the following are true regarding paraphrenia?

1. The risk of a schizophrenic spectrum disorder is higher in families of paraphrenics than in families of adult schizophrenics.
2. Women are particularly vulnerable.
3. The paraphrenic's lifelong personality structure is usually normal.
4. The paraphrenic usually maintains competence in the running of his or her life until the onset of illness in old age.

36.9 The following are characteristic of the clinical picture of depression in the elderly:

1. Somatic concerns are usually prominent.
2. Depressed mood may not be clearly described by the patient.
3. Subjective complaints of memory loss
4. Agitation

36.10 Which of the following are true regarding depression in the elderly?

1. High rates of relapse are common.
2. The elderly are likely to make successful suicide attempts.
3. The prognosis for short-term improvement is good when duration of illness is short.
4. Prognosis is significantly better in patients who do not have evidence of brain atrophy.

36.11 Which of the following are true concerning the use of tricyclic antidepressants in the elderly?

1. The starting dose should be one-half that of a younger patient.
2. They are often used to treat heart block in the elderly.
3. Elderly patients should routinely receive pretreatment electrocardiograms.
4. Doxepin remains the medication of choice for the elderly.

36.12 Which of the following represent modes of treatment for Alzheimer's disease that follow a rational cholinergic model of treatment?

1. administration of oral lecithin
2. administration of physostigmine
3. administration of piracetam
4. administration of hydergine

DIRECTIONS: Each of the following questions consists of lettered headings followed by a list of numbered alternatives. Select the single lettered heading that is most closely associated with the appropriate numbered alternative. Each lettered heading may be chosen only once.

Psychiatric disorders in the elderly

A. Alzheimer's disease
B. Multi-infarct dementia
C. Creutzfeldt-Jakob disease
D. Delirium
E. Normal pressure hydrocephalus

Description

36.13 is characterized by very rapid deterioration and is complicated by muscular atrophy and fasciculations and extrapyramidal involvement. This disorder is thought to be caused by a slow virus.

36.14 is likely to have a sudden onset, a changeable picture, and a stepwise pattern of neurologic decline

36.15 typically results from systemic disorders arising outside of the cranium and is a reversible toxic state

36.16 is progressive in nature and is characterized by an initial loss of the ability to perform "higher level" tasks at home or in the work place and, in the later stages of the disease, aggression, nocturnal wandering, and death

36.17 presents with gait disturbance, incontinence, and slowed mentation

ANSWERS

36.1   The answer is **A**.

The first priority in assessing patients with cognitive dysfunction is a specific inquiry for symptoms of depression or delirium. The diagnostic process should then progress to a history of the symptom. For example, disability that is chronically related to intellectual impairment is a key symptom of dementia. Marked fluctuation of symptoms, depressed affect, or a previous history of depression point more to a depressive process. Subsequent steps in the diagnostic process should involve a physical examination, evaluation of medications, and evaluation of neurological signs of stroke or intracranial mass.

36.2   The answer is **B**.

Persons with chronic, progressive primary and secondary dementias who reside in the community constitute approximately five percent of the general elderly population (age 65 or older). Individuals with these dementias who reside in long-stay institutions comprise another 2.5 percent of the general elderly population (although they make up approximately 50 percent of the long-stay residents). Therefore, most persons with one of these dementias reside outside of institutions.

36.3   The answer is **C**.

The fundamental cause of Alzheimer's disease in not currently known, and there is probably more than one process that underlies this disease process. In surveys of precursors to Alzheimer's disease, head trauma occurs more often than by chance. The presence of amyloid and immunoglobulins in plaques in the brain has led to the suggestion of a brain tissue autoimmune disease. Changes in brain antibody levels and antigens of the histocompatibility system have given support to this avenue of research. Possibly a breakdown in the blood–brain barrier allows access to damaging substances such as aluminum that may give rise to cognitive impairment along the lines of dialysis dementia (although this condition differs in important respects with regard to neuropathology). A slow virus has been sought but has not been identified in Alzheimer's, although such a virus has been found to be important in other neurologic conditions such as kuru.

36.4   The answer is **D**.

Late-onset primary paranoid disorder and schizophrenia share aspects of either their nature, symptoms, or both. The classical form of this disorder is called paraphrenia and is a chronic but not progressive syndrome with an onset in old age and a predominance of paranoid delusions and hallucinations with little or no impairment of affect, volition, or intellect.

The key criteria for paraphrenia have been described as a) onset after 60 years of age; b) paranoid delusions persisting for more than two weeks; c) not being secondary to dementia, delirium, or affective disorder.

36.5   The answer is **A**.

The subgroup of elderly depressed individuals with prominent symptoms resembling dementias is variously referred to as "pseudodementia" or "reversible dementia secondary to depression." This syndrome is discovered in approximately four percent of patients referred for investigation of dementia. These patients tend to recover their normal level of cognitive functioning when the depression is properly treated. Symptoms that characterize pseudodementia are a sudden, acute onset of cognitive symptoms with rapid progression, a history of depression, the presence of depressive symptoms, and the patient's showing excessive concern about cognitive symptoms (truly demented patients usually endeavor to "cover up" their deficits). A detailed neuropsychological evaluation can often be helpful in elucidating, over time, the inconsistent pattern of cognitive dysfunction that is often seen in pseudodementia.

36.6   The answer is **A**.

The dementias are a set of typically chronic syndromes in which the most striking features involve deterioration of memory, orientation, general intellectual and specific cognitive capacities, and social functioning, which arise after normal intellectual maturity has been reached. Consciousness remains clear in this disorder. Although dementias have historically been thought of as being progressive in nature, it is now recognized that it is possible to detect, treat, and reverse certain dementia syndromes.

36.7   The answer is **B**.

In Alzheimer's disease the frequency of microscopically visible senile plaques and neurofibrillary tangles in the cerebral cortex is increased beyond age norms. The plaques enmesh the neuronal terminals with amyloid, and the tangles fill the nerve cells with paired helical filaments. Dendritic processes and spines waste away. However, there is still uncertainty as to whether the neuropathological changes seen in Alzheimer's disease are the cause or result of brain dysfunction. Cholinergic pathways from the nucleus basalis to the temporal lobe degenerate, choline acetyltransferase is decreased, and the production of acetylcholine is reduced. The postsynaptic muscarine receptor sites are not affected.

36.8   The answer is C.

Among families of paraphrenics, the risk of a schizophrenic spectrum disorder is raised, but it is not as high as in families of adult schizophrenics. The risk among relatives is raised for both adult and late-onset types but with some loading toward the latter. It has also been suggested that the mode of genetic transmission in paraphrenia is recessive.

Women are particularly vulnerable to paraphrenia. The lifelong personality of the paraphrenic is usually abnormal, with the patient often being described as being cold-hearted, prone to take offense, and isolated. In spite of an abnormal personality, the paraphrenic usually maintains competence in the running of his or her household until old age.

36.9   The answer is E.

Compared with younger patients, somatic concerns in the elderly with depression are more prominent, and are often elaborated into delusions of disease or of bodily dysfunction. Depressed mood tends to be less prominent in the elderly, with distress being described as feelings of emptiness, anxiety, or unease. Subjective complaints of memory loss are also common. In addition, symptoms such as agitation and nihilistic delusions are also observed.

36.10   The answer is A.

There are exceptionally high rates of suicide among the elderly, particularly among elderly males. In general, elderly patients tend to be serious in their suicide attempts and their first attempt is likely to be their last. Suicide is usually preceded by a clinical depression or by other psychiatric illness. With adequate treatment of the major depression, the prognosis for short-term improvement is good where duration is short. The prognosis becomes poorer if the duration of illness is greater than two years. High rates of relapse are the rule among elderly patients. Although 90 percent recover initially, about 75 percent will relapse over time unless maintained on pharmacological treatment. Evidence of atrophy of the brain does not alter the prognosis for the depression.

36.11   The answer is B.

Antidepressants are often indicated for the treatment of major depression in the elderly. The clinician can use the same medications in the elderly that are used for younger patients. The tricyclic antidepressants, once known to be causes of arrhythmias, are now known to suppress ventricular ectopic beats when used in therapeutic dosages. This action can aggravate a preexisting mild conduction disturbance into a serious heart block. Therefore, elderly patients should routinely receive pretreatment electrocardiograms. Doxepin was once thought to be especially safe for the elderly; however, this drug's relative cardiovascular safety and clinical efficacy remain open to question. In general, starting doses of antidepressants are typically about half of the standard for adults.

36.12   The answer is A.

The specific treatment of Alzheimer's disease has not as yet progressed beyond the experimental stage. Current treatment strategies have recently moved away from combating anoxia toward following a rational cholinergic model. For example, trials of choline in the form of oral lecithin have been used. In addition, physostigmine, arecoline, and piracetam have also been used.

36.13   The answer is C.
36.14   The answer is B.
36.15   The answer is D.
36.16   The answer is A.
36.17   The answer is E.

A very rapid deterioration complicated by muscular atrophy and fasciculations and extrapyramidal involvement is suggestive of Creutzfeldt-Jakob disease.

In multi-infarct dementia, there is usually a more rapid onset than is observed in Alzheimer's disease, and a changeable picture with a stepwise pattern of cognitive decline. In addition, there are often neurological motor signs and asymmetries, the presence of hypertension, a history of signs of stroke, or arteriosclerotic damage at other sites.

Delirium (acute confusional states) states typically result from systemic disorders arising outside the cranium and are reversible: toxic states (such as infections, drug side effects), anoxia, and metabolic or endocrine imbalance. Delirium can also arise from an intracranial process such as an infection or space-occupying lesion.

With Alzheimer's disease, there is a gradual onset and progessive decline in cognitive and social functioning. Alzheimer's disease is an invariably disabling condition that impairs the individual's higher level functioning at work, in handling finances, in finding the way in public places, in shopping, or in self-care. During the later stages of the disorder, simple self-care tasks such as toileting, mobility, dressing, and feeding may be impaired.

Normal pressure hydrocephalus classically presents with a gait disorder, incontinence, and slowed mentation and movement.

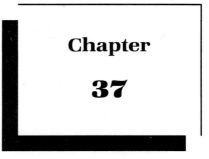

Chapter

37

Community Psychiatry and Prevention

DIRECTIONS: Each of the statements or questions is followed by five suggested responses or completions. Select the one that is the best choice or most complete answer in each case.

37.1 Which of the following statements are true regarding community psychiatry in the 1960s?

    A. It emphasized primary prevention.
    B. It encouraged community activism to change the basic fabric of society.
    C. It involved itself in community, national, and international affairs, poverty, and politics.
    D. It gave high priority to the chronically mentally ill.
    E. It emphasized services to children.

37.2 Which of the following was not an important factor in the deinstitutionalization of psychiatric patients?

    A. aid to the disabled being made available to the mentally ill
    B. the abundance of community resources for the mentally ill
    C. the community mental health centers legislation
    D. the introduction of phenothiazines
    E. the states wanting to shift costs of the mentally ill to the federal government

37.3 Which of the following is not one of the five basic services mandated by the initial community mental health center legislation?

    A. inpatient treatment
    B. outpatient services
    C. drug and alcohol abuse services
    D. partial hospitalization
    E. consultation–education

37.4 Providing psychiatric services in rural areas is impeded by all of the following except:

    A. increased tolerance of deviance
    B. large geographical areas
    C. limited psychiatric services
    D. professional isolation
    E. excessive workload

37.5 Excluding genetic counseling, primary prevention is possible in which of the following conditions?

    A. tertiary syphilis
    B. schizophrenia
    C. pellagra
    D. mongolism
    E. birth injury

37.6 The individual credited with providing the climate for the community psychiatry movement is:

    A. Freud
    B. Charcot
    C. Pinel
    D. Jackson
    E. none of the above

37.7 One of the major issues relating to governance in community psychiatry is:

    A. a tendency for fewer psychiatrists to assume the position of mental health center director

    B. the increasing entry of psychiatrists with administrative backgrounds into community psychiatry

    C. a decreasing interest in treating the acutely ill patient in the mental health center environment

    D. the progressive movement of psychiatrists to more rural settings

    E. none of the above

DIRECTIONS: For each of the statements below, one or more of the alternative answers is correct. Choose answer:

    A   if only 1, 2, and 3 are correct
    B   if only 1 and 3 are correct
    C   if only 2 and 4 are correct
    D   if only 4 is correct
    E   if all are correct

37.8 Principles learned from military psychiatry in World War II include:

    1. the early identification of psychiatric disorders
    2. prompt treatment in the combat zone
    3. active psychotherapeutic techniques
    4. social support

37.9 The original principles of community psychiatry included:

    1. responsibility to the population
    2. treatment close to the patient
    3. comprehensive services
    4. the primacy of psychiatry among the mental health disciplines

37.10 Which of the following is not a problem in treating the chronically mentally ill?

    1. unrealistic expectations
    2. dealing with dependency
    3. providing asylum and sanctuary in the community
    4. not making treatment time limited

37.11 Case management should include:

1. a specific responsibility on the part of every mental health worker involved with the patient
2. monitoring of the patient
3. a psychiatric and medical assessment
4. an individualized treatment and rehabilitation plan

37.12 The knowledge of the psychiatric professional can assist the families of the chronically mentally ill in which of the following areas?

1. helping the family in setting limits with the patient
2. urging the family to support the patient's use of psychoactive medications
3. facilitating an understanding of the biological basis of the illness
4. assisting the family in creating an environment for the patient that strikes a balance between overstimulation and social withdrawal

DIRECTIONS: Each of the following questions consists of lettered headings followed by a list of numbered alternatives. Select the single lettered heading that is most closely associated with the appropriate numbered alternative. Each lettered heading may be chosen only once.

Level of prevention in community psychiatry

A. Primary prevention
B. Secondary prevention
C. Tertiary prevention

Description

37.13 allows patients to regain their normal level of functioning and attempts to prevent further development of the illness
37.14 involves preventing or reversing the sequelae of illness
37.15 involves the actual avoidance of the occurrence of the mental disorder

ANSWERS

37.1   The answer is **D**.

Community psychiatry of the 1960s neglected the chronically mentally ill and instead focused on less sick patients, primary prevention, and community activism in efforts to change the basic fabric of society. This gave rise to criticisms that community psychiatry had branched out beyond mental illness into problems it was not qualified to handle—community, national, and international affairs; poverty; politics; and criminology.

37.2   The answer is **B**.

The stage was set for deinstitutionalization by public outcries about deplorable conditions in psychiatric treatment facilities. This process was accelerated by two significant federal developments in 1963. First, categorical Aid to the Disabled became available to the mentally ill, making these individuals eligible for financial aid for the first time. Second, the community mental health centers legislation was passed. In a later development, Congress passed the Community Mental Health Center Amendments in 1975, which established the principle of continuing federal responsibility for the treatment and prevention of mental disorders. This made community mental health a basic federal responsibility.

37.3   The answer is **C**.

The passage of the Mental Retardation Facilities and Community Mental Health Centers Construction Act in 1963 and the amendment of this act in 1965 provided grants for the initial costs of staffing the newly constructed mental health centers. The centers were defined as requiring five basic services: inpatient treatment, emergency services, partial hospitalization, outpatient services, and consultation–education.

37.4   The answer is **A**.

Working in rural areas can present problems for psychiatrists and for other mental health professionals. They may experience professional isolation and problems of peer support. Also, rural service agencies tend to be understaffed, and the workload may be heavy. These factors may lead to job dissatisfaction and staff burnout. In terms of space, the sheer dimensions of rural service areas can be overwhelming. However, there are also advantages of working in rural areas. For instance, tolerance of deviance may be greater in rural as compared with urban areas. This can work to the advantage of the mental health psychiatrist if the rural social organization is properly used. Consequently, the seriously ill patient may have high visibility, leading to earlier identification by the mental health professional.

37.5   The answer is **B**.

Modern research has increasingly suggested the operation of genetic and biochemical factors in the causation of schizophrenia. The proponents of primary prevention seek to influence the expression of the genetic traits—the actual precipitation of the full-blown illness—through a concentration on alleviation of environmental factors that may trigger the symptoms of the disorder.

37.6   The answer is **C**.

The history of community psychiatry and of the community mental health movement has roots that go back to the 18th century. The individual usually credited with the genesis of this movement is the French psychiatrist Phillipe Pinel. Also playing a role in the development of the structure for the more humane treatment of psychiatric patients were Dorothea Lynde Dix and Clifford Beers.

37.7   The answer is **A**.

One of the major issues relating to governance in community psychiatry is the tendency for fewer mental health directors to be psychiatrists. Instead, psychologists, social workers, and psychiatric nurses have increasingly filled this role. This has come about because of a reluctance by psychiatrists to assume purely administrative roles as well as the considerably lower salary commanded by nonpsychiatrists and the consequent attractiveness of administrative positions to these professionals.

In addition, there has been a growing trend toward the appointment of individuals who have been trained as professional managers. This presents serious problems because individuals who do not have training and clinical experience in the area cannot begin to appreciate the enormity, variety, and complexity of the task of treating the mentally ill.

37.8   The answer is **E**.

Out of the experience of military psychiatrists in World Wars I and II came principles that were to have a significant impact on community psychiatry for the civilian population. These principles were a) proximity (treatment close to the combat zone), b) immediacy (the early identification and treatment of the psychiatric disorder), c) simplicity (rest, food, and social support), and d) expectancy (the expectation of a prompt return to duty).

The principle of treatment close to home has become a major tenet of community psychiatry, as have the principles of early diagnosis and active treatment to effect prompt remission of symptoms and avoid regression. The military experience also demonstrated that psychiatric disorders can often be precipitated by stress and that the identification of stressors can play an important role in the treatment of psychiatrically ill patients.

37.9   The answer is D.

Caplan and Caplan proposed a number of community psychiatry principles that have proved to be useful and valid over the years. The first principle was responsibility to the population. This principle involved the concept of the catchment area or the responsibility of the mental health center for an entire geographic area. Theoretically, a community mental health center should identify all of the mental health needs of its population and formulate a plan to meet these needs. These needs should be determined by both staff and citizens and should take into consideration the cultural background of the population.

The second principle of treatment close to the patient's home grew at least partially out of the military experience. With regard to civilian populations, it has been found that proximity facilitates the patient's utilization of available treatment resources.

The third principle of comprehensive services stressed the provision of a broad range of services such as inpatient, emergency, partial hospitalization, outpatient, and consultation–education.

Another important principle of community mental health is the multidisciplinary treatment approach, which in recent years has stressed the utilization of the unique skills of the different professionals that make up the treatment team.

37.10   The answer is D.

There are a number of problems in treating the chronically mentally ill. First, it is essential that members of the mental health profession have realistic expectations in their clinical work. If the clinician's expectations exceed the functional capabilities of the patient, the result will often be exacerbation of psychosis, dysphoria, and perhaps homelessness. Another problem in treating the chronically mentally ill has been the issue of the patient's dependency. Although psychiatrists may value independence for their patients, expectations for independent functioning must be tempered with the patients' capabilities for independent living, employment, and social functioning.

37.11 The answer is **E**.

A system of responsibility for the chronically mentally ill must be established with the goal of ensuring that each patient ultimately has one mental health professional or paraprofessional case manager who has primary responsibility for the patient. In such a case manager system, each patient would have an individual who would have the appropriate psychiatric and medical assessments carried out, who would formulate an ongoing treatment plan with the patient, and who would monitor and assist the patient in receiving services.

37.12 The answer is **E**.

Psychiatrists can often make use of families' abilities to play an important role in the treatment process. Psychiatrists can help the family set limits and take charge of their households. In addition, the psychiatrist must feel comfortable in enlightening the family on the biological basis of major psychiatric disorders and in urging the family to support the patient's use of psychoactive medication. The psychiatrist can also assist the family and patient in setting realistic goals and in assisting the family in the creation of an environment that strives to strike a balance between overstimulation and social withdrawal.

37.13 The answer is **B**.
37.14 The answer is **C**.
37.15 The answer is **A**.

Secondary prevention or treatment involves enabling patients to regain their normal level of functioning and the prevention of subsequent recurrence of the disorder. Early diagnosis and treatment is the sine qua non of secondary prevention.

Tertiary prevention or rehabilitation involves preventing or reversing the sequelae of illness, that is, preventing disability associated with the illness.

Primary prevention is the actual avoidance of the occurrence of cases of mental illness. Many past and present primary prevention efforts have been attempted through indirect services, as exemplified by consultation to teachers, welfare workers, or the police who have actual contact with the potential patient.

Chapter 38

Administration in Psychiatry

DIRECTIONS: Each of the statements or questions is followed by five suggested responses or completions. Select the one that is the best choice or most complete answer in each case.

38.1 Which of the following is not an important reason for the relative shortage of psychiatric administrators?

    A. greater commitment to treatment among psychiatrists
    B. a view of administration as mere paper shuffling
    C. few role models for young psychiatrists
    D. little academic interest in training psychiatric administrators
    E. relatively low pay in comparison to providers of direct service

38.2 Which of the following is not a reason for a perceived large need for psychiatric administrators?

    A. the increased role of nonpsychiatric professionals in the mental health field
    B. the increased complexity of reimbursement mechanisms
    C. the greater number and effectiveness of treatment interventions
    D. the complexity of delivery systems
    E. the increased involvement of the government in psychiatric decisions

38.3 A four-stage cycle of administrative process has been proposed. Which of the following is not a component of this model?

   A. design
   B. intention
   C. management
   D. evaluation
   E. initiation

38.4 An important area of administrative decision making involves the allocation of resources. Which of the following is the best definition of resources?

   A. the amount of money available to administer a program
   B. either money or a commodity that can be exchanged for money
   C. units of value that can be exchanged for other units of activity
   D. the physical, material goods plus the intangibles of talent in staff
   E. the measurable, concrete units that can be applied toward goals

38.5 Which of the following statements regarding prospective pricing is true?

   A. Prospective pricing involves the projected costs of running a service over a fiscal period, such that individual services can be priced.
   B. Prospective pricing involves a consideration of the customary and usual charges in a given geographical unit in order to determine the limits of the cost transmitted to the patient.
   C. Prospective pricing involves rate determination by the government.
   D. Prospective pricing involves payment in advance of an inclusive fee to cover health costs for the succeeding year.
   E. Prospective pricing involves full specification of fees prior to delivery of services.

38.6 The major budget item in psychiatric treatment programs is:

   A. upkeep of the physical plant
   B. equipment costs
   C. medication costs
   D. support service costs
   E. personnel costs

38.7 Major personnel decisions are best made by:

    A. personnel experts
    B. the chief administrator
    C. democratic vote of staff
    D. the person with clinical responsibility for a given service
    E. consensus among administrators

38.8 Politics is best defined as:

    A. the necessary but unpleasant aspects of organizational activity
    B. the art of successful manipulation
    C. successfully influencing others to give one's own needs priority
    D. the activities involved in the defense of one's own organizational territory
    E. the utilization of resources related to influencing others

DIRECTIONS: For each of the statements or questions below, one or more of the alternative answers is correct. Choose answer:

    A if only 1, 2, and 3 are correct
    B if only 1 and 3 are correct
    C if only 2 and 4 are correct
    D if only 4 is correct
    E if all are correct

38.9 How does the management of human services systems differ from the management of systems with product output?

    1. the amount of utilization of interpersonal relationships in the delivery of services
    2. the ratio of investment to output
    3. the complexity of service versus product delivery
    4. the need for more management skills in product output

38.10 The standard components of job descriptions include:

    1. clarification of major responsibilities
    2. delineation of horizontal relationships
    3. delineation of vertical relationships
    4. description of usual functions

38.11   Which of the following statements regarding performance evaluation is (are) true?

1. It is easier to use performance standards once they have been written than it is to actually write them.
2. Evaluation of performance begins early in the course of employment.
3. Many performance standards in psychiatry may be impossible to state objectively.
4. It is important to have objective criteria for all performance standards.

38.12   To which of the following units is the psychiatric profession is accountable?

1. government
2. the media
3. community
4. other psychiatric services

38.13   Quality assurance involves:

1. systematic evaluation of the adequacy of treatment programs
2. organized steps for enhancing effectiveness
3. organizational procedures to ensure effective change
4. procedures standardized across settings

38.14   Administrative style of the director should include which of the following?

1. insight into his or her own behavior
2. timeliness of decisions
3. knowledge about clinical services
4. integrity

DIRECTIONS: Each of the following questions consists of lettered headings followed by a list of numbered alternatives. Select the single lettered heading that is most closely associated with the appropriate numbered alternative. Each lettered heading may be chosen only once.

Theory of administration

A.   Weber's system
B.   General systems
C.   Matrix system

Definitions

38.15   holds that organizations are related to other organizations in multiple ways and at multiple levels

38.16   is an objective and formal system for reaching goals

38.17   organizes providers into interdisciplinary teams

ANSWERS

38.1   The answer is **E**.

Even though more psychiatrists are being trained now than ever before, there is a current shortage of psychiatric administrators. There are several interrelated reasons for this shortage. Young psychiatrists tend to be more interested in patient care and to have a large commitment to the provision of direct service or to teaching. Administration is not a high-prestige area in psychiatry and is viewed by many as mere paper shuffling. There are few administrator role models for young psychiatrists and relatively more role models in teaching or clinical work. Furthermore, until recently there has been little academic interest in training psychiatric administrators.

38.2   The answer is **A**.

The larger need for psychiatric administrators is the result of technological changes, social changes, and changes in funding arrangements. There is much more complexity in funding arrangements, resulting in increased need to attend to aspects of administration. The greater number and increased complexity of treatment interventions also increase the need for psychiatric administration of treatment provider systems. Therefore, psychiatrists need to assume managerial roles in order to facilitate adherence to clinical goals.

38.3   The answer is **B**.

There are many models of the administrative process. One such model is the four-stage cycle of Design, Initiation, Management, and Evaluation (DIME). Design of the program involves a study of the mission and resources of a service system. Factors influencing the design stage include internal factors such as the ideas of the staff and the results of formal program evaluations. First the mission is defined, then a needs assessment is conducted, and then the resources are identified. Finally the program can be outlined.

The second stage is initiation, in which the staff is educated and reassured regarding the potential changes, and the proposed changes specified in the design stage are implemented. Here, marketing takes place and contacts are made with other programs in order to facilitate interface. The third stage is management. The third stage will determine whether the program will fail or succeed. Here clinical decisions are made regarding the allocation of resources.

The fourth stage, evaluation, actually begins during the early parts of the management stage. A record-keeping and data collection system needs to be designed. Evaluation involves the measurement of the effectiveness and efficiency of the program. Data generated here can be used to improve the public image of the program, understand the underlying cost structure of the program, and measure the continuity and comprehensiveness of the program.

38.4   The answer is **C**.

An important management function related to decision making regards the use of resources. Resources are best conceptualized as units of value that may be exchanged for other units of activity—resources can be concrete, abstract, or symbolic. Resources are collected, invested, and dispersed in relation to the priorities for short-term and long-term goals. There are four general areas of resoures: budgeting and finance, personnel, public relations and accountability, and the law.

Budgeting and finances include the acquisition of monetary credits and the expenditure of money to help achieve goals. A related area is that of marketing. Personnel practices include recruitment, selection, and retention of staff as well as evaluation of staff performance and the requirements of due process. Public relations and accountability revolve around the development and use of power derived from contact with the various constituencies affected by the psychiatric programs. The law relates to resources in terms of mental health legislation and the services that psychiatry can provide to the court system.

38.5   The answer is **D**.

Because of the phenomenal increases in both the costs of health care and the proportion of the costs borne by the government, several systems have been proposed to control and decrease expenditures. One such system is the concept of prospective pricing. This concept involves the advance payment of fees to cover the costs of an individual's or group's health care during the succeeding year. One example of prospective pricing is the health maintenance organization.

38.6   The answer is **E**.

Of all the items in the budget for a psychiatric service, the most expensive is personnel costs. Usually these costs add up to 80 percent of the total budget. Sometimes agencies try to save money by taking advantage of the high turnover common to the area. By instituting a delay in filling open positions, money can be saved. Unfortunately, an undesirable side effect can be a decrement in the level of clinical care. Another money-saving mechanism is that of the line budget. Here, money set aside in the budget for a particular purpose cannot be used for another purpose without higher administrative approval, a situation that delays changes and moves of monetary resources from one area to another. Therefore, if X amount is set aside for nursing salaries, that money cannot be shunted to a salary for occupational therapy until the higher administrators are also convinced of the wisdom of the move, even if that move is viewed as necessary by the unit administrator.

38.7   The answer is **D**.

Major personnel decisions are best made by those people who have direct clinical responsibility for a given program. Staff of the personnel department assist with the decision process rather than direct it. Therefore, it is extremely important for the psychiatric administrator to have a working knowledge of personnel practices, strategies, principles, and procedures. The psychiatric administrator can turn to the personnel staff for advice, but not for direction.

38.8   The answer is **C**.

Politics is generally viewed as a dirty word. This is unfortunate, because far from being a dirty but necessary activity, politics is an important element in improving a care system. However, this importance does not justify dirty activities. The application of politics should be honest, goal directed, rationally planned, and ideologically clear. Perfecting political skills is as important as perfecting other professional skills. A good definition of politics is the art of successfully influencing others to give priority to our own needs. Political activity includes interactions with legislators, court officials, community groups, other health care providers, and personnel within one's own unit.

38.9   The answer is **B**.

Management has several core characteristics, regardless of the setting. However, management of human service organizations, particularly psychiatric service programs, differs from the management of organizations with product output. For one thing, the management of psychiatric programs involves a greater level of complexity in the delivery of the final output. Operations are less likely to be routinized. Another important factor is that there is a very large aspect of interpersonal relations in the delivery of psychiatric services; indeed interpersonal interactions are the core of the therapy procedure. A large amount of emotional response is generated in the delivery of psychiatric services, a fact that is not paralleled in the delivery of product.

38.10   The answer is **E**.

Although job descriptions vary greatly across and among programs, there are a few core or standard components. One of the standard components is a description of major functions that the individual will be expected to perform. Another component is a description of the level of responsibility associated with the position. A description of the vertical relationships involves specifying the person to whom the recruited individual reports and to whom he or she is professionally responsible. A description of horizontal relationships involves the other persons who are responsible to another supervisor. Explication of the vertical and horizontal relationships is needed in order to delineate expectations of accountability. Finally, job descriptions include a description of the knowledge, skills, and experience needed for a given position.

38.11   The answer is **C**.

The performance of an employee begins early in the history of the employment. Objective performance standards need to be stated so that expectations are clearly communicated and that evaluation and fair appraisal occur. Using performance standards may be more difficult than establishing them. Also, it is more pleasant to give positive feedback than to give negative feedback. Despite this difference, it is still very important to provide feedback regarding deficiencies in performance so that performance may be improved. Not to do so for a less-than-productive employee will result in further inefficiency as well as lowered morale in the inefficient person's co-workers.

Many institutions have set procedures for due process. These procedures are facilitated by early notification to the employee regarding unsatisfactory performance. Most times these notifications need to be documented on paper. Furthermore, the response of the employee also needs to be documented on paper.

38.12   The answer is A.

The accountability of psychiatric administrators takes many different forms. Many psychiatric programs are accountable to government agencies, whether federal, state, or local. Heeding the lines of accountability is very important in maintaining good relations with these agencies. It is also important to avoid antagonizing the members of these agencies even when a situation seems to engender such actions. Accountability to the community is also important. Including community factors in the decision process can help ensure that the services provided are consistent with the needs of the community as well as help maintain good public relations and enlist community allies in the struggle to obtain resources.

The media influence public opinion and, by extension, governmental actions. Recognizing accountability to the media can help facilitate favorable impressions of the psychiatric program. The members of the media may often have different goals, but minimizing conflicts with the media has a fairly high priority in determining activities of the administrator. Many psychiatric agencies are accountable to boards of directors or trustees. Although these boards may not have the clinical knowledge that is possessed by the psychiatric administrator, they often have legal responsibility for the actions of the administrators and other employees.

38.13   The answer is A.

Conceptions of quality assurance have broadened greatly in the past few decades. These changes are partly the reflection of an increased need for accountability. Quality assurance is now thought to involve a systematic evaluation of the adequacy of treatment programs, a set of organized steps for enhancing the effectiveness of treatment programs, and an organizational procedure to help ensure that effective change will occur when needed. Techniques involved in quality assurance include program evaluation, utilization review, and peer review. Adequate quality assurance programs help protect patients as well as help prevent embarrassing revelations regarding insufficiencies in the psychiatric program.

38.14   The answer is E.

Administrative style of a psychiatric director affects the overall tone of the program as well as the quality of the output of the program. Successful administrators vary greatly in individual style. However, there are some characteristics that seem to be shared by successful psychiatric administrators.

The administrator can be viewed as a leader. The administrator's behavior should communicate a sense of ethical integrity. He or she should show a commitment to the goals of the program as well as respect for the rights of the patients and respect for the staff. Reliability of the leader is important in fostering a sense of security among the staff. Decisions need to be made in a timely fashion.

An administrator enjoys greater staff confidence when she or he exhibits knowledge regarding the clinical aspects of the program. Of course, the administrator cannot be expected to be more expert than the staff in all areas of practice, but familiarity with different aspects of the program is necessary. The effective administrator has insight into his or her own behavior as well as insight into the behavior of others. The administrator should also model professional collegiality and interdependence by developing structures for acquiring information from frontline staff regarding problem identification and solving. By fostering collaboration among staff, the administrator helps develop common acceptance of program goals. Finally, optimism of the administrator will improve morale of the staff.

38.15   The answers **B**.
38.16   The answer is **C**.
38.17   The answer is **A**.

The sociologist Max Weber developed a careful and logical approach to helping organizations achieve goals. His system is objective and formal. It involves written rules, specification of the relationships between supervisors and subordinates, and formal rules for the organization of the program or unit. He also stressed using the concept of division of labor and the importance of competition.

General systems theory states that organizations are related to other organizations in multiple ways and at multiple levels. This is particularly applicable to psychiatric programs because of their different relations with many different legal, community, and professional organizations. The framework specified by general systems theory is more dynamic and flexible than that specified by Weber's system.

The matrix system is commonly used in contemporary psychiatric care delivery systems. Here the providers of psychiatric care are organized into multidisciplinary care teams. The teams are composed of nursing staff, psychiatric staff, psychologists, recreational and occupational therapists, and other paraprofessionals. The members of a team have responsibility both to the team and to their respective professional units.